"This is a very valuable book. 'Heart Shock or Trauma' was first coined by Dr. John HF. Shen who belongs to our Menghe-Ding Lineage. Dr. Leon Hammer (whom I have been fortunate to know and read his publications) was Dr. Shen's apprentice, and with the advantage of being both a psychiatrist and a Chinese doctor has raised the scope of knowledge to new heights. Ross Rosen's manuscript builds on this information. After reading it I can't help admiring Ross Rosen—without his diligence and wisdom this book could not have been completed. The book shows a full range of levels beyond the ordinary. It offers the reader both an ability to understand the concepts surrounding 'Heart Shock' and also provides detailed explanations of the many healing strategies and treatments. It is worth reading for practitioners or students of Oriental Medicine. I will be recommending this book to TCM doctors in China."

—*Dr. Ding Yie, Chief Physician & Professor, Long Hua*
Hospital affiliated to Shanghai University of TCM

HEART SHOCK

Diagnosis and Treatment of Trauma with Shen-Hammer and Classical Chinese Medicine

ROSS ROSEN

FOREWORD BY DR. LEON HAMMER

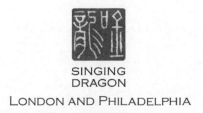

SINGING
DRAGON

LONDON AND PHILADELPHIA

Cover artwork: Calligraphy by Josh Paynter

Images copyright: Figure 1.1, Figures 2.1–2.10, Figure 3.1, Figures 4.2–4.4, Figures 5.1–5.2, Figure 6.1, Figures 10.1–10.2 © Eastland Press

Bullet list on pp.80–81 from *In an Unspoken Voice: How the Body Releases Trauma and Restores Goodness* by Peter A. Levine, published by North Atlantic Books, copyright © 2010b, Peter A Levine. Reprinted by permission of publisher.

First published in 2018
by Singing Dragon
an imprint of Jessica Kingsley Publishers
73 Collier Street
London N1 9BE, UK
and
400 Market Street, Suite 400
Philadelphia, PA 19106, USA

www.singingdragon.com

Copyright © Ross Rosen 2018
Foreword copyright © Dr. Leon Hammer 2018

Library of Congress Cataloging in Publication Data
A CIP catalog record for this book is available from the Library of Congress

British Library Cataloguing in Publication Data
A CIP catalogue record for this book is available from the British Library

ISBN 978 1 84819 373 4
eISBN 978 0 85701 330 9
Printed and bound by CPI Group (UK) Ltd, Croydon, CR0 4YY

Contents

Foreword

Dr. Leon Hammer

From the very beginning of our teacher–student relationship to our subsequent long association as colleagues, I have known Ross Rosen as a careful, creative thinker. For many years he stood out among my students as the one who asked questions and reported clinical observations and ideas in a lively exchange of reflections and viewpoints that informed and inspired me. I still retain a record of these correspondences.

One such observation was the detection of the Leather-Hard pulse in young adults. The Leather-Hard quality, outside of the context of radiation therapy in cancer patients, was new to both of us, and in the early 2000s Ross began detecting it with alarming frequency in patients in their teens, 20s, and 30s. Ross reported these findings to me, and after further corroborating them, in 2009, we published an original article on the early pulse detection of the effect of non-ionizing microwave radiation on the human organism and how to manage it.

For some time Ross Rosen has been one of our most important, successful, and innovative pulse instructors. He also has established one of the most successful practices of Chinese medicine of which I am aware so that all that follows in this volume is grounded not only in a profound study of the classics and current scholarship but also in hands-on practice and a background in the martial arts and traditional Chinese esoteric ritual.

This volume will establish Ross Rosen as a significant Chinese scholar-practitioner of our time and beyond. *Heart Shock* is one of the most thorough texts I have read on any subject in my long career in science. I feel qualified to speak to this subject in particular having been exposed for years to the clinical and conceptual observations on Heart Shock by Dr. John H.F. Shen with whom I apprenticed for many years and recorded them and my own in several published articles.

Ross Rosen has placed this chosen subject, Heart Shock, within that context in his first part of this volume. He has then further and brilliantly expounded Heart Shock, synthesizing it precisely within the context of the human organism's sophisticated defensive system from the Qi to the Blood and Yuan levels as conceived progressively from the Nei Jing to the present as taught by Jeffrey Yuen. I have previously published thoughts regarding "retained pathogens," and Dr. Shen repeatedly mentioned that the "organ depth" on the pulse was further divided. I later identified this as the Blood of Organ depth that identifies qualities representing "retained pathogens" probably in the luo channels and the deeper Substance of Organ depth, identifying "retained pathogens" probably in the divergent channels.

As I read this book aspects of my clinical experience are illuminated. And I find greater comprehension and appreciation of the endless process of intake and excretion necessary to a relatively harmonious existence.

The sections on treatment, or what I prefer to call management, are very illuminating. A phenomenon that I sought explanation for years (until reading this text) was the blood-letting performed by my first teacher of Chinese medicine, Dr. Van Buren. He was first of all an osteopath who adjusted every patient before he did anything else. He would bleed every superficial blood vessel he could find—"spider veins" and even "varicose veins." He did both adjustment and blood-letting with all of the patients, though it was my impression he did less blood-letting with older and more deficient patients. This now makes more sense than at the time when he chose to not explain. I urge the reader to seek out the physiological-pathological events underlying the mechanisms of trauma, something that Ross Rosen provides almost without exception.

Read and learn! Were I a student or someone early in my career I would outline this book and have the outline of indications and needling maneuvers constantly at my side. At least, at my age I could not remember all the diagnostic principles, vessels, points, needling techniques and herbs and the combinations of pathways without considerable assistance. I would also request that Dr. Rosen give workshops where students could have a chance to observe and practice what is recommended in this book, the general principles and specific recommendations. This material is so central to all Chinese medical practice that prospective and current practitioners should make it central to their learning and practice.

A Foreword this short is almost an insult to a volume so profound in knowledge; one that will help alleviate the suffering of mankind and aid the people who minister to them. I offer Ross Rosen my profound apologies and gratitude.

Acknowledgments

About ten years ago one of my regular patients was a successful psychic and medium, even working for the police department helping to solve crimes. One day, after a few months of regular treatments, she asked my permission to reveal her observations of our interactions. Interested, I gave her the ok and she proceeded to tell me how each time I entered the treatment room, an elderly Chinese doctor in a white coat, holding a number of books in his crossed arms, would follow me in and observe my treatment. This was without fail for all of her treatments (and presumably my other patients) over the course of the time I treated her. She described him as very proper, detail-oriented, and learned. She further informed me that some of the books the doctor was holding were, in fact, written by me. The first one was to the profession, of which she said would be an important book that would serve many. The second was to the public/laypeople, and the third, I believe, was to be a children's book. She told me the time was not yet, but that I should start thinking about it, and that in my mid 40s I would write the first book. And so, I did think about it. I thought a lot about it. Mostly, I thought I could not write such a book, that I did not have so much new to say, let alone the time to write it. I sat down a few times and tried in my early 40s. I compiled lots of my information, about 200+ pages worth, and then discarded it.

Over the course of many years and my training and clinical practice in the Shen-Hammer lineage as well as in Classical Chinese medicine as taught by Jeffrey Yuen, I began to merge and synthesize my thinking on the approaches, understandings, and treatments of these two lineages. One such area that I have treated over many years was trauma and Heart Shock. And while this subject is so vast and important, I realized there was no treatise out there covering the perspective of these two lineages. And then I remembered my patient, and the thought of a book on this topic appealed to me. I also contacted her and sent her a picture of Dr. John Shen. While she could not confirm 100 percent, she believed this to be the man who followed me into my treatments. I never met Dr. Shen in person; he passed just before I formally entered into the lineage. But my connection to him always felt strong, and even just the possibility that his spirit follows and guides me inspired me to write the current book, on a topic near and dear to him and the Shen-Hammer lineage. So, my deepest thanks to Dr. Shen for his guidance, and to my patient for inspiring the possibility of this book. And while I cannot guarantee its importance, it has been my attempt to make it of value to the profession.

This book could not have been written without the generosity of Dr. Leon Hammer who has tirelessly shared his information, expertise, love, and friendship with me for nearly 20 years now. I am honored to have his Foreword begin this book, his words being far too generous and very humbling.

Deep gratitude also to Jeffrey Yuen with whom I have taken many dozens of courses over the years, including at the American University of Complementary Medicine's PhD program in Classical Chinese medicine, and through his offices in NYC, and mostly everywhere he travels to teach, as I never tire or fail to learn something valuable from his unique perspectives on Chinese medicine. I hope that I have done his teachings justice in this text.

To my wife, who has always supported and praised my process of learning and cultivating the skills so that I could feel worthy of practicing the healing arts as detailed in the classics. I strive to have a fraction of what she embodies, the ability to heal and inspire simply by her presence and spirit, and I am grateful to have her as my teacher in that regard.

To my children, Ben (the root), Shen (the spirit), and Tatum (the goddess always full of cheer), for giving me the opportunity to experience the full measure of what the Heart can feel.

Thanks to my parents who nearly had a nervous breakdown when I left practicing as a lawyer to pursue a career in Chinese medicine, but supported me anyway.

Thank you to Josh Paynter, my Daoist brother, for friendship since day 1 at Pacific College of Oriental Medicine, and for his valuable insights and comments on this text, as well as sourcing the original Chinese and providing helpful translations. A special thanks for his calligraphy which adorns the cover and for the spirit that it conveys.

Thanks to Brandt Stickley, my good friend and brother in the Shen-Hammer lineage and co-author of a series of articles back in 2007 and 2008 on varied aspects of pulse diagnosis and the lineage. Our constant communications and discussions over the years have inspired me greatly.

Thanks to Bob Heffron, my first teacher in the Shen-Hammer lineage, who invited me to his home in 2001 to study privately after a course at NESA was canceled for lack of enrollment.

Thanks to Phyllis Bloom, with whom I studied pulse after Bob, and who quickly introduced me to Dr. Hammer and accompanied me to Gainesville, Florida, for advanced intensives. Her guidance, encouragement, and friendship have been treasured all these years.

Thanks to those that have assisted in my private classes/teachings on this subject, including the creation of my teaching transcripts which were helpful in constructing this text: Jennifer Sobonski, Ryan Diener, Tracy Soltesz, Yvette Koch, Leslie Aurino, and Liv Ruddy.

Thanks to my friends and colleagues in the Classical medicine lineage as taught by Jeffrey for the selfless sharing of information and knowledge over the years: Jennifer Jackson, and Steve Alpern.

And thank you to Singing Dragon (Claire, Emma, Sean, and the Design team) for your enthusiasm with the project and your ongoing support.

Thank you to John O'Connor and Eastland Press for their generosity in allowing me to use the various pulse images contained throughout this text.

And thank you to my patients for entrusting their health to my care, and working together in the pursuit of healing. You have allowed me to take the theories outlined in this text and create a cultivated practice rooted in our relationships.

Introduction

We are all born with a purpose. And when we live according to it, we can have happy, fulfilled lives. Unfortunately, not everyone is in touch with theirs, and some have suffered traumatic experiences which have cut them off from the wellspring of energy and vitality which comes with living with purpose.[1] This book is an attempt to help those reclaim their heart.

From as early as I could speak, I showed an interest in all things Eastern. I asked to take martial arts classes when just a few years old, well before it was en vogue, and before there were martial arts schools in most communities; there was something drawing me towards it. As with all "arts," what makes it so is putting one's heart into it, finding the spirit through one's passion and hard work. It wasn't long before my interest in martial arts deepened to its foundation and roots in Eastern thought and philosophy, and the dreams and aspirations to learn martial arts and medicine from the ancients in China. But like most of us, life brings us on detours, and we travel on collateral roads instead of the main highway, creating a circuitous, rather than the most efficient, route. And so, as I did not believe that there was an option for a career in the Chinese arts, college, then law school, then practicing as attorney became my collateral. It also took me further from my purpose, clouding the spirit, dampening my fire.

One day sitting in my legal office behind closed doors, eating lunch and trying not to be seen, I came across an advertisement for the Pacific College of Oriental Medicine (PCOM) in the *Village Voice*. An instant epiphany and light bulb resurrecting my heart, I immediately called for an application, applied, interviewed, got accepted, and quit my job, only to start PCOM within a couple months. Back on the highway, my heart was awakened.

What does it mean to have one's heart awakened? What does it mean to have "heart"? To wear one's heart on one's sleeve? To put one's heart into one's actions? To get to the heart of the matter? The amount of expressions associated with it makes it abundantly clear how vital and important the Heart is to our existence. The Heart is what animates us, gives us joy, allows for our expression, provides purpose, and drives us towards our destiny. But these capacities can falter or become damaged. Certain experiences can create this damage, and we must learn to recognize and treat it appropriately.

Years ago I was amazed to learn that trauma, even trauma that happened while in utero or during the birthing process, could be detected on the radial pulse. That there were signature pathognomonic findings that left their imprints on one's being indefinitely after a traumatic event, preventing healing. I discovered that it was possible to determine the timing and specific nature of said trauma (e.g., cord being wrapped around throat during delivery). Prior to my studies with Dr. Leon Hammer and Jeffrey Yuen, I had attributed these seemingly magical abilities to mystics and shamans who were outside of the realm of science and reasoning, so I was delighted to discover that these were in fact skills I could cultivate and incorporate into my practice. And I have observed that understanding the nature and timing of patients' traumas with such specificity facilitates an intimacy between patient and practitioner that fosters a healing dynamic that is essential to a successful patient–practitioner relationship.

So it is curious, and somewhat tragic to me, that so few of us are offered tools for accessing such critical information. My journey led me to a few specific lineages of Chinese medicine. I was lucky to discover the first one upon graduating from Chinese medical school, and it required significant time and cultivation to fully embody. There are many roads and choices a new practitioner can make upon graduating; tons of weekend courses and certificates to be received, but not necessarily an overarching paradigm to structure one's knowledge. When confronted with all these options, I chose to dedicate my time and efforts to building a solid foundation, foregoing the myriad things to focus on the two (Shen-Hammer and Yuen), in search of the one (the essence of Chinese medicine).

In early 2001 I began formally studying and practicing within the Shen-Hammer lineage. I learned to feel pulses with the renowned Dr. Leon Hammer and would meet for four days a few times per year to hone my skills and see patients with him and the other certified teachers within the lineage. The detailed nature of the pulse system has some 28 pulse positions and 90 pulse qualities, some which have been added by me and Dr. Hammer over the time period I have been associated with him. The beauty of this system is that it is constantly evolving as it reflects changes in our lifestyles and environment, and how we humans adapt to it, and the pathologies it creates. Not only does it demonstrate the relative yang of the more cosmopolitan urban populations, for example, but it can also reveal a tendency to carry your cell phone in a particular pocket. It can turn up a shared quality among a population plagued by particular environmental toxins or even reveal the healing impact of a favorite pet, or a dietary shift.

To understand the pulse positions and qualities is to access and understand processes, environments, and constitutions and how those things interact, and, using that information, I have been fortunate to work with Dr. Hammer (a renowned psychiatrist and doctor of Chinese medicine and only disciple of Dr. John Shen) in helping the system evolve. Part of adaptation requires a constant questioning, broadening, and refocusing of the lens we use to see and treat our patients. In 2005, with exposure to the teachings of Jeffrey Yuen, my lens was further enhanced and simultaneously focused. His spiritual/Daoist background and transmission of vast information on Chinese medicine added another layer of insight to the information that could be gleaned from the pulse. I began reading all of the transcripts that were available on a multitude of different subjects and had a real appreciation for how these teachings enlarged the paradigm I had become accustomed to. I began more formally studying Classical Chinese medicine within this lineage in 2006 after being admitted to the American University of Complementary Medicine's Classical Chinese Medicine PhD program. And being in a suburb of NYC, I have been fortunate to take part in many dozens of courses, as well as year-long programs, Jeffrey has offered here in my backyard.

Book structure

It is from this background and extensive study that this treatise evolved. *Heart Shock* is an attempt to demonstrate some of the paradigms and structures of Chinese medicine that I have learned and synthesized from these two prolific lineages. This book is intended to be a process, not the final word on the subject of trauma, or on the vastness of possibilities that Chinese medicine offers. It's an approach to understanding Chinese medicine and to treating any and all diagnoses and conditions, not solely Heart Shock and trauma as the title would suggest. Rather, it uses the concept of trauma to present multi-faceted lenses through which to view any ailment, as well as a process for moving between these different lenses and seeing their interrelationships. This "conceptual fluidity" is an essential and important tool in understanding Chinese medicine as a whole. Very different from an "anything goes" or shot-gun approach, it presupposes a strong foundation in multiple perspectives and lineages.

While focusing on Heart Shock and trauma, I would like to present this "conceptual fluidity" model by first detailing the specific theoretical underpinnings of each lineage and each lens within the lineages. For example, each channel system is a distinct approach to understanding physiology and pathology. Looking through the lens of the divergent channels will yield different information than the sinew meridian or luo vessel lens as it orients one differently in thinking with regard to progression of illness, resources, and psychological perspectives, and overall how one perceives oneself and one's illness. To know each individually is crucial to seeing the interplay between them and even more so to being able to combine them and their principles into a graduated treatment plan and strategy.

On Heart Shock

While the concepts associated with the diagnosis and treatment of Heart Shock and trauma originate from a variety of places, I would like to focus on the lineages that I am most familiar with—the work of Dr. John HF Shen (who coined the term "Heart Shock") and Dr. Leon Hammer (Shen-Hammer lineage), and Classical Chinese medicine as taught from the oral lineage of Jeffrey Yuen. Some of my greatest insights and successes within my own practice have resulted from the synthesis of ideas from these lineages and I hope to demonstrate how the two can be combined to allow for a more complete diagnostic understanding as well as more holistic treatment strategies.

There are many descriptions of "shock" and other types of emotional disturbances and traumas from classical terms, and they can fit neatly through the lens of the Shen-Hammer lineage. Dr. Hammer enlarged the scope of Dr. Shen's material based upon his training and expertise as a psychiatrist and his observations over decades of treating patients coming in with disorders having their roots in trauma. As a psychiatrist, Dr. Hammer had the opportunity to observe the longer-term impact of various traumas and was able to integrate his understanding of Chinese medicine and pulse diagnosis into this body of work. Over the years I have experienced that the vast majority of patients exhibit some degree of what we now refer to as Heart Shock. Our pulses collectively confirm which traumas and insults we continue to carry around with us and give practitioners a way to track progress within a treatment plan. Whether they are aware of the trauma or not (many times people are not), this comprehensive system of pulse diagnosis is immensely useful in dealing with the stubborn issues that often block the effective resolution of chief complaints and persistent symptoms.

Jeffrey Yuen's teachings have proven to be another critical resource, particularly with regards to providing treatment principles that align with the diagnostic parameters presented by the Shen-Hammer pulse system. Yuen's insights into the Channel System approach are very useful in determining the best method and modality of treatment for any given patient and/or depending on the practitioner's lens and belief system. The particular dynamics of the patient's presentation revealed by pulse diagnosis can readily direct practitioners towards effective treatment plans within specific channel systems. I will present an overview of the dynamics of each collateral (sinew, divergent, luo, and 8 extraordinary) as well as how each of them can have a role in treating trauma. Each channel system has its own set of psycho-emotional components as well as specific pulses that reveal underlying activity.

This book will also examine different types of herbal approaches, including some of Drs. Shen and Hammer's own formulas as well as Classical herbal approaches that fit within this model, including herbs that associate to the channel systems. I will also briefly discuss some additional Classical concepts and treatments, including a couple from Ge Hong and Sun Si-miao and the use of the 13 Ghost points (including their herbal equivalents). And lastly, I will present some options for the use of essential oils to treat Heart Shock as oils have a direct impact on the brain and our emotional regulation centers within, as well as our constitution. As such, they offer an opportunity to make both quick and profound changes to patient psyches as well as deeper yuan qi dynamics. To conclude the discussion, I will present a couple of my own case studies to demonstrate the approach of tying all this information together.

This book is by no means the final word on this vast subject, but rather my understanding and explication of it. I welcome feedback and discussion to further the positive impact that treating trauma can have on our collective patients.

A note on capitalizations

The Chinese medical concepts of the organ systems and the Western anatomical organs share the same English names and translations. In order to properly differentiate them, when I am referring to the Western anatomical organ there will be no capitalization. When discussing or referencing the broader Chinese medical energetics (which includes the wide-ranging functions and attributes as well as the anatomy), I will capitalize said organ.

Abbreviations

Throughout the text, abbreviations will be used to refer to the various channel systems, as well as acupuncture points. These abbreviations include:

Organ systems/channels:

Lungs: LU

Large Intestine: LI

Stomach: ST

Spleen: SP

Heart: HT

Small Intestine: SI

Bladder: BL

Kidney: KI

Pericardium: PC

Triple Burner: SJ

Gall Bladder: GB

Liver: LR

Channel systems:

Sinew meridians: SM

Luo meridians: LM

Divergent meridians: DM

Eight extra meridians: 8x

Other abbreviations:

Nervous system tense: NST

Nervous system weak: NSW

Digestive system weak: DSW

Dragon Rises, Red Bird Flies: DRRBF

Windows of the Sky points: WOS points

External pathogenic factor: EPF

Any additional abbreviations will be noted in the body of the respective chapter, noting it in parentheses as "(hereinafter…)."

A note on the words *Heart Shock*

Heart Shock as used in this text will refer to the systemic instability resulting from trauma and its sequelae. When referring to the title of the book, it will be italicized (*Heart Shock*).

PART I

DEFINING
HEART SHOCK

CHAPTER 1

Heart Shock

Traumatized Emperor, Chaotic Empire

What is Heart Shock and why is it so important?

Heart Shock[2] refers to a systemic instability, and to some degree chaos, resulting from life insults or traumas. It is crucially important because a vast majority of patients (and people in general) present with some manifestation or symptomatology consistent with this diagnosis. Traumas associated with Heart Shock can occur early in life or they can occur later in life—key determining factors being how those traumas are perceived by the individual, as well as the person's age and level of development, maturity, and stability at the time of the shock/trauma. Not all shocks are created equal. Some are more significant than others, and individual constitutions vary considerably, creating the need to weigh all the variables as we interpret our findings. The Nei Jing Su Wen states:

> The channel, blood and energy of a man will be affected and changed by terror, fright, anger, fatigue… Under these situations, if one has a strong body, his energy can be dredged, and his sickness can be recovered; if his body is weak, the evil energy will hurt the body in the wake of it.[3]

"Shocks" can be physical traumas, like accidents and injuries, or they can be purely emotional in origin. They can be localized injuries and/or major, systemic attacks. Regardless of scope and severity, all physical traumas have an emotional correlate. For example, someone who gets into a car accident may experience significant physical repercussions, but the emotional shock of that incident will have a lingering and profound impact as well.

The instability that results from the shock is termed "Heart Shock" not because it exclusively affects the Heart, but because the Heart is the epicenter of impact. The Heart is considered the Emperor (or Empress) in Chinese medicine, so instability to the Emperor will affect the entire Empire. This is true of any systemic insult of this nature, and is how it can become an obstacle to long-lasting and effective treatments.

Su Wen Chapter 8 discusses the vital role of the Emperor:

> As the Heart is the monarch in the organs, it dominates the functions of the various viscera, so when the function of the Heart is strong and healthy, under its unified leadership, all the functions of the various viscera will be normal, the body will be healthy and the man will live a long life, and in his life long days, no serious disease would occur. It is just like the condition in a country when the monarch is wise and able and all the work in various departments are in concert, the country will be prosperous and powerful, but when the monarch is thick-headed, that is, when the function of the Heart is incapable, the mutual relations between the viscera in the body will be damaged, the body will suffer great injury to affect one's health and the length of life. In a country, the political power will be unstable and every thing in the country will be out of order. It is advisable for one to pay attention to it greatly.[4]

This translation addresses the concept of instability and demonstrates the elevation of the Heart as the Emperor. Thus, anything that significantly impacts the Heart and creates a scenario where the Heart is incapable of performing any of its functions will lead to chaos. The Heart and other organ systems have multiple interrelationships, and every organ system relies on the Heart for stability, for proper circulation of blood, and for movement of the shen through the blood, and on the spirit to keep things calm and anchored. One of the primary manifestations of Heart Shock is this lack of grounding. This instability creates a barrier to treatment unless corrected.

Many practitioners are aware of the five element/constitutional model of JR Worsley, which refers to different types of blocks. Dr. Hammer has also delineated a number of "blocks" that need to be addressed, either concurrently or prior to other diagnoses. Heart Shock is a major one. The idea is that, in order to fully resolve any condition, you must first remove these obstacles that interfere with the healing mechanisms of the entire organism. Otherwise, treatment runs the risk of failure, or at best only temporary symptomatic relief.

When it comes to trauma, chronology matters. Generally speaking, the earlier in one's life a trauma occurs, the more significant its impact. Many patients are surprised to discover that a trauma from decades ago can contribute to subsequent and seemingly unrelated symptoms and suffering. A trauma that occurs prior to the age of maturation impacts the entire process of maturing. Cycles of 7 and 8 (tian gui) are affected. Growth and development become stunted. An early life trauma impacts the Heart/Kidney axis and subsequently interferes with the distribution of yuan qi. Furthermore, trauma hampers overall circulation, preventing blood from properly nourishing the organ systems and extremities, weakening the adrenals/Kidney yang, and promoting an overactive nervous system. These systems become increasingly taxed over time so that the sequelae of an early trauma can be debilitating later in life.

Physical trauma

From a physiological perspective, physical trauma restricts peripheral circulation of qi and blood. Following a traumatic injury, peripheral blood vessels constrict to increase blood flow to the center of the body.[5] Emotional trauma and shock create the same effect. The idea is that, when you have a particular trauma or something is very suddenly shocking to the system, the body contracts, drawing its resources inward. For example, if you hear a gunshot at close range or someone slams down on the table all of a sudden, you are likely to recoil and tighten inward. This occurs as a protective measure—essentially it is the Heart sending yin, qi, and blood into the internal aspects of the organs to preserve their function.

As yin and blood are drawn towards the center of the body, we start to see a disconnect between the yin and the yang. Without yin to anchor it, yang will "float" upward. Following a traumatic event, the heart rate becomes elevated and blood and nourishment are driven toward the center of the body to protect it. This pathodynamic is really basic physiology. It's a protective measure, not really "pathology," as in essence it is "ecology."

Although the effects of minor trauma are likely to be limited to local circulation, that circulatory impairment can have a broader impact and make the area more vulnerable to other conditions. When we experience a major trauma, the circulation of qi and blood is affected systemically. Ultimately this drains the qi, yin, and blood of the Heart. The Heart then attempts to compensate for this decrease in circulation by working harder and harder to overcome the stagnation. Over time this taxes the Heart. It is very similar to the dynamic of over-exercise (which we will cover in more detail in Chapter 2). When we start to make the Heart work harder, we need to finance that level of activity and that level of vigilance from somewhere. Over time the additional strain on the Heart depletes resources. Dr. Hammer continually points out that Heart Shock affects every cell in the body. Diminished circulation eventually results in a decrease in the essential nutrients that the blood provides, and an increase in waste products within the blood, putting additional strain on the systems that help with detoxification.

As stated earlier, all major physical traumas also cause an emotional shock to the Heart. There's always the emotional correlate, so we cannot simply focus on treatment of a particular injury. Many traumas can date back to conception, pregnancy, and even to the birthing process itself. Traumas related to Heart Shock encompass in utero events, the health of the fetus, the health of the mother during gestation and pregnancy, the integrity of the mother's circulation, and any kind of shock or traumatic event that impacts the mother during pregnancy. Modern birthing practices have become medicalized. Although birth is a natural process, we now commonly hook women up to tubes and pump medication through their systems, using tools like forceps and introducing drugs like pitocin/oxytocin to speed up the delivery. These things tend to intensify the birthing process, often introducing pain and additional stress, and can be considered shocks and traumas to both the mother and the baby.

There are many predisposing variables—the mother's constitution, her circulation, the integrity of the baby during the gestation process—that can affect the level of an infant's capacity to tolerate some of these interventions. Not every baby born in a hospital will undergo Shock, but a large number are vulnerable to enduring problems resulting from the now commonplace use of drugs and forceps. Furthermore, pregnancies now frequently occur later in life, when the constitutions of the mothers are often compromised. Rather than giving birth in their 20s, many women are having children in their 30s and perhaps 40s. This can have a significant impact. What rises to the level of Heart Shock in one person may not rise to the level of Heart Shock in someone else, so the varied aspects of constitution, lifestyle, physiology, and circumstance must be accounted for.

Within the context of Heart Shock, one must also look at what happens during the bonding process early in life. In general, the earlier the trauma, the greater the impact. This is because, early in life, the Heart and Kidney axis have not fully been formed;[6] those systems have not yet matured. Therefore, they tend to bear the brunt of the imbalances, causing a stunting in development.

In terms of physical trauma, the principal short-term issue is pain. But this pain often becomes chronic. This happens when the healing process is impaired because of a weakness and taxation on the Heart and circulation. Symptoms like migrating joint pain often result from the decreased circulation. Over time this deficit can lead to different kinds of structural defects, which often manifest as pain and discomfort in other parts of the body as well.

Once the Heart's capacity to circulate blood and nourishment is impacted, we start to see changes in all the different tissues and structures that rely on that blood and nourishment for support; areas of the body become deprived. It can be helpful to imagine health as a beautiful garden and the body as having a system of interconnected hoses which are used to bring nourishment and fluids to that garden. If you start to get kinks in those hoses, you will start to see diminished resources and water flowing to those corresponding areas. In these areas of limited access, you would eventually see that the flowers and plants dry out, wither, and decay. This is similar to what happens internally when improper blood flow fails to properly nourish the muscles, tissues, and sinews. Bones and joints are not as highly vascularized as some of the other tissues, so they tend to deteriorate more quickly and be more profoundly impacted.

As the pattern progresses, manifestations of impaired circulation and taxation on the Heart will include things like insomnia and other sleep disorders. We may also see "shen disturbances"—variations of anxiety, depression, and other mood and panic disorders—because we are dealing with the stability of the Heart, the Emperor, which also governs the patient's emotional life.

Consequently, the ups and downs of these mood swings can impact the Triple Burner[7] and its ability to regulate temperature. Some people emotionally feel "hot and cold"—going from one extreme to the other, from mania to depression within the bipolar continuum. These problems are more likely to result from traumas that occur earlier in life, before the maturation of the different organ systems.

Some of the things I commonly see that are frequently overlooked are the chronic fatigue syndrome and fibromyalgia presentations. These are often perceived as "mystery illnesses" and people often wonder where these diagnoses come from. Over the last few decades there has been an explosion of these diagnoses. It is really a collection of symptoms that tends to just get lumped into these categories of fibromyalgia and chronic fatigue because the Western medical community doesn't have a clear understanding of the pathomechanisms behind these symptoms. However, when you cross-reference this population of "chronic fatigue" sufferers with those presenting with Heart Shock, a strong connection arises.

As a practitioner in a suburban town with well-funded athletics programs, I often see patients suffering from concussions and post-concussion syndromes. Concussions readily and frequently rise to the level of Heart Shock and trauma. They exemplify many aspects of trauma—all the different types of soft tissue injuries and stagnations of blood and circulation to the tissues. The head becomes even more of a concern, since it will impact brain function. Systemically, the impact will create more taxation on the Heart and more stress on the circulation. More waste will be created internally and emotional instabilities are more likely to take place. Head injuries often rise to a higher level of severity, and result in significant qi and blood stagnation, warranting treating the Heart as a primary component of the treatment plan. I can attest to how quickly someone can respond to treatments, especially if the concussion is of a fairly recent origin. Repetitive concussion is common in athletes, and this requires a longer healing process as well as increased number of treatments. In any scenario where someone's getting repeated injuries, it's important to stop the activity that's causing the injury to allow for proper healing. However, our current athletic system, which prioritizes the game over the individual, is often unsupportive of a prolonged healing process. Furthermore, symptoms often disappear before the underlying mechanisms are resolved, creating a strong vulnerability for further injury as well as the sequelae of Heart Shock symptoms to progress and become more severe.

To reiterate, Heart Shock can be physical as well as emotional, and when physical injury rises to the level of Heart Shock, there will be an emotional correlate that occurs at the same time as the initial trauma. Beginning from this event, and worsening over time if no intervention takes place, is impairment to the circulation. A patient who has had a concussion, depending on the patient's level of maturity and the strength of their constitution, may heal with proper time and rest, but in many cases, people simply become less symptomatic and assume they have healed without examining all the other dynamics that result from the injury itself. A Western doctor may do an MRI or a CT and look at what's going on structurally and, if nothing is revealed on the imaging, may conclude the injury is gone. But this does not address the taxation on the Heart, nor does it consider the impact to the nervous system or how that nervous system hypervigilance is impacting the sinews/muscles/tendons, how it has impacted the adrenals, the Triple Burner mechanism, blood stagnation congesting the tissues, etc. These are some of the things that we want to factor into a complete healing process. As practitioners treating the sequelae of Heart Shock, it is imperative to create a strategy which factors an understanding of all the levels of diagnoses included within Heart Shock, not just the appearance of healing via the disappearance of symptoms.

The impact of traumas can last for decades, long after the initial injury has seemingly healed. Treating trauma goes well beyond the sports medicine approach of patching someone up so that they can get back on the field or court again. In Chinese medicine we are charged with creating health and nourishing life, as well as well-being and longevity (yang shen). To do so requires understanding the underlying root causes and the myriad manifestations that are created as a result. In treating those with injuries that have risen to the level of Heart Shock, we cannot simply remove a symptom and send them on their way. At the very least, they are vulnerable to another injury, and most likely future illness, as the dynamics of Heart Shock continue to create future pathology. As we embark on our relationship with these patients, we must educate them on the impact of their lifestyle and activities on their healing process, and engage them to make the necessary changes and commitments in service of their health.

Countless patients have come in over the years with a variety of injuries that can seem pretty straightforward, but a thorough evaluation often reveals critical information about the nature of the injury, the underlying constitution, and often a diagnosis of Heart Shock acting as a systemic block to healing. Discussion always takes place to explain the mechanisms preventing the healing process, and for athletes, often it requires time away from the training regimen until the condition stabilizes. After a trauma, the Heart needs to be strengthened, yin and blood need to be nourished and secured, the nervous system relaxed, the adrenals and Kidney yang anchored, etc. Without taking these (and other) strategies into account, one can create more damage to the tissues, and long-lasting injuries can, and often do, result.

A recent patient sought my help five months after she experienced a head trauma. The patient, 34 years old, woke up in the hospital the following day with significant pain, headaches, face numbness, dizziness, palpitations, low blood pressure, and numbness in her tongue. She was put on a week of anti-seizure medications and vicodin. Five months later she still felt weak and faint, facial numbness, and pain in her head, as well as significant anxiety. Heart Shock was a major component of her presentation, but from a more detailed evaluation, prior traumas were revealed which set the stage for her constitutional weakness and vulnerability. All of these significantly impacted her body condition, leaving pronounced instability and chaos ("Qi Wild," deficiency, as well as circulatory deficits). Her case study can be found in Part III of this book.

Emotional trauma

In terms of emotional shock, as a general rule, daily stress primarily affects the Liver, but shock affects the Heart.[8] Over time, as the Liver gets impacted by daily stress, it will eventually impact the Heart as well. The weaker the Heart is, the greater the impact; it is especially vulnerable to the heat that builds up in the Liver and rises to the chest, and the impact of blood stagnation[9] that will impair circulation to the Heart.

A basic ecological impact of emotional shock is that it provokes the protective mechanism of the Pericardium.[10] It also creates vasoconstriction of the peripheral circulation and the emptying of Heart yin as part of the recoil action, which drives yin and blood towards the interior of the body in an attempt to maintain circulation to the vital organs. This basic dynamic helps explain why in the Shen-Hammer lineage Sheng Mai San (Generate the Pulse Powder) is one of our base formulas that are modified to treat shock. Sheng Mai San nourishes Heart yin and astringes the Heart. It is typically modified by removing ginseng (Ren Shen) and adding American ginseng (Xi Yang Shen), the latter being stronger in terms of its supplementation to Heart yin. This becomes the base for understanding the primary treatment strategies, and, like many of the Imperial Academy formulas, serves as a teaching example from which one can modify, adding and removing herbs as needed and warranted from the other attending diagnoses. Abiding by the treatment principles (to be discussed in Chapter 3) is necessary to ensure the restoration of qi and yin to the Heart, otherwise separation of yin and yang and circulatory chaos ensues.

Heart Shock is a diagnosis of systemic instability. Since the Heart controls the mind, chaos tends to be expressed in our patients' lives as a chaotic lifestyle and often as mental instability.[11] Dr. Hammer compares this phenomenon to "a ship without a captain." He explains that the "Hun flies and the Po scatters all" (this concept will be discussed in more detail later in the text), and Su Wen Chapter 39 talks about shock "scattering the qi." And as the classics do mention fright (see the section about Classical references), its elaboration on all the varied mechanisms and treatment strategies is lacking. This chapter will flesh out these concepts in significant detail, and the remainder of this book is dedicated to its further understanding and treatment.

A lesser psychological consequence of shock becomes the tendency towards obsessive thinking. A common finding with a diagnosis of Heart Shock is a Hesitant pulse wave (see Figure 1.1), which is reflective of someone who is obsessively thinking about a particular subject, often that subject being trauma.

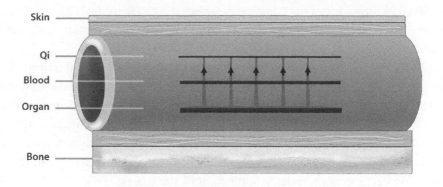

Figure 1.1: Hesitant pulse
Reproduced with permission from Eastland Press

Dr. Hammer has also stated that the protective measures of the Pericardium that cause vasoconstriction are accompanied by Heart qi and blood stagnation (which can translate to coronary artery stagnation if not treated properly).[12] Stagnation over time produces excess heat and, as a compensatory response to that heat, the body will start to accumulate dampness. The dampness is the body's attempt to quell heat and put out the fire, but as heat and dampness mix together they create phlegm. When found in the left distal position (Slippery pulse), this can create "Phlegm Misting the Orifices," often associated with mental, emotional, and psychiatric disorders. Many of those suffering Heart Shock will suffer signs of this, including depression and other mood disorders, as it impacts one's capacity to perceive clearly. Opening the orifices, therefore, becomes a very important component of treating Heart Shock. We must allow for the patient to perceive things differently, for as with all things, our perceptions create our reality.

With trauma, the triggering event alters our perceptions and our expression of yuan qi. The Triple Burner's dissemination of yuan qi up the Bladder channel and depositing its yuan qi into the shu points is how the constitution unfolds. This is often impacted from trauma which alters the dissemination. Treatments will be discussed later for rectifying this, including the use of the Window of the Sky points, jing-well points, and other acupuncture and herbal approaches to opening the portals.

According to Dr. Shen, the failure of the Heart to move qi and blood creates an intractable preoccupation with vengeance.[13] Heart blood stagnation, which he referred to as "Heart Small," also includes the propensity to lifelong fear, as part of the mechanism creating the stagnation has its root in trauma.

Further complicating this picture, if Heart Shock is left untreated, the yin and blood supply to the nervous system innervations of the Heart can become impaired, leading to fibrillations and electrical problems.[14] This process creates a vicious cycle in which increasingly diminished Heart function leads to decreased peripheral circulation. (From the Classical perspective, the Heart deals with peripheral circulation, whereas the Pericardium deals more with systemic circulation into the chest and throughout the Heart itself.)

The physiological effect of emotional trauma is the same as a physical trauma. With emotional trauma, the Heart affects the circulation rather than circulation affecting the Heart from physical trauma. With both physical and emotional trauma every cell in the body can be affected and there are decreasing nutrients and increasing waste products. It should be noted that the emotional component of a physical trauma can often be worse than the physical trauma itself. People can suffer more from the fear and psychological aspects than the actual extent of the injury.

The symptoms of Heart Shock are diverse, but some common ones are related to emotional lability and mood changes. One of the hallmarks of someone who has undergone a significant trauma or multiple traumas is that their life becomes chaotic so that everything around them seems as if it is falling apart. These people are always trying to keep things together and they always seem flustered. They can feel like they are on a roller coaster ride emotionally, with constant ups and downs and highs and lows. One minute they are stressed, the next minute they are happy. As their moods shift often, so does their energy, feeling hyper, then emotionally and physically tired. As Heart qi becomes weakened, depression can assert. As Heart yin gets impacted, and the separation between yin and yang occurs, anxiety and panic disorders are likely. Being easily stressed is a very common symptom related to taxation on the nervous system and the hypervigilance that ensues. The Heart is responsible for maintaining the shen, and its relationship with the hun; disturbances from trauma often include insomnia and dream-disturbed sleep, commonly with nightmares and vivid dreams and/or a lack of calm and peacefulness during the nighttime hours. Palpitations and other types of electrical problems in the Heart with rate and rhythm issues are also likely to occur.

Fatigue is another common symptom. Heart Shock is regularly overlooked as a source of fatigue in modern Chinese medicine, although it frequently occurs with Heart symptoms. Western medicine makes the connection more readily when looking at an elderly population with a higher incidence of heart disease, but I see a broad spectrum of patients in my practice experiencing fatigue from improper circulation limiting sufficient blood and oxygen to the tissues. As I mentioned earlier, when peripheral circulation is diminished, stagnation ensues, allowing waste products to accumulate in the system. This further hampers the body's ability to recover energy and feel adequate supplies of energy throughout the day.

Mental confusion is common especially when we see phlegm misting the orifices and, as mentioned earlier, there is often some type of dysfunction impacting perception after traumas.

Worry is also a common symptom. Patients often obsess about their trauma and the likelihood of something bad happening again. Distorted perceptions and changes to the sensory portals post trauma tend to amplify these feelings of worry and fear.

In children there is often fearfulness and nightmares, creating an inability for kids to sleep peacefully throughout the night. This can provide an important clue to parents that something traumatic was potentially perceived.

Wandering joint pains commonly occur after a trauma, especially if weakened Heart qi is diminishing circulation to local areas post physical trauma. It can also simply result from the impact to the Heart and its subsequent inability to govern the blood circulation.

Common symptoms of Heart Shock

- Emotional lability
- Mood changes
- Feeling flustered
- Feeling like one is on an emotional roller coaster
- Depression
- Anxiety
- Panic disorder
- Hypervigilance
- Insomnia and dream-disturbed sleep
- Nightmares (especially in children)
- Fatigue
- Mental confusion
- Worry
- Wandering joint pains

There are many other symptoms that can be discussed in terms of Heart Shock, but those listed above are the most common. Symptoms common with patterns of Heart qi deficiency, Heart yin deficiency, Heart blood deficiency, and Heart Qi and blood stagnation are all possible and likely.

Classical references: Terror—Chaos, rebellion, paralysis, and frozen yang

From a Classical perspective, fear, shock (kong 恐), and fright (jing 惊) can create a number of dynamics. First, fear can have the nature of freezing the qi-yang and creating immobility. This paralysis is often seen with extreme traumas where people feel unable to respond or react; the fight/flight mechanism being only two of the three options from experiencing trauma, the other leaving one frozen. This can happen physically where one feels incapable of moving, or emotionally with an inability to contact one's feelings, or emotional numbness. There are many examples of this in nature, and Peter Levine cites a number of them in *In an Unspoken Voice, How the Body Releases Trauma and Restores Goodness* (2010). He states:

> When an organism perceives overwhelming mortal danger (with little or no chance for escape) the **biological** response is a global one of paralysis and shutdown. Ethologists call this innate response tonic immobility (TI).[15]

Levine aptly notes religious and mythical expressions of this tonic immobility in the stories of Lot's wife being turned to a pillar of salt when disobeying orders to not look back on the destruction of Sodom and Gomorrah, Medusa turning those who match her gaze into stone, the Greek god Zeus invoking terror and paralysis in his enemies, and the indigenous peoples of South and Mesoamerica who treated this paralysis (which they called "fright paralysis" and "soul loss") with shamanic healing.[16] He goes on to mention, and we will discuss more later, how humans often become fixated in this paralysis and become incapable of re-engaging in present life. From the Chinese medical perspective we can view this as an imbalance between the Hun and the Po, and I will discuss treatments for this later in this text.

Levine and Dr. Hammer both discuss how wartime traumas impacted soldiers on the battlefield. Terms like "soldier's heart" and "shell shock" depict the devastating impacts with symptoms such as anxiety and panic disorders, uncontrollable shaking, arrhythmias, night terrors, and the inability to psychologically move on from one's traumatic experiences. Being frozen in time…

But, as we will discuss within this text, any trauma prevents the opportunity for growth as well. As we heal from the specific traumas we have faced, we learn more about ourselves, our resilience, our priorities, and what really matters to us in life. Building on the Medusa analogy, Levine notes a second version of this myth wherein Perseus collects a drop of blood from Medusa's wound in two vials: one giving the power to kill, the other the power to heal and renew life. So, too, with the treatments offered by Chinese medicine. We are uniquely gifted with tools to tap into our patients' deepest essence to help them resurrect their spirit and destiny. And Hexagram 51 attests to this when it states:

> When Quake [Thunder] comes, people shiver and shake, but then they whoop it up with talk filled with laughter.[17]

Legge's translation is in accord:

> Zhen (gives the intimation of) ease and development. "When the (time of) movement (which it indicates) comes, (its subject) will be found looking out with apprehension:"—that feeling of dread leads to happiness. "And yet smiling and talking cheerfully:"—the issue (of his dread) is that he adopts (proper) laws (for his course). "The movement (like a crash of thunder) terrifies all within a hundred Lu:"—it startles the distant and frightens the near. "He will be like the sincere worshipper, who is not startled into letting go his ladle and cup of sacrificial spirits:"—he makes his appearance, and maintains his ancestral temple and the altars of the spirits of the land and grain, as presiding at all sacrifices.[18]

And in essence, this hexagram sets forth the very thesis of the current book: that on the other side of trauma and shock, if managed correctly, are freedom, joy, and happiness. The I Jing is the Book of Changes, and Chinese medicine is predicated on the Daoist notion of change, on non-attachment, and being rooted in the moment, maintaining flexibility, non-judgment, constant movement, and adaptability to present circumstances. Heart Shock patients have lost this ability, and the strategies set forth herein are meant to restore it.

As with any experience, an experience of shock must be transitory and fleeting, as health requires constant movement. Concepts such as "flowing water never decays" or "moss doesn't grow under a rolling stone" reflect what we know from Chinese medicine: health is a dynamic process that requires the free flow of qi and blood and the balance of yin and yang. Rooted in Daoist philosophy, we cannot become fixated on our experiences, or desiring a particular future; we must remain open in the present moment. So, too, is the case with traumas. We call upon many defensive and adaptive mechanisms to deal with the severity of these situations, but, they too, must be transitory to allow us to return to the present moment and not become stuck/frozen in the past event. In many situations, our survival may rely upon this. Levine discusses this in relation to animals on the Serengeti where a cheetah leaps on a gazelle which collapses to the ground in a state of "fear paralysis" upon imminent death despite that it may be uninjured at the time of collapse. Animals often enter this altered state of consciousness when there is no possibility of escape and many believe that this can prevent or ameliorate the pain and suffering of an untimely demise by creating a numbing or dissociated state. So, for one who is frightened and must be ready to fight or flee, muscles become tense and readied; for one who approaches a certain death, one becomes flaccid and numb and dissociated.[19] This Flight (escape), Fight (can't escape), Freeze (frightened/frozen), or Fold (collapse/dissociate) happens in varying degrees in different individuals depending on the severity of the traumatic experience and the patient's constitutional and available resources and adaptive strategies, and they can implicate different levels of energetics (channel systems) that must be engaged in order to successfully treat. But, no matter which strategic system is employed, it becomes crucial to move this individual into the present moment and engage them in the here and now.

Second, fear can create a rapid descension of qi by weakening the Kidney yang. This is commonly seen in children who wet themselves when frightened, but has also been seen in the cases of shell shock as mentioned above wherein soldiers will lose control of their bowels in the trenches.

> [W]hen one is in terror, the energy will be bogged down…[20]

> When one is in terror, the refined energy will be declined, and the decline of the energy below will cause obstruction of the upper warmer, as the energy cannot reach the upper warmer, it will return to the lower warmer, and the energy stagnation will cause fullness and distension of the lower warmer. It is called "unstableness and descent of the energy."[21]

> Excessive terror may hurt the Kidney.[22]

> When one has excessive terror, it will injure the Kidney.[23]

Third, shock (kong) and fright (jing) often have an impact on the Kidney qi by creating chaotic movement. The Su Wen and Ling Shu instruct us:

> When one is in excessive terror, the beat of the heart will cause him to feel like helpless [sic], it seems that his spirit and mind have nowhere to rest, and his misgiving has nowhere to stop. So, it is called the "confusing of the energy (qi)."[24]

> Excessive terror and pondering cause the wastage of Yin energy to become unstable of the patient.[25]

> Excessive terror causes the unrestraint of the refined energy due to the unrest of the spirit.[26]

> Excessive terror and pondering will injure the spirit, when the spirit is hurt, one will not be able to control himself…[27]

> [T]error and anger cause the excitation of the spirit…[28]

> When a man is invaded by cold, he will be disquieted and restless like being on alert [jing], his spirit and energy excrete outside [fu-float] and his Yang energy becomes unstable.[29]

We might see such symptoms as inability to sleep, fainting, etc. It also can create neurological symptoms from weakening the Kidneys and allowing for exuberant Liver yang with wind with such symptoms as seizures and convulsions, vision and sensory decline, and somnolence and narcolepsy, as the Liver "is liable to fright."[30] We may also see a desertion syndrome. The analogy of the gazelle on the Serengeti is but one example of many that occur in nature.

Fright also prevents the Lung qi and yin from properly descending and anchoring to the Kidney as a result. This dynamic can create an excess of qi in the chest leading to symptoms like hyperventilation. And when Lung yin cannot descend, turbid fluids can be retained in the chest, creating phlegm as well as phlegm misting the orifices of the Heart.

> [W]hen the lung energy is in prosperity (yin overabundance), one will dream of being frightened and crying.[31]

Fourth, an unresolved shock tends to affect a person to his core, meaning the yuan qi level. The shock as a wei qi energetic (external environment) becomes displaced and begins to move towards the yuan level. Often this is done via the divergent meridians (discussed more in Chapter 7). As it reaches the yuan level, the 8 extraordinary meridians become involved and we see a contamination of the jing-essence. As mentioned above, the yuan qi is disseminated via the Triple Burner mechanism and deposited into each meridian via the Bladder shu points. A physiological correlate to the constitutional disposition of someone being a wood person or a metal person is determined by how much yuan qi deposits into the associated shu point. Often in trauma we see a displacement of this constitutional yuan qi into other points as a compensatory measure. So, the individual who was normally quite independent and self-assured pre-trauma can become reclusive, fearful, and increasingly vulnerable post trauma from this displacement of yuan qi being impacted from the event.

Fifth, fright creates a block preventing the proper communication between the Heart and Kidneys. Palpitations, insomnia, anxiety, etc. often result with this imbalance.

> When one is in excessive anxiety, his heart will be injured and his spirit will become dull, the energy will be stagnated and fails to circulate. So it is called "stagnation of energy."[32]

> [E]xcessive joy may hurt the heart, but terror can overcome the overjoy.[33]

And lastly, shock can create rebellious qi.

> The excitation of moods like overjoy, anger etc. [including anxiety and terror from the preceding paragraph] may damage the viscera, so it hurts the vital energy of man.

Violent rage makes the vital energy flow reversely and force the blood to run upwards and causes blood stagnation above, as a result, the Yin is hurt. Violent overjoy causes the vital energy to slow down and descend, as a result, the Yang is hurt.[34]

When the patient…becomes frightened and restless as if someone is going to arrest him, it is the syndrome of the evil energy in the gallbladder, and the disorder of the vital energy will affect the stomach; when the bile is overflowing, there will be bitter taste in the mouth, when the stomach energy reverses up, the bile will be vomited.[35]

One of the most common manifestations of this would be running piglet disorder. Chapter 8 of the Jin Gui Yao Lue states, "Bentun [running piglet qi], vomiting of pus, fright and fire-evil are four diseases caused by fright."[36] Or we may see symptoms like migraines, coughing, vomiting, etc. as a rebellion or reflection of one not liking the world the way it is, or that it has seemingly become, post trauma.

Correlations to the channel systems

As we look at the dynamics above, what we see is a number of correlations to the Classical channel systems. First, we have the fright acting as an external event confronting our wei qi and nervous system. The recoiling action of a sudden shock and the tension and armoring and/or activation of the muscles (fight/flight/freeze response) call to action the sinew meridians. Initially, this event confronts the taiyang (BL and SI) in its activation of the fight/flight/freeze muscles, but if it's not resolved, the condition becomes chronic, weakening the taiyang and impacting other sinew channels as well. We will discuss these dynamics in Chapter 4.

Second, in many individuals the wei qi is not strong enough to confront the trauma directly, enabling it to move internally like a pathogen. Depending on the type of trauma, and the condition of the individual, the luo vessels may be called upon to quiet the impact and put it into a state of latency. When that system is not fully able to do so, we see classic luo vessel symptoms like emotional and shen disturbances, pain, and/or rebellious qi. Further discussion of the luo channels will take place in Chapter 5.

Third, a severe trauma that overwhelms wei qi may move aggressively towards impacting the organs themselves. In that case, the divergent channels become activated to help translocate this pathology away from the organs and towards the bony cavities, using available resources to surround it like a blanket. As resources are consumed and latency begins to be lost, we see symptoms such as arthritis and bi-syndromes and inflammatory conditions taking place. The Su Wen discusses this bi-syndrome in relation to the Liver:

> The symptoms of the hepatic bi-syndrome are: being frightened. The symptoms of the hepatic bi-syndrome are: being terrified often when sleeping at night…[37]

More on the divergent channels in Chapter 7.

Fourth, some traumas shake us to our core, directly impacting the deepest parts of us. Running piglet qi, for example, affects the Heart, Liver, and Kidneys and the pathway of its ascent is via the Chong mai. This is likely in children or when the trauma is severe enough. The trauma begins to contaminate the jing-essence itself and alters the dissemination of yang qi. The Ling Shu states:

> When the excessive terror is not relieved, it will injure the essence of life…[38]

This is reflected in the dynamics of the 8 extraordinary meridians. See Chapter 8 for more information on the 8 extraordinary meridians.

Even Zhang Zhong Jing in his famous Preface to the Shang Han Lun noted how those struck by illness can be perceived as traumatic, causing one to tremble and despair:

> [When they then] suddenly suffer [an attack of] evil wind qi and [consequently] develop an extraordinary illness, meeting misfortune and disaster, [they] tremble and shake. Abandoning their integrity, they lower themselves to grovel before magical healers. Declaring [their] helplessness, [they] attribute [their misfortune to fate ordained by] heaven, with hands tied, they accept defeat.[39]

What follows in this text is meant to create a lifeline to those in need, unshackle the bonds, and provide hope while moving past trauma and into the mysteries and wonder of the present moment, and beyond.

CHAPTER 2

Heart Shock Presentation

Etiology, Signs, Symptoms, and Aggravating Factors

Signs of Heart Shock generally take precedence over symptoms as they are a more accurate barometer of the imbalance. Not everyone will experience symptoms, some will be unaware of them, and others will fail to report them. This is especially true for psycho-emotional symptoms, as there is unfortunately still stigma surrounding psychological diseases. Many patients are reluctant to admit to any form of psychological illness. Others are simply out of touch with what is happening in their bodies. So the signs of Heart Shock become very important as they allow practitioners to perceive these issues directly without questioning the patient. As an added bonus, this helps to create an immediate bond and heightened level of intimacy that may otherwise take months of treatments to form. Often, simply mentioning that the pulse (or other sign) is highly suggestive of trauma (or depression, anxiety, fear, etc. as these all show up on the pulse) opens the door to a discussion of these often painful subjects. It also removes the stigma from the clinical setting by approaching it in a non-judgmental and caring way.

Signs refer to the information that we as clinicians can perceive objectively. There are pathognomonic findings that can substantiate a diagnosis of Heart Shock even in the absence of symptoms. Symptoms are, of course, helpful to flush things out and prioritize your treatment (e.g., to choose the specific acupuncture points or channel systems or herbal strategies or the oils that you could use or the food that you would suggest), but it's the signs that are the most important aspect of making the diagnosis.

The first thing we can observe on the pulse after a trauma is an elevated rate, or a Rapid pulse. The degree to which the pulse will elevate is in direct response to the significance and the severity of the trauma, as well as the overall body condition and constitution of the patient. So a vulnerability in the Heart system can cause a significant jump in heart rate in someone who experiences even a minor trauma versus someone who is very robust experiencing a more severe trauma.

> Yellow Emperor said: "Good. But these are not what I want to know. I want to know why can some people enjoy a long life even when they encounter great misery and great fright to have terrible moods, they remain healthy and not being injured even encountering the bitter cold or scorching heat, but some other people can by no means to evade

disease even when they stay in the room sheltered from wind without any stimulations of deep sorrow or great fright?"

Qibo said: "The five solid and the six hollow organs are the places where the exogenous evils retain, when one's five solid organs are all small, the disease contracted will be light, but this kind of people often pay attention to worrying things which will inevitably cause them to become grieve; when one's five solid organs are all large, he will be slow in doing things, and he can hardly become sorrowful. When the position of the five solid organs are all high, one will crave after something high and far-reaching which is out of touch with reality; when the position of the five solid organs are all low, one will be weak-willed to rest content with remaining under others. When the five solid organs are all firm, one will not contract disease; when the five solid organs are all weak, one will not divorce from the disease. When the positions of the five solid organs are upright, one's disposition will be gentle and amiable; when the five solid organs are slanting, one will be harbouring wicked intentions, hankering for stealing, and his words are fickle."[40]

Here, the Ling Shu instructs us to consider our patient's constitution and body condition. It must be factored in to have a full understanding of the implications of shock. With regards to rate, there is not a set rate to suggest a severe trauma versus a minor one. However, other factors on the pulse will help make this determination. (We will discuss normal healthy heart rates in the following section.) Rate must always be measured against the specific nature of the patient's constitution; but it's important to remember that a Rapid heart rate always creates some degree of taxation on the Heart. Anytime an organ system works harder than it needs to, it will consume some of its energy, and that energy requires financing.

One critical factor that determines whether one's experience will rise to the level of trauma and lead to Heart Shock is whether or not the initial elevated rate returns to normal quickly after the event. Peter Levine notes this too in *In an Unspoken Voice*, where he cites the findings of Dr. Arieh Shalev's 1998 Israeli study from an emergency room:

> Of course, most patients are upset and have a high heart rate when they are first admitted to the ER, since they are most likely there as victims of some terrifying incident such as a bus bombing or motor vehicle accident. What Shalev discovered was that a patient whose heart rate had returned to near normal by the time of discharge from the ER was unlikely to develop posttraumatic stress disorder. On the other hand, one whose heart rate was still elevated upon leaving was highly likely to develop PTSD in the following weeks or months.[41]

The Heart's ability to return to its normal rate depends largely on the protective measures surrounding the Heart, including the Small Intestine's ability to quickly clear excess heat, the Pericardium's adaptive strategies, and the Triple Burner's self-regulatory functions. As Peter Levine states:

> In general, the capacity for self-regulation is what allows us to handle our own states of arousal and our difficult emotions, thus providing the basis for the balance between authentic autonomy and healthy social engagement.[42]

> This capacity for self-regulation holds the key for our modern survival—survival beyond the brutal grip of anxiety, panic, night terrors, depression, physical symptoms and helplessness that are the earmarks of prolonged stress and trauma.[43]

Maintaining an elevated rate over time will gradually consume the qi of the Heart, ultimately causing the heart rate to slow.

The other pathognomonic finding is a Rough Vibration over the whole pulse (see Figure 2.1). The intensity of the Rough Vibration will give us a sense of the severity of the trauma. This quality is rated on a scale from 1 (minor) to 5 (severe). The level and intensity of that vibration provides information about severity, and the timing and depth at which we feel the Rough Vibration can offer additional clues. A Rough Vibration that is only perceived at the superficial aspect of the pulse (Qi depth) generally indicates a fairly recent trauma. If it is moving down to the middle depth (Blood depth) or the deepest aspect (Organ depth) and throughout the pulse, we can be certain that this trauma is such that it has been affecting the person for a much longer period of time, especially if it's on both left and right wrists. Sometimes the Rough Vibration from the trauma may only start on the left-hand side and then make its way down the depths and onto the other side. So, one must assess the quality of the vibration, the intensity of the vibration, and the location (sides and depths) of the vibration. Smooth Vibrations are also common with Heart Shock, and while not diagnostic of trauma, often occur as a sign of worry.

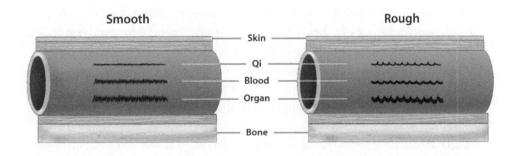

Figure 2.1: Vibrations
Reproduced with permission from Eastland Press

From a Classical perspective, a Rough Vibration often signifies the involvement of the 8 extraordinary vessels. We will discuss more about these pulse shapes and qualities in Chapter 8, but essentially, when vibrating, these pulses are reflections that one has been shaken to their deepest core and the pathological impact remains active. Different channel systems reflect differing layers of energetic refinement, and there are particular signatures that reveal their movements. This is clearly seen, for example, in the needling techniques for different channels. The 8 extraordinary channels are accessed via a shaking or vibrating needle technique. The idea being that they are the deepest and most dense level of energetics internally and therefore require a stirring up via shaking/vibrating to be properly accessed and awakened. This is done slowly if the intent is to nourish and supplement, and quickly if the intent is to sedate or drain. (The sinew meridians deal with wei qi; this is a more hyperactive movement, and its energetics are accessed with more circular and spiraling techniques. The luo vessels deal more with the ying layer and their needling is done via lifting and thrusting. The divergent channels are mediating the wei and yuan levels and are needled with a three-time method of accessing the wei level with circular/spiraling movements, then moving to the yuan level with vibrating techniques (needling techniques will be explored in each chapter).)

What we know from Chinese medicine, and is reflective of our own understanding and experiences, is that when we are really scared or anxious we have a tendency to shake and tremble. We can also feel cold. Both of these responses demonstrate an impact to the yuan level. Not surprisingly, when one experiences a significant trauma, there is also this autonomic response of shaking or trembling.

> When it [the Kidneys] is reversed, shiver occurs…[44]

And it is not just humans who have this innate response, but our friends in the animal kingdom as well. In *In an Unspoken Voice*, Peter Levine cites numerous examples, including: wild animals trembling when confined, during sexual encounters at climax, shaking/trembling during spiritual practices, and even in certain lineages of qigong and yogic practices. He states:

> All of these "tremblings," experienced in diverse circumstances and having a multiplicity of other functions, hold the potential for catalyzing authentic transformation, deep healing and awe.
>
> These gyrations and undulations are ways that our nervous system "shakes off" the last rousing experience and "grounds" us in readiness for the next encounter with danger, lust and life. They are mechanisms that help restore our equilibrium after we have been threatened or highly aroused. They bring us down to earth, so to speak. Indeed, such physiological reactions are at the core of self-regulation and resilience.[45]

Shaking and vibrating can be mimicked by our needling techniques as mentioned above, and they can also happen spontaneously during treatments, as many practitioners can attest to having patients twitch or shake while relaxing on the table during an acupuncture session. I can recall some of my own experiences that many would consider highly traumatic that left no imprint of Heart Shock. One notable one included a shattered nose at age 11 from being hit accidentally with a hockey stick. The impact and injury were not traumatic as I was used to a lot of rough play and injuries, but having the nose set and packed in a doctor's office in an hour-long procedure without anesthesia was. I remember focusing all my energy on maintaining stillness while gripping the table with both hands as tight as I could. The pain was intense, but I refused to make any noise other than some deep grunting as I bore the discomfort with every bit of will power I could muster. After the procedure was over, I was left on the table and began violently shaking. I asked no one to touch me and I shook for approximately 30 minutes until my body calmed down on its own accord. I did not have the knowledge at that time to understand the importance of this shaking, nor did I check my heart rate, but I imagine the release helped bring my body back to homeostasis, that my Triple Burner mechanism had restored my physiology. And, like anything else, even our worst experiences can be meaningful and beneficial. Again, Hexagram 51 of the I Jing states:

> When Quake [Thunder] comes, people shiver and shake, but then they whoop it up with talk filled with laughter.[46]

> When Quake comes, there is danger, and this one, alas, loses his cowries… He sets forth without any response or support, and wherever he goes there is not shelter for him. As awesome severity holds great sway here, no one takes him in, and he has to move about without any provisions. Although he repeatedly crosses over strategic high ground, he surely will come to grief through exhaustion of resources and will not last more than seven days.[47]

> Quake comes, so this one is anxious and distraught, his gaze shifty and unfocused.[48]

Wilhelm's understanding of this Hexagram is similar. He states:

> The fear and trembling engendered by shock come to an individual at first in such a way that he sees himself placed at a disadvantage as against others. But this is only transitory. When the ordeal is over, he experiences relief, and thus the very terror he had to endure at the outset brings good fortune in the long run.

Shock comes and makes one distraught
If shock spurs to action
One remains free of misfortune.

There are three kinds of shock—the shock of heaven, which is thunder, the shock of fate, and, finally, the shock of the heart. The present hexagram refers less to inner shock than to the shock of fate. In such times of shock, presence of mind is all too easily lost: the individual overlooks all opportunities for action and mutely lets fate take its course. But if he allows the shocks of fate to induce movement within his mind, he will overcome these external blows with little effort.[49]

When looking at the level of severity of a trauma, we can assess the rate and the Rough Vibration (intensity, quality, depth) by factoring in the patient's current age as well as the age of the traumatic event (if the patient knows). For example, if someone is 30 years old and they have a heart rate of 60 but they have a significant Rough Vibration over their whole pulse and some arrhythmias, we can be fairly certain that that trauma was something that happened decades before. Why? Because that is an unusually low heart rate for a 30-year-old and it would take many years for the heart rate to slow to that pace. We could surmise that he experienced the traumatic incident as a young child, which would have prompted his heart rate to jump into the 90s, if not above. Over time it would have weakened the Heart, and the heart rate would have eventually slowed down as Heart qi was consumed. An additional clue is the presence of an arrhythmia. Typically, for there to be rhythm changes on the pulse, the trauma would have happened prior to the age of 15 or the age of maturation. (This is dependent on physical state and the robustness of the Heart qi at the time of trauma, so it is possible for someone to experience a trauma later in life and still create an arrhythmia if the Heart qi was depleted.)

A Flat pulse (see Figure 2.2) occurring in the left distal position is another quality that would be reflective of Heart Shock and trauma. This quality indicates that a trauma occurred when a person was very young, was in a very weakened constitutional state at the time of impact, or that the trauma was of overwhelming intensity. In a Flat pulse, the sensation is only found in the deeper depth of the left distal position, tucked under the scaphoid bone. It feels like a very squashed/flattened pulsation, devoid of any waveform.

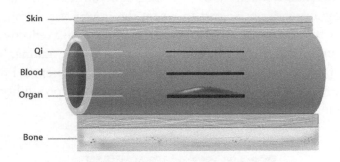

Figure 2.2: Flat pulse
Reproduced with permission from Eastland Press

The Inflated quality (see Figure 2.3) is also another sign of trauma when found on the left distal position. This pulse feels like a fully inflated balloon with a constant level of pressure no matter what depth you are pressing on; it doesn't give way as you exert more pressure. The Flat pulse's opposite, the Inflated quality indicates that the event occurred when the person was relatively robust. It is a sign that there is significant trapped qi in the Heart and chest. The Inflated pulse is frequently found in patients who were stuck in the birth canal during the birthing process, while the Flat pulse results from the umbilical cord being wrapped around the baby's neck during delivery.

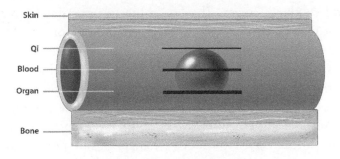

Figure 2.3: Inflated pulse
Reproduced with permission from Eastland Press

While not pathognomonic of trauma, additional findings on the pulse can include the Tight pulse (see Figure 2.4). This can reflect the emotional and/or physical pain that often accompanies trauma. With physical pain, you may find it in a specific area of the body anatomically related to where the injury was sustained. A Tight pulse found over the entire superficial aspect of the pulse is also reflective of nervous system tension and a state of hypervigilance that is created post trauma. It reflects the constant state of readiness that comes from being constantly prepared to encounter some traumatic event, or the worry that is engendered from the possibility of suffering an additional trauma.

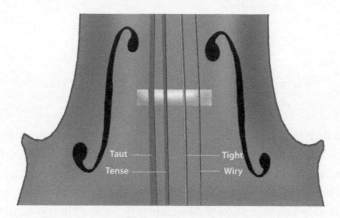

Figure 2.4: Taut-Tense-Tight-Wiry pulses
Reproduced with permission from Eastland Press

More on the pulse: Rate and rhythm issues

Some of the more common features of trauma as reflected on the pulse include the host of rate and rhythm changes. The first thing to understand when looking at rhythm is that it is reflected throughout the entire pulse. From the Shen-Hammer perspective, rate and rhythm are found over the entire pulse, not just in one position or another. This is because they reflect systemic problems and as such we need to recognize that they are affecting the Emperor. In terms of rate alone, the Shen-Hammer lineage measures it with a clock creating the same reading regardless of position (with some possible exceptions[50]). From a Classical perspective, we can have different rates in different pulse positions (changes in rate per patient's breath, or specific qualities interpreted as impacting rate), so, in that case, it is going to reflect issues in the organs/channels we find it in.

As stated above, the Heart is the Emperor, and everything within the Empire will be impacted by rhythm issues. As it impacts the Heart/Emperor, we will also see an impact to the mind, as well as the emotions and the nervous system, due to its intimate relationship to the Heart. Classically, the Heart controls the mind, and a lot of the stability of our emotional life comes from the stability, strength, and integrity in the Heart itself. As a result, where rhythm is impacted, stabilizing the mind, spirit, and Heart, as a unit, is required.

Rhythm is always reflecting the Heart, but that doesn't negate other relationships as well. From a Classical perspective the Lungs play a role in the movement of blood, which is governed by the Heart. This relationship is founded on the Lungs' governance of wei-defensive qi. Wei qi is a major driving force behind the heartbeat as well as the rhythm as it governs smooth muscle contraction. The Heart is a smooth muscle, and the integrity of wei qi in relation to the Heart creates a healthy rate and rhythm. Anything interfering with wei qi can potentially impact the Heart's rate and rhythm. This is commonly seen with childhood febrile diseases where wei qi is called upon to confront an external pathogen, creating a fever and also causing an elevated heart rate. (Wei qi deals with the peristaltic activity in the gut as well, another smooth muscle area which will be discussed in Chapter 4.)

The Lungs' role in respiration and the evenness of our breathing mechanism is also significant in relationship to the Heart and its rhythm. Holding breath, not breathing evenly, shortness of breath, tightness in the chest, or restrictions in the diaphragm can interfere with, and impact, heart rate and rhythm, making it important to assess the role of the Lungs and the wei qi.

A problem with rhythm, as a marker of systemic instability, constitutes one of the most critical diagnoses and, as such, becomes a priority in treatment, either taking precedence over, or currently combined with, other strategies and immediate interventions. According to Dr. Hammer, integrity of rhythm is the single most important aspect of pulse diagnosis and a significant indicator of cardiac functioning and the state of health of the Heart system.

Looking at rhythm, a number of parameters help to classify and characterize its significance. First is whether or not we are experiencing skipping of beats (Interrupted or Intermittent) or whether we are experiencing speeding up and slowing down (Changing Rate at Rest).[51] This latter quality is different from counting a rate of 60 beats per minute and then counting again for another minute and finding 70 beats per minute, which is not technically a rhythm or rate issue (though it still may be diagnostic of other instabilities of the Heart in other capacities).

To further differentiate, we want to know:

1. Does the change occur at rest?
2. Is the rate measurable?
3. Are there missed beats?
4. If there are missed beats, are they consistent or inconsistent?
5. How often does the irregularity occur?
6. If there are no missed beats, is there a changing rate?
7. If there is, is it occasional or constant?
8. What is the degree/severity, i.e., how large or small is the shift?

According to Dr. Shen, all rate and rhythm changes involve Heart function and are intimately connected to the nervous system. When we are looking at the nervous system we are looking at wei qi to some degree. We're also looking at yuan qi and jing-essence, as it's partly a combination and communication between the Kidneys, Kidney yin-jing-essence, and its regulation over the central nervous system mediated in terms of movement and circulation by its counterparts, the Bladder and Small Intestine. The taiyang energetics have a responsibility and role in maintaining, at least from a sinew channel perspective, all of the muscles and innervations of the nerves. But, we also must consider wei qi and a zang-fu perspective, and that would include the Lungs and Liver. The Lungs regulate the movement of wei qi to the surface/skin, and the Liver circulates wei qi to and through the peripheral nerves and the musculature: sinews, muscles, tendons. And as mentioned earlier, when we undergo stress it impacts the Liver, creates heat, and harasses the spirit, mind, and Heart. It can also impact and stress the adrenals, as well as the taiyang, it being the outward manifestation of the shaoyin relationship.

Instability in the nervous system can be a reflection of either weakness, or the excessive stirring, of the jing-essence, which impacts and destabilizes the Heart in its association to the mind, the spirit, and the emotions. This creates a vicious cycle wherein the instability of the Heart causes further imbalances in the nervous system. Constant stress causes adrenaline release. One gets tight, armored, and enters the fight/flight/freeze response. It makes one nervous, panicky, and fearful, further feeding tension, creating the renewed need to stimulate adrenaline release. This stimulates the Heart. The rate increases, rhythm may become affected, and the cycle ensues. These interconnections require that the Heart, nervous system, and adrenals be treated simultaneously.

Over time, the symptoms of emotional instability will increase both in frequency as well as severity. Any of the varied rate and rhythm issues may become manifest with chronic stress and resultant instability in the nervous system. This cycle enervates the Heart as well as the nervous system energetics over time.

Rhythm issues tend to have an etiology before the age of 15, or the age of maturity (which can vary with constitutions and life circumstances), as there is less stability in the Heart and the nervous system (rooted in Kidney energetics). While there are exceptions, generally, if someone has an arrhythmia, there was some trauma prior to that age. Oftentimes rhythm issues involve traumas that happened either in utero, during the birthing process, or early in one's life. And, the more consistent the arrhythmia, the earlier or greater was the triggering event.

Constitutional Heart qi deficiency will also predispose one to all different types of arrhythmias, and as such can make a trauma that much more severe. Scarlet fever, for example, can weaken the Heart, lead to rheumatic heart disease, and create more significant changes. When there is underlying qi deficiency, the rate tends to be more Rapid immediately after the shock and in the initial stages, later tending to slow down. When there is an acute stress or one experiences a secondary trauma, it will exacerbate and take advantage of the deficiency, increasing the rate significantly.

The different types of arrhythmias include the following.

"Changing Rate at Rest" pulse

This pulse tends to speed up and slow down and is noticeable within a relatively short period of time. The cadence is changing but it's not dropping any beats. The interpretations depend on a few factors. If it's occasional, this is a Heart qi agitation: a nervousness in the Heart creating some instability. If it's consistent throughout the evaluation, as well as over multiple examinations, it signifies Heart qi deficiency. When shock is the etiology, and the constitution is strong, the left distal position can have a very Tight quality in the center of the position; when it's weak it tends to be more of a Feeble (see Figure 2.5) quality in the left distal position.

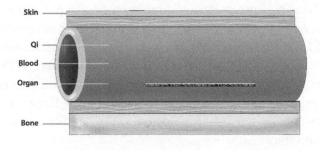

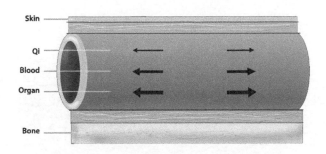

Figure 2.5: Feeble pulse: early stage and as it progresses
Reproduced with permission from Eastland Press

Heart qi agitation has multiple etiologies: excess heat from qi stagnation, yin deficient heat, and mild shock or trauma (which will also create a Rapid rate). Large changes reflect more severe Heart qi deficiency, often creating Heart blood deficiency, especially when there's prolonged worry. Large changes are often seen in people with borderline psychological states, and those who exhibit mental and emotional instability. If there is a constitutional Heart qi deficiency and someone is working beyond their means, for a period of time we can sometimes see a larger Changing Rate at Rest.

Symptoms related to the Changing Rate at Rest are consistent with some that are typical with Heart Shock. Emotionally, people tend to feel as if they're on a roller coaster ride, their mind racing out of control. They tend to feel moody, constantly changing their minds; they find it hard to focus, and tend to doubt themselves; they experience palpitations. Their self-esteem and self-worth can be low; they are generally agitated and nervous, experience anxiety, and their lives are marked by turmoil. They have trouble sleeping, and tend to wake up tired in the morning, generally experiencing fatigue and a feeling of impotence in their lives. All of these symptoms become more profound and more severe with larger changes in rate and, not surprisingly, tend to signify a more profound triggering event.

When the Changing Rate at Rest gets more pronounced it signifies a moderate Heart qi deficiency and all of the symptoms show an increase in severity. Palpitations and shortness of breath come on exertion. We might see spontaneous or excessive sweating, or even a cold sweat as it goes towards yang deficiency. We will also see more coldness in the extremities from improper circulation. Patients tend to talk excessively as they're not able to contain their emotions. There's a higher degree of emotional vulnerability and lability. Edema in the hands and face may present; circulatory function shows impairment.

Typically, along with this pulse the Changing Intensity and Amplitude pulses show up (see Figure 2.6). As an overall measure of stability, amplitude (measure of yang) and intensity/substance (measure of yin) should be consistent.

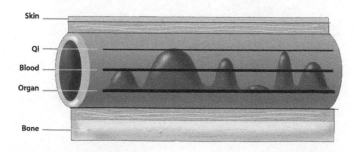

Figure 2.6: Changing Intensity and Amplitude pulses
Reproduced with permission from Eastland Press

Interrupted and Intermittent pulses

Rate Measurable: When the rate is measurable with missed beats we have two qualities called Interrupted and Intermittent. The Interrupted quality is one that misses beats on an irregular nature (e.g., 3 beats, then 5 beats, then 7; it's not consistent). This reflects moderate-to-severe Heart qi deficiency, and if it's occasional it can also reflect qi agitation of a milder nature and qi deficiency.

The Intermittent pulse misses beats on a regular schedule and suggests a greater degree of qi, blood, and yang deficiency. Patients often complain of oppressive chest pain, more fatigue, and shortness of breath with exertion. It is difficult to lie down, and their bodies tend to be cold, especially the limbs. If only occasional, of course, it is less severe than when consistent.

Rate Not Measurable: When the rate is no longer measurable, the severity is increased. When it's missing a beat and has no regular cadence and you can't even count because the pulse is so chaotic, it's a very serious situation. And when the pulse becomes Hollow (see Figure 2.7[52]) at the same time, meaning that the middle/blood depth is not present (or is significantly Reduced Substance (see Figure 2.8)), it requires immediate interventions.

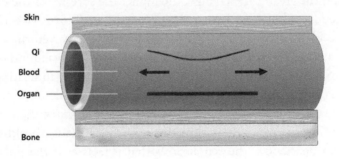

Figure 2.7: Hollow pulse
Reproduced with permission from Eastland Press

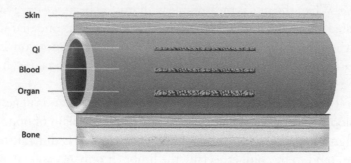

Figure 2.8: Reduced Substance pulse
Reproduced with permission from Eastland Press

Pseudo-arrhythmias

Pseudo-arrhythmias are qualities that feel like arrhythmias, but aren't. Two have been mentioned already, the Changing Intensity and Amplitude pulses that reflect varying force/substance and amplitude/height of the beats. These pulses are a sign of Heart qi deficiency, and the greater the change, the higher the severity of the deficiency.

Another pseudo-arrhythmia is the Hesitant pulse/waveform (see Figure 1.1 in Chapter 1). The Hesitant wave actually has no perceivable waveform and gives the impression of faltering and balking in between beats. It is always found on the whole pulse and Dr. Shen considered it the mental "push pulse," indicating obsessive-compulsive behavior, and the tendency to ruminate or think on a single subject incessantly. As many people who suffer Heart Shock are stuck in their traumas, it is a pulse that manifests commonly within this population. It is a mild-to-moderate sign of Heart yin deficiency. The sensation is that it feels as if the pulse is coming straight up and down, hitting your finger without creating any rolling movement, so it doesn't maintain the same type of contact with the fingertips as a normal one. As such, it feels to balk or falter, hitting all three fingers at the same time.

Along with the Hesitant waveform, it's not uncommon to also see a Smooth Vibration (see Figure 2.1 earlier) over the whole pulse revealing a tendency for constant worrying. As mentioned earlier, sometimes a Slippery (see Figure 2.9) quality shows in the mitral valve position or even the left distal position showing phlegm misting the orifices, with clouded and confused thinking. When Slippery shows up in the mitral valve position it's usually a sign of incompetence of the mitral valve with some type of regurgitation and the mitral valve prolapsing. These are all signs of weakness and qi deficiency in the Heart, and one which even Western medicine correlates to anxiety and panic.

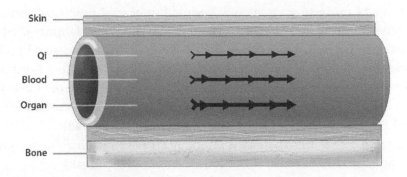

Skin

Qi

Blood

Organ

Bone

Figure 2.9: Slippery pulse
Reproduced with permission from Eastland Press

Rhythm in the Classical Chinese perspective is similar, mostly using different nomenclature, e.g., Knotted and Hasty instead of Interrupted and Intermittent, and also considering rate. A quality that Jeffrey Yuen discusses is the "Not Rested" pulse. This is basically a combination of traits which encompass the above rhythm qualities within the Shen-Hammer lineage. What he discusses is a pulse that hits the finger with varying strength and substance (i.e., Changing Intensity) as well as jumping to different heights (i.e., Changing Amplitude). The third aspect of the Not Rested quality is one that changes tempo (i.e., Changing Rate at Rest). So, essentially, the Shen-Hammer lineage differentiates each of these three aspects as a different pulse quality. The interpretation is also similar as these pulses are found in patients who are unsteady emotionally, often with some type of shen disturbance or lack of groundedness.

More on rate

Classically, where deviations to the normal rate were found, it would relate to either hot or cold conditions. But, nowadays, deviations from the normal rate are more often a sign of problems that are well beyond hot or cold problems, and tend to be associated with Heart and circulatory issues. From the Shen-Hammer perspective we are looking at the entire pulse where rate is reflecting a systemic issue. In this lineage, we assess the rate for a full minute with an automatic watch with a sweeping second hand (with quartz movements, often practitioners are lulled by the ticking and find lots of rates of 60 bpm). We are not measuring it according to someone's breath as we would in Classical pulse (this provides different information).

The table below depicts normal resting heart rates for different age groups. (As always, we must also factor in the uniqueness of the individual.)

Dr. Shen		Dr. Amber	
Age	**Rate (bpm)**	**Age**	**Rate (bpm)**
Birth to 4 yrs	84–90	In embryo	150–160
		Upon birth	130–140
		1st year	115–130
		2nd year	100–115
		3rd year	90–100
4–10 yrs	78–84	4–7	85–90
10–15 yrs	78–80	8–14	80–85
16–40 yrs	72–78	Adolescence	85–90
40–50 yrs	72	Adulthood	75–80
50+ yrs	66–72	Old age	60–75
		Decrepitude	75–80

The information in this table provides an important barometer from which to gauge patients' heart rates in order to determine the health of the Emperor. What the table reveals is an understanding of nature. As an embryo is forming and as the heart is developing, a heart rate is approximately 150 or 160 bpm. During the birthing process and the first year the pulse starts to slow a bit. As a child moves into his second year of life this continues, and as one reaches the bulk of adulthood (ages 16–40, prior to decline), that rate hovers in the low-to-mid 70s. As we age, the heart rate declines, and in old age it beats in the 60s.

What this clearly reveals is the cycle of life, of yang. When we're just being formed, and early in our lives, our yang is at its newest. We have the most vitality and the most yang in the Heart at that time. As we get older and as we utilize this energy/qi/ yang of the Heart over years and decades, eventually the heart rate slows, as work is financed from its storage. And as this continues over time we put more taxation on to the Heart so that it slows, eventually stopping when we die. We are only alive so long as our Heart is pumping blood, qi, nourishment, and resources to all the organ systems in the body that require it to thrive and function. If our Heart is beating slowly, it suggests less yang and subsequently less circulation of blood, oxygen, and nutrients to the tissues.

This is also very relevant to those who exercise excessively, getting their resting heart rates down into the 50s or lower. This places great taxation onto the Heart causing the rate to slow down, diminishing Heart functioning. It's not an uncommon scenario for athletes to have early stages of arthritis, joint pains, and muscle ache; have numbness and tingling, and circulatory problems; have labile emotions and tend to get depressed; have sleep disorders, insomnia issues, and falling and staying asleep; and so forth. These are the early signs of Heart yin, qi, and blood deficiency. Sweat is the fluid of the Heart, released from a steaming of the blood, causing the release of fluids out the exterior to cool down. This taxes the Heart qi and blood over time, causing the blood to dry and become thicker and more viscous. This makes it more difficult for the Heart to push and circulate blood, requiring more energy and taxing the Heart, eventually slowing down its rate. This can result in Heart blood stagnation and problems in the coronary arteries.

The important thing to understand about these normal resting rates, combined with the knowledge that trauma elevates heart rate, is that over time this elevated rate taxes and weakens the energetics of the Heart. The Rapid pulse, over time, is going to weaken the qi, yin, and blood of the Heart.

The Bounding quality is also common in trauma. Similar to Rapid, it has the sensation of running away, faster than the actual rate. It is associated with extreme anxiety and panic, but can also be felt in someone who has high fever, especially when in a weakened condition. I feel it in those who have experienced a recent Heart Shock or trauma and occasionally in someone who is experiencing acute pain.

Trauma, emotional or physical, will initially cause an elevation of heart rate. If the coping mechanisms that protect the Heart (Small Intestine, Pericardium, Triple Burner) haven't fully matured, or are insufficient due to constitution, lifestyle, etc., the ability of the Heart to return to homeostasis becomes impaired. This sets the stage for the sequelae of Heart Shock and its disruption of physiology systemically. Children, or those who are vulnerable or in weakened states, become increasingly susceptible to the negative impacts of Heart Shock or trauma.

Physical trauma will also result in the elevation of heart rate. Additionally, it causes qi and blood stagnation to the periphery, increasing circulatory demand and taxing the Heart, eventually succumbing to qi deficiency and a Slow rate.

The Rapid rate can also be due to "Nervous System Tense," an increased hypervigilance in the nervous system that requires a constant output of adrenaline and a constant need to be on guard and armored. Nervous system tension is a common etiology in our fast-paced industrialized modern world which creates constant secretions of adrenaline, lack of sleep, overworking, and an overall inability to rest and recharge the batteries.

The Slow heart rate is primarily associated with diminished Heart functioning and circulation of blood rather than cold. It typically signifies Heart yang deficiency, often from a trauma many years before that weakened the Heart over time. It can, however, also be from poisoning or exercising beyond one's energy, or later-stage arteriosclerosis, and/or chronic diseases, etc.

Besides rates that are Rapid or Slow, Heart Shock can present with wide variations of rate. For example, in the beginning of the evaluation the pulse can be one rate, and 20 minutes later at the conclusion of the pulse assessment it can be markedly different. This can be a significant finding and usually reflects a patient who is very worried with a backdrop of Heart deficiency and a certain degree of instability.

Rate on exertion

Another aspect of assessing the Heart via pulse in the Shen-Hammer system is measuring the rate after exertion. After completing the pulse evaluation, the patient is asked to stand up, and while we hold one wrist, he swings the other ten times vigorously, then stopping, as we count the rate for ten seconds. That number of beats is multiplied by six to determine the beats per minute and is compared to the resting heart rate. A normal increase is between 10 and 15 beats per minute, ensuring the Heart's proper response to the energetic demands placed upon it. Outside of this parameter is considered pathological. The chart below details the possibilities and attending diagnoses.

Rate (bpm)	Finding
10–15	*Normal*
>15	*Heart Blood Deficiency*
15–20	Mild
21–25	Moderate
26–30	Severe
31–40	Very Severe
Above 40	Extremely Severe
Stays same or rises by <10	*Heart Qi Deficiency*
Decreases	*Severe Heart Yang Deficiency*

An elevation above 15 beats per minute is a sign of Heart blood deficiency. Heart qi deficiency is diagnosed if the rate stays the same or rises less than 10 beats per minute. If it drops below the resting heart rate, that is severe Heart yang deficiency. Usually those people tend to have overt Western medically defined heart diseases and are symptomatic with shortness of breath, tightness in the chest, oppression in the chest, difficulty lying down, etc. It is common to see the entire gamut of these possibilities with Heart Shock patients, depending on patients' constitution, severity of the trauma, how long ago the trauma occurred, and any other pre-existing Heart conditions or vulnerabilities.

Rate from a Classical model

From a Classical Chinese medical perspective, speed is assessed in relationship to the breath of the patient. A Rapid pulse is suggestive of heat (and occasionally a tendency towards bleeding) impacting the fu/hollow organ/channel. A Slow pulse reflects activity of the zang organ and indicates cold and hypoactivity.

Besides a pulse that is Rapid as defined per breath, there are also other qualities that can be considered Rapid, including the Flooding and Robust Pounding qualities. They are Rapid based on their "rate of arrival."[53] In the Shen-Hammer system multiple qualities are distinguished to signify heat and overworking of the system. Robust Pounding is one and has the sensation of hitting the fingers with an accelerated feeling. The Flooding quality/waveform (see Figure 2.10) is generated from the deeper aspects of the position, but at its apex, instead of finishing off the second half (yin half) of the sine curve, drops off precipitously. In the Shen-Hammer lineage, it is a sign of an infectious process.

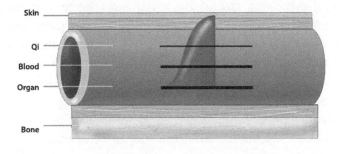

Figure 2.10: Flooding Excess waveform
Reproduced with permission from Eastland Press

From a Classical perspective we can consider all these qualities as Rapid. In fact, we may even feel one or more of these qualities in discrete positions and not over the entire pulse. With Classical pulse one is feeling the pulse with all three fingers simultaneously and certain positions may demonstrate a Robust Pounding or Flooding quality and not the others. This is another way of differentiating speed, and it becomes significant to help us determine where exactly the heat/hyperactivity or cold/hypoactivity originates from as the sequelae of traumatic experiences.

From this Classical perspective any pulse position or depth evidencing greater than 4 beats per breath would be considered Rapid, as follows: 5 beats slightly Rapid, 6 beats Rapid, 7 beats very Rapid. For Slow, less than 4 beats is Slow, as follows: 3 is Slow, 2.5 very Slow (measured by counting 5 beats per 2 cycles of breath). It is important that the breath is in relationship to the patient, not practitioner, to assess the relativity of heat and cold.

In the clinic, this requires a constant shifting of perspectives from Classical to Shen-Hammer. An example of how this can play out is where one might have a Rapid pulse in a given position relative to the breath but yet only be clocked at 50 beats per minute. Assuming we have the other signs of Heart Shock on the pulse (e.g., Rough Vibration, Hesitant wave, Changing Rate at Rest), we can consider this a Heart qi deficiency (50 beats per minute), but also evidencing that perhaps the heat/urgency/excitation from that shock is being played out in a particular organ system.

If the patient's breathing is slow, potentially a wei qi deficiency (and Lung deficiency) is reflected. Because, in this context, rate is a relationship between beats and breath, rate not only affects/implicates the Heart. If a pulse of 50 beats per minute was not impacted by nourishing Heart qi, one must look to nourishing Lung qi or wei qi in its relationship to cardiovascular movement and smooth muscle contraction. Some of these treatments from both an acupuncture and herbal perspective may overlap (e.g., Gui Zhi/Cinnamon Twig, or Ren Shen/Ginseng).

Another way of perceiving rate is that speed is a reflection of the amount of excitement, animation, or urgency that a person feels about themselves, their life, about what they're experiencing, and about what they perceive their future to be. A Rapid pulse reflects a heightened state of urgency. A Slow pulse reflects a person who is hesitant or perhaps unwilling to engage in certain aspects of life. Understanding cold and heat as metaphors to one's temperature and one's temperament in this way adds another layer of sophistication to our relationship with patients. Perceiving a sense of the urgency or heightened animation/nervousness/anxiety in our patients allows us to cultivate the patient–practitioner relationship and delve into emotional and psychological root causes, creating further intimacy and enhancing trust, aiding the overall treatment.

These concepts and metaphors can be further understood according to Five Element/Phase relationships.

Wood: The wood element provides directionality in moving us towards things we want in our lives. A healthy pulse here would show someone being animated, engaged, and driven in their life. With regard to trauma, a Rapid pulse here may be the result of trying hard to overcome and ignore one's past, suppressing it, creating stagnation and resultant heat which over time consumes their qi, weakening them, and perhaps even depriving them from cultivating certain other areas of their lives. They become hypervigilant and obsessed with pursuing goals so as to not feel the pain of the past. A Slow pulse may be found with someone who is lacking drive, depressed, and unmotivated. Trauma may create an inability to move away from the past, creating lethargy and a lack of animation.

With wood's energetic being upward and outwards, we know one aspect of the Liver's role is responsible for discharging or detoxifying. When the Liver is over-burdened by toxins, or if the Liver is constantly required to process and move things out of the system because our lifestyles are too toxic or stressful, this adds to our need to become hypervigilant. This can impact our ability to modulate what Dr. Hammer considers to be one of the cardinal aspects of the Wood phase, the ability to advance as well as retreat. In *Dragon Rises Red Bird Flies*, Dr. Hammer discusses the Liver's necessity to retreat, go inward, store blood, and regenerate. Where the Gall Bladder's movement of the yang aspect would be to move into the world and animate and achieve things and become very goal oriented and driven, it must be balanced with its nurturing counterpart. And so, if we don't have that capacity to move internally and retreat and go inward and nourish ourselves, then life becomes very taxing. Causing the body to work overtime will create a Rapid pulse and/or some variation of the stagnant pulse (e.g., Tense) as it is forced to constantly detoxify stress. Understanding these pulses allows us to reframe for our patients so that they can slow down and find nourishment.

As the eyes are the portals of the Liver, the hypervigilance so common with Heart Shock creates a need to constantly look ahead and view the future. As we will discuss later, this creates tension around the eyes and the heat and overworking of constantly trying to look and perceive threats from all around us. The "retreat" that Dr. Hammer speaks of would be better served by turning those eyes more inward into the upper, middle, and lower dan tian via meditation to replenish.

Fire: The Fire phase should have a very slightly Rapid pulse as the nature of the Heart is to be animated and excited about life. The Emperor is about conquering, about being on a quest, and having desire for engaging on that quest and living out one's curriculum in life. But, like anything else, it can become excessive and distorted by all the desires in life creating excess joy (mania, hyperexcitation). One loses the ability to moderate wants and the pulse becomes more Pounding on the moderate depth, and we start to see it at the 3 and 6 beans of pressure as well, reflecting the body's inability to internalize and cultivate nourishment. The Fire phase is about relationships, about needing to connect. This Pounding reflects an imbalance in the need to constantly engage outside stimuli and desires with the inability to quiet one's shen and achieve contentment.

Slow pulses here reflect a withdrawal, a pathological lack of fire/interest/desire to engage in life or to create or nurture relationships.

Both of these pulse configurations are very common with traumas, depending on how the patients perceived and responded to said trauma. In some, there is an elevated need to connect, and even a loss of boundary, creating an inability to prevent oneself from sharing too deeply or caring too much—the proverbial wearing one's heart on one's sleeve. Others withdraw completely from outside life, considering it threatening and painful.

It should be noted that each of these pulses can also combine with the Slippery pulse, demonstrating an alteration of perception and lack of clarity in the shen. With a Rapid pulse the Slippery aspect often creates a dian kuang presentation with psychosis and aggression. With a Slow pulse we may see clouded, sluggish thinking and confusion, amongst other things.

Earth: On the moderate level we would expect the Stomach to be slightly Rapid in relation to the deep level, reflecting the Spleen, especially after eating. Other than that, Rapid here will reflect a hyperactivity in the need to process too much stimulation. The Stomach is responsible for processing and assimilating thoughts and emotions, and it is the channel (from a Primary channel perspective) that allows for internalization, typically at the level of the throat. When the stimulation becomes excessive, we become hyperactive, with racing thoughts and agitation. As the energy becomes stuck in the head, we may see a lot of stagnation in the jaw with an inability to move and thoroughly chew our ideas to a point where they can become fluid enough to internalize into the inner domains of the body and be transformed into something that nourishes ourselves. We see clenching and grinding, headaches, etc. This can impact sleep as the wei qi cannot fully enter the chest peacefully.

Slow pulses here reflect an inability to separate the pure from the turbid with accumulation of dampness. We gain weight, and become lethargic, overly sensitive, and perhaps clingy in our relationships. Overwhelmed with too much stimulation, one can shut down, and we see a breakdown in the processing and assimilation of thoughts and ideas. We get trapped in our heads. Our narratives become stuck, replaying and reliving the same ideas and events (traumas) over and over again.

Metal: The Metal phase and the Lungs deal with wei-defensive qi. As such, issues of vulnerability, individuality, and protection become highlighted. It is interested in purity and deals with assigning value, especially in terms of self-worth. Rapid pulses here reflect someone who always feels as if they have to fight and defend themselves; they feel they must be constantly on guard against some perceived outside threat. Often this person is anal, uptight, and self-righteous.

Slow pulses here reflect an inability to defend and a person who is often a target to be taken advantage of. Their lack of self-worth leads to a feeling of exaggerated vulnerability and often perversities from difficulty letting go of unnecessary things in life.

Water: The Water phase is about nurturing and quietude. It's about accepting one's life, destiny/curriculum, and path taken. A Rapid pulse in the Kidney position reflects a progression of someone's inability to accept or surrender to their life. Dissatisfaction can create a need to burn through some of their jing faster because they're trying to create something different, akin to creating alchemical change. Rapid pulses here can also reflect a state of hypervigilance and overworking of the system in response to fear, i.e., someone still in the fight/flight/freeze response.

Often a pulse in the Kidneys can be simultaneously Slow and Rapid. Slow in relation to the breath and Rapid in terms of its Pounding or rate of arrival. Here, we see the impact of hypervigilance and constant readiness and adrenaline post trauma, creating taxation on the Kidney yang. If the Kidney pulse is also Tight, this suggests it is trying to hold on to its essence. If it's very Tense, the patient is lacking acceptance of his/her life. The patient becomes resistant to their destiny, and stagnation of their qi and eventually jing develops. This impacts the dissemination through the Triple Burner mechanism, preventing animation of their spirit as well as creating toxicity. That stagnation, of course, creates heat which exacerbates the Rapid pulse and impacts the relationship of the Kidney to the Liver, as the Liver's drive and ambition is financed by Kidney yang. If the Liver is unable to retreat because it's constantly on the move, constantly feeling goal oriented and wanting to do everything and achieve everything that creates a demand on the Kidney yang to finance that activity and adrenaline increases. Adrenaline gets metabolized in the blood, governed by the Liver, so a Rapid pulse develops in the Liver as well. Over time, this develops into yin deficiency, with irritation and burn-out.

Additional pulse findings

In addition to the above, there are many other pulse findings that are often the result of traumas which will be discussed throughout this text. Many are dependent on the uniqueness of the patient's terrain at the time of said trauma. These can include: Spinning Bean pulse in the left distal position, the depth of which can clue the practitioner in to the timeline (the deeper the pulse finding, the longer ago in history the trauma occurred), systemic Empty and other Qi Wild pulses (Dr. Hammer's *Chinese Pulse Diagnosis: A Contemporary Approach* should be referenced for more information on these pulse configurations), Scattered pulse in the left distal and/or proximal positions, Muffled pulse (representing stagnation of qi, blood, and fluids in anatomical areas that have been traumatized, such as via surgeries and/or injuries, as well as the result of emotional stagnation), and the Diaphragm pulse (with suppressed emotions, e.g., betrayals, divorces), etc.

It is common with trauma that the Heart-Kidney axis becomes affected. One can determine Heart-Kidney communication via Classical pulse diagnosis. One way to do so, is to press all three pulse positions on the patient's left wrist to the 9 beans of pressure, then pump down on the proximal position a bit deeper, and then pump down on the distal position. One is looking to see that this movement causes the proximal position to be pushed upwards, reflecting communication. To determine if the Heart is expressing its shen, one presses on the patients left wrist at the distal position down to 9 beans, then pumps the proximal, then the middle and lifts up slowly on the distal. The distal position should feel something push up against it as it rises to the 3 beans of pressure. (One will discern with experience that there can be many gradations within these.)

Facial diagnosis signs of Heart Shock
Eyes: Seeing the world differently—A distorted lens

Eyes: For the eyes,[54] we assess under the lower eyelid. With the patient looking forward, we use our thumb to gently press below the lower eyelid to reveal its underside. In a healthy state, we should see discrete vertical red lines.

> *Physical trauma*: For a physical trauma, on the side the trauma was experienced, there can be a red horizontal line at the base. Oftentimes, we see changes here; for example, with toxicity we tend to see lack of uniformity as well as varying colors, including a brownish color. This can happen even with Heart Shock as a major etiology due to accumulation of waste products resulting from the stagnation associated with it.

> *Emotional trauma*: With emotional trauma we may see a confluence of these vertical lines and/or increasing redness relative to the amount of heat (excess or yin deficiency) present.

Other characteristics of the eyes are that they may show confusion or spaciness post trauma, and it is very common to see a hollowness in the eyes. Alternatively, one can see very pronounced glare reflecting shen disturbance.

Face color: Carrying your trauma wherever you go

Face/Complexion: The complexion is another way to diagnose Heart Shock. With trauma the facial color turns blue-green, often prominent around the mouth (typical if the shock happened earlier in life), or additionally on the temples (if the shock happens a little later in life), and/or the entire face may manifest this blue-green color (if the trauma was exceedingly severe).[55]

This is becoming increasingly common to see in children for a number of reasons—most prominently, birthing practices have become "medicalized" to the extent that most women are induced with medications such as pitocin, which increases the intensity of uterine contractions, they are given a host of other pharmaceuticals during the delivery period, and the use of forceps and other such procedures is widespread. Additionally, moms giving birth later in life, the potential for diminished jing-essence, and circulatory and Heart deficiencies impacting the quality of circulation to the placenta also play a part in creating a greater likelihood of shock being experienced.

Comparing hand and face: Comparing the color of the face and hands is another way we can look at diagnosing trauma. When the face is redder than the hands, it tends to be a scenario where the Heart is affecting the circulation. This occurs more when we are looking at a primary emotional shock. When the hands are redder and the face is paler, it tends to be more when the circulation is affecting the Heart. Usually this is when the root cause stemmed from a physical trauma rather than an emotional trauma.

TONGUE SIGNS WITH HEART SHOCK: TRAUMA
MAPPED ON THE ORIFICE OF THE HEART

Physical trauma: Where one has experienced physical trauma, we tend to see a long-lasting ecchymosis or purple blister on the same side of the body where the trauma happened.[56] Oftentimes you can see it anatomically related to where the injury was experienced.

Emotional trauma: With emotional trauma, the tongue tip often displays raised red spots and it can also be a little contracted and pointed. A purple color can eventually pervade the entire tongue from the blood stasis and poor oxygenation that's taking place.

A very common presentation includes a midline crack that extends from the middle of the tongue and reaches to the tip. The depth of this crack will also point to its severity. And often we will see an increasing redness along this crack, as well as the tip, with increasing severity and more acute presentations. Where there is also phlegm misting the orifices, we can see a yellow sticky/slimy coating near the front tip. The tip can also display red raised petechia or roughness from Heart fire and/or yin deficiency respectively.

Other diagnostic signs of Heart Shock and trauma
Hand and palm diagnosis: How one handles stress

Chinese medical palmistry is a subject all in itself; however, there are a few diagnostic signs that are easy to notice when one knows what to look for. First, one needs to be oriented to the anatomy and reflexology of the palm. The basic features are presented in Figure 2.11.

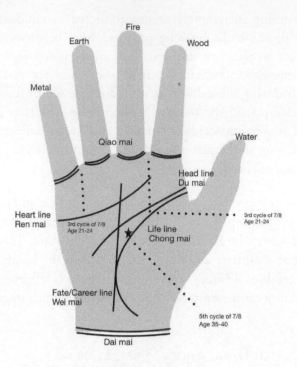

Figure 2.11: Palm diagnosis

Looking at the above figure, the Five Phase orientations are present, as are the 8 extraordinary meridians, along with a basic mapping of the patient's age and the cycles of 7 and 8. The top line on the palm is related to the Ren mai from an 8 extraordinary meridian perspective, but also considered to be the Heart line. The junction of the Heart/Ren mai line and the space between the fourth and fifth fingers is associated with the third cycle of 7 and 8, or roughly 21–24 years. Looking at the life line, that is associated with the Chong mai, and the third cycle of 7 and 8 is at the junction of the index and middle fingers, and the fifth cycle is located at the junction of the life line and the center of the palm. Using this mapping, we can identify markings on the palm and also date their occurrence.

One type of marking that presents with trauma is stars, which look like "***" located on the line one is assessing. Stars are commonly seen on the Heart/Ren mai line, and where on this line they are found, we can date the occurrence based on the reflexology discussed above. The more stars and the darker and deeper they are, the more severe the trauma. They represent intense accumulations of blood/phlegm/qi/yin/yang. On the Heart/Ren mai line, they can represent early life traumas like molestations, etc. When this is the etiology, one may also see paleness in the area reflecting the lower jiao (later signs including infertility and obstetric/gynecological problems), with hormonal issues being reflected in the water moon and hypothenar eminence moon area. Islands can also be found on these lines as well as the life/Chong mai line and look like "φ" or "--¢--." They suggest deficiencies, and if the islands are darker, it suggests shock. Grids can also show up on these lines, and look like "#," reflecting leakage of qi and rebellious qi (we might see luo vessel pathology with these signs: see Chapter 5). Bracelets are another sign that tend to show up on the wrist crease, and they reflect pathology that has been suppressed/repressed into the Dai mai with traumas, major disappointments, and memories that one cannot let go of. The Qiao mai and Wei mai are also mapped here and can point to additional 8x vessel pathology from trauma (see Chapter 8). To help determine what one is struggling with, we can look to other areas (e.g., metal mound and sadness, Pericardium 7 area with fear of failure and anxiety/panic, life line and fear of death, etc.). The life line can also manifest with breaks along the pathway often from traumas that interrupt the flow of one's life, altering it from that point onwards. Dating it based on its location can confirm other findings from the pulse, etc.

Abdominal diagnosis

As with palm diagnosis above, the abdomen is a complex system of diagnostics, and my goal is not to present much instruction on it, but rather to point out some simple confirmatory diagnostic information related to trauma. One of the main findings that I correlate with trauma is a significant guarding of one's abdomen. Many of these patients will always have a hand covering their upper abdomen over the area of Ren 14–15, and when the hand is moved away to palpate or needle a point, it quickly returns once the area has been evaluated or needled. With palpation, these patients tend to tighten their abdomen and have a hard time relaxing it when asked to do so. Breathing through this area is also often strained, and these patients tend to breathe more with their chest than their diaphragm.

Aggravating factors

With a foundation of Heart Shock as a systemic diagnosis, assessing its severity is warranted. For one, the severity of the trauma is going to increase the intensity of the impact of that trauma on the physiology and also on one's psychology. Those whose injuries are more intense will have greater likelihood for more demonstrative signs and symptoms. And as mentioned earlier, the age or the level of maturity, and the level of the integrity of resources available to the individual at the time of trauma, will also play a significant role. The more mature one is, the stronger the organ systems are, and the greater the likelihood it is that they will find their way back to homeostasis very quickly. If we have sufficient resources to bring to bear on the trauma then we can resolve that trauma quicker than someone with diminished resources. Someone who is extremely blood deficient with severe blood stagnation, experiencing emotional lability, anxiety/panic, and dream-disturbed sleep, will require more time to reach resolution.

One's physical and emotional condition at the time of trauma is also very significant. If the individual is physically robust they are going to have an easier time rebounding. If they are emotionally labile to begin with, or tend towards Heart imbalances and psychological conditions, whether they are anxiety or panic disorders or other types of depressive states, and then experience trauma, it's going to be more difficult to treat and will require more time. An awareness of these factors is important to provide reasonable time frames and expectations.

Pre-existing Heart Shock is also significant in terms of the magnitude of what a patient will experience post trauma. Each subsequent shock and trauma will increase the severity because the body will already be suffering compromised functions as a result of the prior insults. Similarly, any weakness or vulnerability in the Heart will make one predisposed to a higher level of severity of trauma.

The condition and integrity of the nervous system will determine the nature and severity of the symptoms experienced. If the nervous system is weak or compromised, we will see symptoms more related to the psychological level; if the nervous system was strong at the time of the trauma, symptoms tend to be more somatized, creating physical symptoms. Dr. Hammer has discussed with me his experiences in the war and how his fellow troops handled the extreme stresses and trauma associated with it. Those who had compromised nervous systems experienced anxiety, panic disorders, and psychosis; those with strong nervous systems tended to get other types of physical problems, including digestive problems.

Any weakness or vulnerability in the Kidneys (our root) will also predispose one towards more severe Heart Shock. The Kidneys are our shock absorbers; they secrete cortisol and adrenaline and are responsible for our fight/flight/freeze response, which gets called into action when we experience a trauma. The stronger the Kidneys, the more able a person is to handle whatever demand is put on them. Those with very weak Kidneys tend to be "nervous system weak" individuals with heightened symptoms post trauma.

Additional aggravating factors

Additional factors which will increase the severity of a traumatic event include the many life factors that can destabilize one's physiology. People who have experienced environmental deprivation (lacking clothing, proper shelter, or access to clean water/food), overworking (especially in one's early years, e.g., child laborers), and overexercising (which weakens the Heart) are going to make the constitution more vulnerable, i.e., less stable. Excessive lifting strains the Heart and chest, creating stagnation of qi and blood in the diaphragm, and impacts the functioning of the Heart itself. Substance abuse, as well as exposure to toxins, will impact the Heart, Liver, Kidneys, etc. and will weaken the constitution as well as the nervous system and impact the blood circulation.

Vaccines can also impact the severity of trauma and, in fact, can be a trauma themselves. From a Chinese medical perspective, vaccines are introducing pathogens directly into the body (via intramuscular injection and occasionally via inhalation) and bloodstream. This demands a response. Often the vaccines contain adjuvants like mercury and aluminum, which initiate strong immune reactions that can be overwhelming and extremely toxic. In certain individuals this creates wei qi hyperactivity, Liver wind, high fevers, neurological reactions, ADD/ADHD symptoms, and even autism. This puts significant burden on the system and often calls into action the divergent channels and/or 8 extraordinary meridians to put it into a state of latency. In order to create latency we need to divert resources; this means taking resources that would normally be performing normal day-to-day functions but instead are being sequestered to contain a pathogen somewhere in the body. If those resources cannot be brought to bear to a particular trauma or shock when needed, then we become more vulnerable to the impacts of different types of stressors and traumas.

Heart Shock etiology

The types of events that can rise to the level of being traumatic are too manifold to list separately, and as stated earlier, what becomes traumatic for one person may not for another, depending on level of maturity, emotional state at the time of the event, constitution, etc. But, there are some events that pretty consistently create the objective signs (pulse, face, tongue, etc.) of trauma. Those discussed here are only some of the most common and do not preclude others.

Dr. Hammer has described, and I have consistently corroborated, that emotional shock to the mother during pregnancy affects the fetus in utero. It has been shown to alter cortisol and adrenaline levels as well as corticosteroids in the mother which are transmitted through the placenta. As Fisher mentions:

> The RH amygdala…comes on line between 5 and 6 months in utero, the same time that fetal movement begins. From that time on at least, the fetus can feel fear, and this fear is the fear of the mother in her loud, chaotic environment, external or internal. The fetus can hear her pounding heart and the angry voices, and the fetus will register the blows the mother takes. All the fetus can do in this gestational period and in early post-natal times is to react. There is no safety in these wombs.[57]

Other shocks[58] to the fetus include of course things like physical traumas to the mother during gestation and/or delivery; placenta previa, which can often diminish circulation and nutrients to the fetus; drug abuse by the mother; prolonged vomiting, which can impact growth and development in utero during critical times; or illnesses like toxemias (eclampsia, HELLP syndrome). Being born premature will also presuppose insufficient resources and lack of nourishment to the fetus in utero and also suggests a lack of maturity in one's organ systems (i.e., diminished resources).

C-sections, high forceps, cord being wrapped around the neck, and different types of abnormal presentations like breech birth are all early shocks that will impact the Heart and circulation (as well as oxygenation to the baby), nervous system, as well as Kidney essence.

Early life traumas tend to create Water phase defects and negatively affect the balance and harmony between the Heart and Kidney axis. They tend to be some of the more severe and significant types of shocks and traumas that can create the whole spectrum of the different disorders that we can see, ranging from mental retardation to developmental mental disorders, including autism and spectrum disorders such as sensory integration problems.

Other types of trauma include the loss of a parent or caretaker, or the loss of a loved one through death or separation, especially in childhood when that bonding and nourishment is so crucially needed. These losses profoundly affect the Heart and call to action its protector, the Pericardium, to create a host of adaptive responses, including the stagnation of qi and blood.

> When one is sorrow-stricken greatly, his heart and its tissues connecting to the viscera will become strained, the lobes of the lung will become swelling up, the upper and middle warmer will be obstructed, and the heat inside will remain retaining. So, it is called the dissipation of energy.[59]

Withdrawal is another possibility which Dr. Hammer describes as an adaptive response to protect one's feelings. This becomes "Heart Closed" (Dr. Shen's Heart qi stagnation), and when it occurs in childhood it leaves a permanent challenge with certain interpersonal relationships throughout one's life.

Often when these traumas occur early in life, they are repressed (common with people who have been physically abused and/or raped). Depending on the type of treatment strategies employed, memories may re-emerge during treatments. Knowledge of the channel systems (discussed in Part II) will help determine whether or not a patient can handle a particular strategy and which approaches and/or channels systems will need to be utilized to move the trauma without the memory/emotions being triggered. As many patients simply cannot handle the memories and reliving of these traumas (that's why they are still suffering), we may need to assert latency until they are stronger and have more resources to bear, or release it in a way that doesn't move through the psyche (ying/blood level).

As we mentioned earlier, certain physical traumas can trigger Heart Shock. Traumatic injuries, car accidents, sports injuries, concussions, spinal injuries, etc. can all rise to this level.

Different types of deprivation, disappointment in love, divorces, and all types of betrayals of intimacy (e.g., husbands and wives cheating, etc.) can set the stage for significant Heart Shock.

All the varied types of abuse will also trigger a Heart Shock condition: physical abuse, sexual abuse, mental-emotional abuse, and bullying and intimidation. These are all shockingly commonplace and impact a wide majority of our patients. My intake form for new patients is seven pages long, four of which question birth history, parent health, early life, and trauma, as a recognition of the importance of these factors on constitutions, vulnerability, etc.

Wang Qing-ren

Wang Qing-ren, a practitioner in the Qing dynasty (1768–1831), did a lot of dissection; he was influenced by Western medicine and the cross-section with Chinese medicine, in particular blood stagnation. Within his conceptions of the Heart and circulation, he authored a lot of herbal formulas for invigorating blood. His work speaks to the Heart being the Emperor, and having systemic impacts on physiology, as all relies on Heart qi, blood, oxygen, nutrients, and resources for their own energy and survival.[60]

The model that Wang Qing-ren gives us is of interest in Heart Shock. He describes the different chambers of the Heart as reflecting different energetics (see Figure 2.12). The right atrium reflects the shaoyin and the dynamics of Kidney yang returning to the Heart—Kidney yang supporting Heart yin by moving blood back to the Heart. This movement helps set the rate and rhythm. As blood returns back to the Heart it returns to the right atrium, then to the right ventricle, represented by taiyin (Spleen/Lungs), which then moves that blood to the Lung organ system and pulmonary arteries. The Spleen helps manage the blood, so here we see taiyin's role in maintaining blood pressure. The taiyin provides connection to cardio-pulmonary circulation, picking up oxygen and then circulating it to the left atrium under the auspices of shaoyang (Gall Bladder/Triple Burner mechanism). Here we invoke the ability to clear heat in the blood as heat consumes qi (and oxygen was just retrieved from the Lungs). Of note is that the left side of the Heart is typically where we see the majority of damp heat accumulations and plaques/cholesterol building up. The Gall Bladder and Triple Burner mechanism move the blood to the left ventricle, taiyang (Bladder/Small Intestine), which is the yang counterpart to the Heart itself as well as all the yang in the body coming from the Kidneys and adrenals. When there's heat in the Heart, it is cleared via the Small Intestine and Bladder. Here the taiyang displaces heat as it circulates the blood and oxygen throughout the body. The greatest yang has the most force to pump and push everything out so that the circulation gets to the rest of the body. This descending trajectory can also be analogous to the Chong mai.

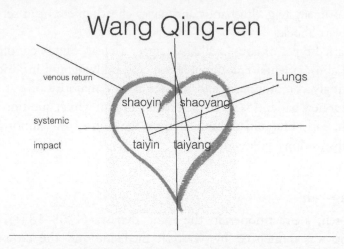

Figure 2.12: Wang Qing-ren Heart chambers

Valves are also situated between these chambers, allowing for linkage. The tricuspid is situated between the right atrium and ventricle, the pulmonary, mitral/bicuspid, and aortic. These valves also can show up on the pulse in the Shen-Hammer pulse system and can help determine which aspect is impacting the Heart. An example is a current patient with congenital defects in the pulmonary valve. Her doctors have been recommending surgery for many years to which she is unwilling. Focusing on the taiyin energetics as well as treating the Heart in general has kept her asymptomatic for the decade I have known her. Her last visit to the doctor as well as a transesophageal echocardiogram (TEE) revealed increased integrity to the valve, and that the valve aperture had decreased in severity from a 4 out of 4, to a 1.5 out of 4.

Wang Qing-ren's model gives us further information in understanding the dynamic in the Heart's movement of blood and how rhythm and rate can impact not just the Heart itself but potentially implicate all of these organ systems, requiring them to work harder over time with eventual taxation. We will discuss more about Wang Qing-ren with some of his formulas in Chapter 5.

CHAPTER 3

Heart Shock Diagnoses and Treatment Principles/Strategies

Thus far I have provided a framework for the understanding of Heart Shock, some of the objective signs that signify it (e.g., pulse, tongue, facial diagnosis, etc.), and its pathodynamics, etiologies, and aggravating factors. In this chapter, I will begin to structure this knowledge and present the many diagnoses and the treatment principles and strategies involved. Some have been alluded to already in the prior discussions, but here they will be fleshed out. Heart Shock is a large concept, an umbrella under which multiple systems are evidencing turmoil. While it is a systemic diagnosis, it has a few primary systems that it impacts more than others. The following discussion will be my attempt to break down this larger diagnosis into its disparate parts, with an understanding that, in clinical practice, all of these parts must be considered and treated simultaneously, as they are all always at play within the Heart Shock patient. As stated in the Shen-Hammer pulse lineage, "big things are big," referring to the fact that qualities that appear over the larger segments of the pulse (e.g., rate, rhythm, uniform qualities) reflect systemic processes.[61] Things that are happening systemically and are more pronounced generally have a greater diagnostic import and should be the focus of one's immediate interventions (there may of course be exceptions, such as instabilities, infectious processes, etc.). We will discuss more of this later in the text (as well as prioritizing interventions), but it's instructive to note that as you treat the roots you also treat the branches. Focusing on the root diagnoses of Heart Shock typically has the most profound impacts.

Root diagnoses

Heart

First, we must treat the Heart. Heart Shock as a diagnosis includes Heart yin deficiency. We discussed the recoiling action that takes place when we experience a trauma in earlier sections. Heart yin deficiency is initiated by a rapid and pronounced movement of yin that drives itself internally, creating a separation with the Heart yang which becomes hyperactive and now begins to float and scatter. It no longer remains rooted by the Heart yin/Heart blood. This hyperactivity begins to manifest with the Rapid heart rate, boost in adrenaline, nervousness, pounding heart, and even sweat, reflecting a leakage of Heart qi-yang. This requires us to assess the integrity of Heart qi as well as Heart blood, Heart yang, and also Heart qi and/or blood stagnation.

The Pericardium is involved with vasoconstriction as one of its protective measures, contributing to qi and blood stagnation in and around the Heart and often restricting movement of the diaphragm. The diaphragm is the link between the chest and the abdomen, often regulated by the Liver and the jueyin relationship to the Pericardium and Heart. And as the link to the chest and the home of the shen, it allows for emotions to be magnified (or dulled). Qi and blood stagnation are often created here to lock in and compartmentalize the pain of trauma away from our memory. The Liver not only controls the diaphragm, but also the sinews, tendons, and muscles. This qi and blood stagnation impacts not only the chest/diaphragm, but also the peripheral circulation (as mediated and assisted by the jueyin pair, Pericardium).

> When the patient is being frightened again and again to cause obstruction
> of the tendons, his disease is due to numbness.[62]

Thus, the Su Wen alludes to this obstruction syndrome in the tendons, but also the numbness, which here has the two-fold meaning of being caused by blood stagnation and also the psychological component from the trauma. As the shen resides and circulates in the blood, stagnating the blood keeps us from experiencing the trauma. The mechanism of stagnation invokes heat/mobilization as an ecological response to moving the stagnation, and should the stagnation be too great, or the individual too deficient, we begin to see dampness and phlegm being produced as compensation to quell the heat. Over time, this creates phlegm misting the orifices and the sensory portal and perception problems that are ubiquitous in Heart Shock patients.

Nervous system

Second, we must treat the "nervous system." Trauma creates nervous system tension in all its varied forms, including hypervigilance. The nervous system as discussed by Dr. Shen includes many different aspects of physiology, and can (and should) be looked at from multiple lenses. From a zang fu perspective we can talk about it as the Liver. The energetics of the Liver include how it regulates the movement of wei qi and blood to the sinews, muscles, and tendons. Post trauma, we see the Liver using this protective measure to armor the body. When we experience the fight/flight response the body tenses up and it mobilizes blood into the sinews and larger muscles to prepare for the fight/flight response.

Adrenaline also kicks in as the Kidneys regulate the prima materia of the nervous system. From a sinew meridian perspective this is mediated via the shaoyin-to-taiyang relationship. As the protective measures of the Heart and Pericardium become impacted, the adrenaline does not shut down properly and continues to be secreted. Adrenaline gets metabolized in the blood and stored by the Liver, so we start to see hyperactivity in the Liver to accommodate this. This creates tension and concomitant heat which may create muscle tension, pain, spasms, and tightness in the neck, muscles, and calves—the larger muscle groups that are responsible for that fight or flight response along the Bladder and Small Intestine sinew channels.

From a divergent meridian perspective we can look at the Bladder channel in terms of its capacity to take yuan qi and convert that into wei qi. Dr. Shen also likened it to the nervous system and the taiyang energetics by noting that it regulates the "faster and lighter" moving energies. Essentially, from a channel perspective, this is the taiyang and the Bladder channel from a divergent and sinew meridian perspective being financed by yuan qi or the Kidney (shaoyin). Of course, the Heart is the other half of the shaoyin energetics, and we have already discussed the Heart's intimate relationship to the nervous system.

Yuan qi converts to wei qi to support the fight/flight response and its sequelae. This further develops into nervous system tension, hypervigilance, armoring, and the resulting tightness and pain. As wei qi homes to the chest, Heart palpitations and an inability to relax (both mind and body) are common. The inability of wei qi to internalize results in insomnia and disturbed sleep patterns, where it may take a long time for one's body to settle down, and when it does, only allowing a light sleep, with the patient waking often as the wei qi keeps externalizing from the adrenaline release, hypervigilance, and inability to root yang qi.

From another perspective we can say that there's not enough Liver yin-blood to buffer and cool the adrenaline surge and nourish and contain the Hun. An ability to do this irritates the Liver as well as harasses the Heart and shen. As the Ling Shu states, "The Liver stores the blood, and soul adheres to the blood. When the Liver energy is deficient, the mood of terror will occur…"[63]

Approaching the concept of the nervous system with the conceptual fluidity noted in the Introduction is important for understanding the complexity of its dynamics. Dr. Shen was a Classical practitioner trained in the Shanghai College of Chinese Medicine as well as an apprentice within the Ding family lineage. He was well versed in the Classical concepts, yet still used Western terminology such as the "nervous system." My understanding of this was not that he was trying to simplify the concept or to suggest a 1:1 correlation with Western concepts, but rather to find a way to relate to the Western mind while still retaining all the concepts inherent in the understanding of what constitutes the nervous system from all the concepts we discussed above in terms of wei qi, yuan qi, sinew meridians, and taiyang and shaoyin energetics, the divergent meridians in terms of how they mediate both wei and yuan, as well as the energetics of the Liver system.

Moving fluidly between models, the Liver (jueyin with the Pericardium) governs the peripheral circulation. And as such it also mobilizes blood and circulation to the sinews and muscles to prepare for action and movement. As mentioned before, the Kidney yang is secreting adrenaline in response to the stress/fear. This adrenaline gets metabolized in the blood, governed by the Liver. The Liver takes the cue of heightened stress/fear/urgency and mobilizes its stored blood to the muscle channels for action. But as we noted before, with Heart Shock patients, the stress is always perceived to some degree. It does not desist after the event that triggered it does, but persists into the future, rewiring the nervous system to constantly be on guard. This creates constant activity for the Liver which must perpetually move its storage to the muscles. Over time, this creates considerable armoring and tension in the fight/flight muscles and also taxes the Liver organ system. One of the more common findings on the pulse with Heart Shock is to find a Thin Tight pulse over the Qi depth and a very Tight pulse in the left middle position reflecting the Liver. This is a sign of a "Nervous System Tense" condition.

The nervous system and the mind

The integrity of the nervous system is the primary factor in the etiology of all psychological disorders. No matter what the stress may be, if the nervous system is vulnerable, there will inevitably be psychological conditions. If the nervous system is strong, the stress is more likely to produce physical disorders rather than psychological, especially if another "system" or organ is at risk. However, powerful stressors may overpower even the strongest resistance.

There are essentially two basic kinds of nervous system disorders: nervous system tense and nervous system weak, each of which can be further differentiated. The principal symptom signifying nervous system tense is an ongoing tension that may or may not be related to a particular life stress, often found with tension uniformly over the entire pulse and a Thin Tight pulse at the Qi depth. A further differentiation can be made between a constitutional type, and that derived from lifestyle. Nervous system weak, a constitutional condition, is often found in a person who has a lifelong history of neurasthenia, one whose symptoms are always changing and who is highly vulnerable, unstable, and easily disturbed or stressed, and also subject to constantly fluctuating allergies. The disorder does not represent illness as much as physical and mental instability and vulnerability to illness. Nervous system weak can be differentiated on whether the weakness is mostly in the yin, yang, or qi of the Kidney organ system as the nervous system in essence is analogous to the marrow/brain/ central nervous system and governed by Kidney organ system energies.

The Heart also has a close association to the mind, nervous system, and one's emotional state, and instability here can cause an emotional roller coaster, including significant depression (lack of joy-type), anxiety and panic disorders, manic states, depersonalization, and dissociation. On a physical level, as the Heart governs the circulation of blood and nutrients to the entire bodymind, a wide array of symptoms can present, including arthritis and other circulatory disorders; gynecological disorders, including pre-menstrual syndrome, endometriosis, and the like; infertility; chest pain, palpitations, and cardiac disease; insomnia and sleep apnea, etc.

Similarly, when this takes place over periods of time, we see the resulting depletion to the Liver with the whole gamut of qi and blood deficient findings on the left middle position pulse: Thin pulses (blood deficiency), Reduced Substance pulses (see Figure 2.8 in Chapter 2; qi and blood deficiency), Feeble pulses (see Figure 2.5 in Chapter 2; qi-yang deficiency), and most importantly the Empty pulse (see Figure 3.1; reflecting significant deficiency and instability/chaos ("separation of yin and yang")).

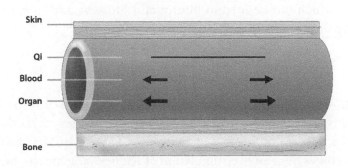

3.1a: Empty pulses: Early stage

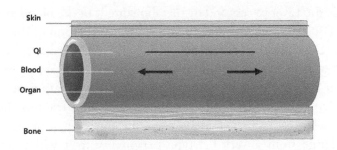

3.1b: Empty pulses: Middle stage

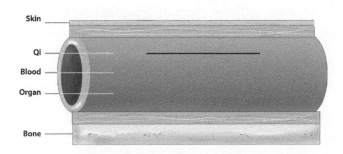

3.1c: Empty pulses: Late stage

Reproduced with permission from Eastland Press

The conceptual fluidity as represented in this book is a necessary component to understanding the nervous system, but it is also important to understand how all these differing lenses can come together to provide the most complex understanding of all the concepts surrounding Heart Shock and Chinese medicine as a whole. Moving seamlessly through different models/lenses/lineages gives us tremendous freedom to choose treatment strategies and the treatments themselves. Of course, one must stay true to the basic principles inherent within any concept, but there is much overlap which can be used to inform and broaden one's perspective, and an understanding of the nervous system is but one example.

Kidneys

The third major component is addressing Kidney qi-yang as well as the Triple Burner mechanism. Hyperactivity of the nervous system can be viewed via the taiyang wei qi aspect of its deeper counterpart of shaoyin yang/yuan qi. The financing of the hyperactivity comes from an overstimulation of Kidney yang in response to the fight/flight/freeze response initiated by the traumatic event. The Kidney qi deals with the secretion of adrenaline and cortisol and is the shock absorber in the body, adjusting to stress in the body until the threat subsides (or is perceived to subside). In trauma patients, this threat is perceived to persist and adrenaline continues to be released. This demands the Liver to respond by metabolizing it in the blood as we mentioned, but also the Triple Burner, which regulates the dissemination of that yuan qi via the ladder of life (Du mai), depositing yuan qi into the Bladder back shu points.

Identifying someone as a wood/Liver person, a fire/Heart person, or an earth/Spleen person is because of the disproportionate dissemination of Kidney yuan qi to those particular back shu points. As the experience of trauma often changes the perception of what has happened in one's life, this dissemination can become altered. One may change from a very fire-type personality to a withdrawn, very fearful personality as the yuan qi dissemination becomes displaced, no longer reaching as abundantly into the fire element. Understanding this shift is important as it allows for an opportunity to correct the displacement, or potentially create a chosen one.

As with most diagnoses and conditions, the treatment of Heart Shock can be as varied as the styles of different types of practitioners. Because of this, the most important things to understand are the major impacts and sequelae of this diagnosis so that one can begin to craft one's own strategies and treatments that are most comfortable for oneself as a practitioner as well as considering the needs of the patient. The three primary impacts as discussed are crucial to that understanding.

Heart Shock primary impacts

1. The Heart, including the circulation as well as one's emotional stability.

2. The nervous system and all its relationships to wei qi, sinew channels, muscular armoring and hypervigilance, taiyang/shaoyin relationships, the Liver, and Kidney yin nourishment of the central nervous system (cortisol) and yang (adrenaline).

3. Kidney Yang/adrenals (fight/flight response) and the Triple Burner mechanism.

Secondary diagnoses

With anything that has primary impacts, there are also secondary effects that result from it. This is especially the case with Heart Shock as it is a systemic diagnosis that impacts and destabilizes all of physiology. As the Heart is the Emperor, anything that impacts him/her will have far-reaching implications. For the Heart itself, many of those impacts can create other Heart imbalances. Reference has already been made to Dr. Shen's Heart patterns,[64] and any of these diagnoses can present themselves depending on the particular individual experiencing the shock. It is very common to find significant degrees of Heart qi deficiency, Heart qi stagnation, including the more severe Heart Full/Trapped Qi in the Heart (especially when the patient is strong or where there has been trauma to the chest or a major upset like the loss of a loved one which kicks in the protective measures of the Pericardium), and Heart blood stagnation (from traumatic injuries or where the peripheral circulation has been taxed and/or weakened over time).

Another secondary impact relates to the sensory portals and perception. Here, a big component is the presence of phlegm. Phlegm misting the orifices is a common phenomenon post trauma. As a person experiences a trauma it impacts the way he perceives as it becomes influenced from the new lens of the trauma. Imagine someone who is very carefree and never had an experience of being scared or concerned, and one night walking by herself she gets mugged. Consider how that may color her perceptions about walking at night again or how she may perceive her safety or the level of threat from the outside world. How might her personality change from this experience? How will this trigger bodily reactions and sensations of fear, agitation, armoring, hypervigilance, and tension, and a narrative of needing to be concerned for her safety and protection? How will that change the health and perceptions of the portals (which are a direct reflection of the health of the organs that regulate them)? Consider how that will impact her eyes. One's eyes and their clarity are going to be determined by a large degree by the health of the Liver. As all this Liver blood is now being shunted to the fight/flight/freeze muscles to maintain the mental hypervigilance, how will this impact what she sees? How will that change the tension around her eyes as she's constantly searching for a potential threat? Opening the portals and strengthening and clearing the orifices is a necessary strategy which also strengthens the organs and allows those organ systems to come back to their full state of health and security. Indeed, clarity of one's perceptions is perhaps one of the most important characteristics of a healthy person, and a primary goal within Daoism itself to obtaining the Dao. Laozi's *Scripture of Constant Clarity and Stillness* speaks to this:

> *Fū rén shén hao qīng ér xīn rǎo zhī*
> The shen prefers clarity, yet the mind disturbs it.
>
> *Chéng qí xīn ér shén zì qīng*
> Clarify the mind and the shen will become clear on its own.
>
> *Wèi huà zhòng shēng míng wéi dé dào*
> The transformation of phenomena is called obtaining the Dao.
>
> *Zhòng shēng suŏ yǐ bù dé zhēn dào zhě wéi yŏu wàng xīn*
> The reason people do not attain the Dao is because the mind is delusional.
>
> *Wéi yŏu wàng xīn jì yŏu wàng xīn*
> If the mind is delusional, the spirit will be unsettled.[65]

As does the Nei-Yeh, *Inward Training*:

> The Way fills the entire world.
> It is everywhere that people are,
> But people are unable to understand this.
> When you are released by this one word:
> You reach up to the heavens above;
> You stretch down to the earth below;
> You pervade the nine inhabited regions.
> What does it mean to be released by it?
> The answer resides in the calmness of the [Heart]-mind.
> When your [Heart]-mind is well ordered, your senses are well ordered.
> When your [Heart]-mind is calm, your senses are calmed.
> What makes them well ordered is the [Heart]-mind;
> What makes them calm is the [Heart]-mind.
> By means of the [Heart]-mind you store the [Heart]-mind:
> Within the [Heart]-mind there is yet another [Heart]-mind.
> That [Heart]-mind within the [Heart]-mind: it is an awareness that precedes
>   words.
> Only after there is awareness does it take shape;
> Only after it takes shape is there a word.
> Only after there is a word is it implemented;
> Only after it is implemented is there order.
> Without order, you will always be chaotic.
> If chaotic, you die.[66]

Heart Shock secondary impacts

1. Heart: all the varied Heart patterns, especially Heart qi deficiency, and Heart qi and blood stagnation.
2. Sensory portals: phlegm misting the orifices and all sensory perception issues.

Primary treatment strategies

With the primary and secondary impacts of Heart Shock identified, the next step is to formulate treatment strategies. The first strategy we want to contemplate with someone who has experienced Heart Shock is the need to nourish Heart yin and anchor Heart yang. The Heart yin has retreated internally and has been taxed, while the Heart yang has been excited and moves recklessly without the ordering of Heart yin. This separation of yin and yang creates the fundamental instability within the Heart Shock diagnosis and as such becomes our first order of business to correct.

Within this primary impact, we must address the concomitant secondary effects if present. They include the possibilities of Heart qi deficiency, Heart blood deficiency, Heart qi stagnation (and potentially Heart Full/Trapped Qi in the Heart), and Heart blood stagnation (Heart Small). One needs to address these aspects simultaneously as nourishing when there is stagnation can be counterproductive and worsen an already precarious condition. We must also remember that strength of Heart qi is required to invigorate blood. One cannot successfully invigorate blood if there is not enough Heart qi to do so, and attempting this without strengthening Heart qi can become very taxing to the Heart. If invigoration of Heart blood is required, there must be sufficient Heart qi to do so. If there's not, then we need to implement a different strategy, whether that be to "move" blood, which relies on the Lung qi, or to "break" blood, which will rely more on Kidney yang. (But most likely if Heart qi is deficient and we can't invigorate then we're not going to be able to get to the next level of breaking blood with the Kidney yang energetics.) We can concurrently nourish Heart qi while invigorating blood, however.

The second strategy is calming the nervous system. Based on our understanding of the nervous system, this can be approached in multiple ways depending on the lens in which we decide to view this system. This can invoke a sinew meridian perspective to relax the muscles. It can be tapping into the shaoyin and Kidney energetics of nourishing yin to calm and regulate the nerves and the mind. It can utilize a divergent meridian approach to mediating wei and yuan levels. It can adapt a zang fu approach and focus on the Liver organ system in its capacity of storing and mobilizing the blood to the sinews as well as its dominion over the peripheral circulation. We can also nourish and regulate Liver yin and blood to access and calm the Hun. All these strategies will be discussed in more detail later in this text.

The third strategy is calming and settling the spirit and communicating Heart and Kidneys. Heart and Kidney communication is the axis of fire and water, the fulcrum that everything else revolves around. We need to make sure that we are creating stability between these two fundamental north and south poles.

Our fourth strategy is to strengthen and anchor Kidney yang and regulate the Triple Burner mechanism and its dissemination of yuan qi. Kidney yang must be sufficient to either warm the frozen qi or to provide enough foundation for consolidating back to the lower warmer. Only when we are no longer leaking yang/adrenaline and we have sufficient reserves can the Triple Burner adequately disseminate. Here, we are bringing back the sunlight into the depths of ming men to rekindle the spark of life.

Our fifth strategy is to ensure the opening of the orifices and the sensory portals. As discussed earlier, trauma colors our perceptions and how we view ourselves, the world, and our relationship to it. Healing requires a shift in this perspective and a clearer mirroring of our true inner nature. As Dr. Bessel Van Der Kolk says in *The Body Keeps the Score, Brain, Mind, and Body in the Healing of Trauma*:

> We have learned that trauma is not just an event that took place sometime in the past; it is also the imprint left by that experience on mind, brain, and body. This imprint has ongoing consequences for how the human organism manages to survive in the present.
>
> Trauma results in a fundamental reorganization of the way mind and brain manage perceptions. It changes not only how we think and what we think about, but also our very capacity to think.[67]

The above are the primary principles and strategies that we must be mindful of. It is not always necessary to address every single one of these treatments. That will be determined by the uniqueness of the case presentation and which diagnoses are present. For instance, if you are palpating the pulse and you notice a Rough Vibration, but the heart rate is still within the normal range and the Heart pulse is relatively robust and strong, you may not need to nourish Heart qi but you may decide to invigorate blood more strongly as a result. Typically, invigorating the blood becomes part of every treatment plan because Heart Shock will always impact the shen, and as the spirit resides in the blood, one of the body's ways to handle trauma is to stagnate the blood to prevent reliving and remembering the painful events. The trauma itself is like a pathogen that lodges itself into, and stagnates, the blood and shen. Invigorating the blood helps to release the shen and begins to rid the trauma itself.

It can be very helpful to think of trauma as a pathogen. As with pathogens, we either need to create a strategy for eliminating it or establish some means of making it latent. That will be determined by the integrity of the individual patient and the strength of her resources. It is not advisable to treat with protocols or in a vacuum. Recently, a colleague contacted me asking what to do when, after releasing someone's divergent channel, the patient experiences palpitations and anxiety/panic disorder with dissociation. First, it is important to recognize that wrong treatments can create pathology. In this case, a releasing treatment should never have been employed as the patient did not have the resources to warrant it. Bringing this patient's pathology back into remission would be required in order to quell these symptoms. The next step would be to build up the resources until such time as the pathogen can be safely released.

Heart Shock primary treatment strategies

1. Nourish Heart yin and anchor Heart yang.
   a. Strengthen Heart qi and/or blood.
2. Invigorate blood (and qi).
3. Calm the nervous system.
4. Calm the shen and communicate Heart and Kidneys.
5. Strengthen and anchor Kidney yang and the Triple Burner mechanism and its dissemination of yuan qi.
6. Open the orifices and sensory portals.

Thus far I have delineated a number of discrete diagnoses that Heart Shock incorporates and set forth the primary strategies to address them. But, there are also numerous other diagnoses that can attach themselves to, or manifest concurrently with, Heart Shock and can be incorporated into treatment. The idea with my approach to treatment is that we want to craft a treatment strategy that encompasses as complete a picture as we can, with the understanding that Heart Shock is a block and a systemic problem that must be addressed for any other treatments to be effective. But, there is no reason why we cannot incorporate other elements into these diagnoses and treatments. Many of the secondary issues that arise can seamlessly be integrated into our strategies.

The first is if there is trapped qi in (or out of) the chest. That would include the Flat pulse or Inflated pulse that we discussed in Chapter 2. Additionally, we often see a Diaphragm pulse reflecting obstruction between the upper and middle burners. It often reflects suppressed anger and frustration and even the transmutation of tender feelings when one has been betrayed by a loved one. This build-up of tension creates a tremendous amount of stagnation in the chest and diaphragm and must be freed up to allow for proper movement between the three burners. If we cannot connect chest to abdomen to pelvis, we limit our success in the treatment.

Second, we can combine other diagnoses in the chest and upper burner, such as Lung qi and/or Lung yin deficiency. As we will see later in the text, many of the herbal strategies employed will concurrently augment Heart and Lung qi/yin. And as cardio-pulmonary circulation is so intimately connected, addressing any other types of stagnation in the chest or Lungs can be included within our strategies.

Third, we often look to address any weakness and/or stagnation in the middle burner. The integrity of the Spleen qi is instrumental in creating stability and groundedness and must be utilized to break down and assimilate any internal medicines given. As such, ensuring that there is no Stomach qi stagnation and that the middle burner is open is of crucial importance. Additionally, we must rely on the integrity of the Spleen and Stomach to create more energy and resources for our patient. As we will be tapping into wei and ying levels during our treatments (to be discussed infra), we must ensure that the source of wei qi production is intact. And, we must be able to ascend the pure yang of the Stomach. As mentioned earlier, to create a state of latency/dormancy for our symptoms, one of the strategies is to ensure that the Spleen and Stomach are strong. Should we try to release and clear the pathology, we will also rely on the Spleen and Stomach in its capacity of providing sufficient fluids.

We also know from Chinese medicine physiology that one of the jobs of the Spleen is to ascend its essences up to the chest to create more blood. An additional crucial energetic dynamic is that as we ascend this substance to the chest it is also utilized to counterbalance and quell/pacify Heart fire. With Heart Shock, Heart yin and yang are in need of communication, and quelling Heart fire is an important strategy. The ascension of the red substance by the Spleen assists in this process and helps to nourish the Heart, much like the herbal formula Gui Pi Tang (Restore the Spleen Decoction), which brings blood to the Heart to calm the shen while strengthening and nourishing the Spleen itself.

Heart Shock secondary treatment strategies

1. Regulate qi in the chest and diaphragm.
2. Nourish Lung and wei qi; move Lung qi and release wei qi stagnation; free the po to live in the moment.
3. Strengthen and harmonize Spleen and Stomach and restore the center; boost center qi; quell Heart fire.

In *In an Unspoken Voice* Peter Levine sets forth his treatment strategies for approaching patients with PTSD. They are surprisingly similar and include:

a. Establish an environment of relative safety.
b. Support initial exploration and acceptance of sensation.
c. Establish "pendulation" and containment: the innate power of rhythm.
d. Use titration to create increasing stability, resilience, and organization. Titration is about carefully touching into the smallest "drop" of survival-based arousal, and other difficult sensations, to prevent retraumatization.

e. Provide a corrective experience by supplanting the passive responses of collapse and helplessness with active, empowered, defensive responses.

f. Separate or "uncouple" the conditioned association of fear and helplessness from the (normally time-limited but now maladaptive) biological immobility response.

g. Resolve hyperarousal states by gently guiding the "discharge" and redistribution of the vast survival energy mobilized for life-preserving action while freeing that energy to support higher-level brain functioning.

h. Engage self-regulation to restore "dynamic equilibrium" and relaxed alertness.

i. Orient to the here and now, contact the environment, and re-establish the capacity for social engagement.[68]

All of these nine strategies have some correlation to what I have delineated above from a Chinese medical approach, albeit with different language and accompanying energetics. While the first two strategies Levine discusses have some rooting in the patient–practitioner relationship,[69] there are energetic equivalents within Chinese medicine. Creating relative safety can be likened to our first strategy of nourishing the Heart's yin. Yin is substance; it is resources. It helps to calm and creates a feeling of safety and stability. It quells and anchors the hyperactivity of the wandering yang. As it anchors, it also helps us to be more in contact with our bodily sensations; it helps bring one back from a state of dissociation and allows us to begin to process our feelings and sensations. Jeffrey Yuen has stated that the Pericardium gives options (adaptive responses), but it is the Heart that gives hope.[70] By nourishing Heart yin and anchoring Heart yang, we once again provide the bodymind with the capacity to connect to itself and regain the possibility of wholeness.

Establishing pendulation and containment and using titration (Levine's third and fourth steps) is within Chinese medical purposes akin to balancing the need for strengthening qi and invigorating qi and blood versus the need to nourish and calm. This is an important concept and has a few relationships within Chinese medicine. The first is related to concepts of the divergent meridian energetics and the ability to assess the integrity of the individual's landscape and inner terrain to determine the appropriate strategy of releasing trauma or quieting it down and putting it into a state of latency/dormancy. To release the pathology/pathogen, we need to ensure sufficient resources. In general, we must make sure we have strong Lung/wei qi, and sufficient Lung and Stomach yin to provide passage, and we must be able to clear the heat/irritability/anxiety that has been suppressed/repressed, as it became an internal pathogen. If any of these capacities are insufficient, releasing pathology to the surface will exacerbate the condition and aggravate any signs and symptoms. We must then choose to create latency by nourishing yin and blood, slowing down the movement of the pathogen and blanketing it, guiding it to the deeper aspects of physiology, and nourishing the center to keep strong and stable.

From Dr. Hammer's perspective, we must be very aware of the balance between advance and retreat. Discussed in relationship to the Wood phase in DRRBF, it is equally applicable to any situation in which we need to be mindful of the expenditure of our resources, or where moving in only one direction (forwards, backwards, or stagnation) can be detrimental. It is imperative to balance the yang/moving/pumping/action with the yin/resting/relaxing/nourishing. We will discuss more about this concept in Chapter 6. But, essentially, the idea of advance and retreat, ebb and flow, expansion and contraction, and systole and diastole demonstrates a yin–yang relationship and the idea that all things eventually change. Faith in this endless transition helps one to bear the difficulties in life with an increasing grace. Along with this concept of modulation we must also be creating new experiences. Dr. Hammer has often stated that one cannot undo a traumatic experience; the experience will always be there. But, one can, however, dilute it.[71] Dr. Van Der Kolk shares similar views when he summarizes Maier and Seligman's results in reorienting traumatized dogs after being electrocuted.[72] In this experiment, despite the removal of any danger, the traumatized dogs had to be repeatedly dragged out of their cages to teach them to escape. This prompted Van Der Kolk to question whether those who have experienced traumas actually found some refuge in the familiar, and that new physical experiences were partly required to regain a sense of control and move on from their traumatic experiences.[73] As positive experiences increase, the power of the trauma decreases. And the more positive experiences, the better the Triple Burner can disseminate yuan/yang qi.

Another concept Dr. Hammer speaks on often relates to containment. The ability to create stagnation (temporarily) is an important one. This is often mediated by the Liver's role in shutting down or restricting the movement of the diaphragm. The chest is where emotions are amplified prior to expression. With the diaphragm restricted, emotional expression is often impacted. This can often serve us as we need to create stagnation at specific times. For example, when one is being reprimanded by a boss or superior, it would not be beneficial to lash out and jeopardize one's employment. Instead, the emotions are suppressed, and hopefully one can move that energy in a safer way in the near future. According to Dr. Hammer, and confirmed by my experience, many people are unable to contain their emotions by suppressing them temporarily. Our collective Livers are so overburdened, toxic, and deficient that they have lost the capacity to contain. While so many in my profession diagnose pathologies of Liver qi stagnation, what we are finding more and more is that we can no longer create Liver qi stagnation and pathologies are increasing at exponential rates. In the context of those who have experienced Heart Shock, we see varying degrees of abilities to contain the pathology. Some have utterly lost this ability, and their symptoms tend to be the most difficult to contain. Others are stuck within their stagnations, trapped in their internal terrain with no foothold to crawl out of it. And others are teetering right on the edge of losing containment and moving too quickly to a point of releasing their traumas, which can open up a Pandora's box. Mediating this balance requires the Liver to be strengthened as well as balancing the yin-nourishing aspects with the yang-moving aspects of treatment. Often when there is pathological suppression and containment, we will see a Diaphragm pulse. This manifests as an Inflated quality (see Figure 2.3 in Chapter 2) as one rolls a finger between the cun and guan positions, the feeling as if the pulse inflates and pushes the finger up a hill. This Diaphragm pulse can reflect anger and the suppression of tender feelings in cases of betrayal (Dr. Shen often referred to this as the "Divorce Pulse"), but can also be directed inwards, suppressing guilt, shame, and tremendous frustration. The inability to contain and create Liver qi stagnation typically manifests with a host of deficient findings on the pulse in the left middle position, the most significant quality being the Empty pulse (see Figure 3.1 earlier) signifying chaos and a separation of yin and yang. This Empty quality in the left middle position also represents a significant compromised ability to handle stress, often manifesting in feeling overwhelmed, inability to recover one's energy, depression, agitation, and potentially despair. For me, it becomes a marker on the integrity of the healing process with a host of nervous system pathologies. And as the Liver regulates the diaphragm and the circulation to the chest and breast, it is also a finding seen with, and for me a marker of, breast cancer when found with other qualities in the Special Lung Position (which reflects not just the Lungs, but also the chest and breast).

Providing a corrective experience and empowering defensive responses relates to the Pericardium (Heart Protector) and its ability to utilize higher-level adaptations. Strengthening the Emperor and its ministers within the fire element, we allow for additional tools to be accessed, including more appropriate expressions and verbalizations.

Separating the conditioned associations of fear and helplessness from the immobility response of our Chinese medical approach would be working with the Kidneys and Triple Burner mechanism. One of the integral aspects of treating trauma is to reassert the patient's proper dissemination of yuan qi to allow them to return to their original nature to live out their destiny. Breaking the cycle of fear and immobility to encourage the Triple Burner's dissemination of yang qi is essential. This needs to be done closely with titrating the response to prevent an adrenaline rush or immobility response.

Levine's seventh step is to resolve hyperarousal and, from our perspective, this means working on calming the nervous system. Often here we will be mediating the need to clear nervous system tension with calming the nervous system, depending on the integrity of the patient's constitution. And at this stage we may see the spontaneous shaking and trembling or muscular fasciculations as the body resets and discharges internalized tension and fear. From an acupuncture perspective this can take a number of forms, whether it be accessing the divergent meridians with the three-time needling technique to stir up the yuan level and bring it to the wei level for release, or tapping into the sinew meridians, or even approaching the Liver and Lung's relationship to wei qi. Regardless of the approach taken, it is a potential opportunity to utilize wei qi to thrust out the pathogen.

Step eight involves restoring self-regulatory functions and equilibrium. Here we look at the re-establishing of the Heart–Kidney axis and restore proper communication.

His last step is to orient to the here and now and allow for social engagement. From our Chinese medical approach we are correlating that with opening of the sensory portals, harmonizing the Hun and Po, and allowing the Emperor to once again reside in, and engage with, the present moment. Once we have reoriented to the present moment and unblocked the proper dissemination of yuan/yang qi within the Triple Burner mechanism, we have stability/security/peace/safety firmly established and rooted within the Water phase/element and the Fire phase can once again engage in new experiences with a renewed sense of belonging and contentment. At this point we are further diluting negative past experiences with the creation of new meaningful ones. As Sri Aurobindo states:

> We were never meant to look behind, but ahead and above in the superconscious light, because it is our future, and only the future can explain and heal the past.[74]

> It is not that past that impels us, but the future that draws us and the light above that gradually pervades our darkness—for how could darkness ever have created all that light?[75]

Additional Chinese medical treatment strategies

As Heart Shock has its primary impact on the Heart, it tends to manifest for many as a form of shen disturbance. As such, we can look at some traditional strategies (some of which were set forth by the Imperial Academy) that have been employed in the treatment of shen disturbances to further round out our strategies in the treatment of Heart Shock. Many will overlap from our previous discussion, and as such, I will list them without much elaboration.

Strategies for shen disturbances

1. Calm and settle the shen.
2. Tonify original qi to nourish the shen.
3. Clear heat from the Heart and Pericardium.
4. Nourish Heart yin.
5. Invigorate blood (move or break).
6. Communicate Heart and Kidneys.

7. Open ming men and disseminate yang qi.

8. Strengthen the Spleen and deal with any phlegm or food stagnation.

9. Clear heat (blood heat, damp heat, internal heat).

10. Anchor the Liver.

11. Open the portals.

12. Uterus and brain connection.

One of our main strategies here is calming the shen. Within calming the shen (an shen) we can quiet the shen (qing shen) or stabilize the shen (ding shen), which involves the Kidneys and an anchoring of the spirit back down. Quieting or calming the shen utilizes the Liver to send its blood up to engender Heart qi to nourish the Heart and spirit. The heaviness of the Liver blood comforts the Heart and shen.

Additionally, we want to also clear any heat from the Heart and Pericardium that may be harassing the spirit. And as we discussed above with our Heart Shock strategies, in treating shen disturbances we also want to work on nourishing Heart yin as well as invigorating the blood (or moving and breaking the blood as appropriate). And then also we look to clearing other sources of heat that may be disturbing the shen such as blood heat, damp heat, or internal heat (e.g., Stomach fire and dian kuang syndrome).

We also want to adopt an overall strategy of nourishing the blood and enriching the yin in order to soothe the patient and build additional resources. The heaviness of the blood is also calming (like giving the patient a big hug), and where the Liver (which has a tendency to be exuberant) is hyperactive (especially with the presence of neurological symptoms), we want to use heavier medicinals and strategies to anchor Liver's yang, pacify the Liver, and potentially extinguish any wind. Pacifying the Liver also helps bring in the Kidney-water energetics to assist with anchoring. Often the use of heavy minerals, thorns, and horns can be used along with bitter herbs to allow for proper descension, some of which also have strong portal-clearing functions. Many of the herbs we use to nourish blood are seeds (e.g., Suan Zao Ren/ jujube seed, Bai Zi Ren/biota seed, etc.), which impact the shen. They are being planted into the soil of one's consciousness, creating the potential for more blood and nourishment to grow.

Boosting the yin also assists with working on the patient's self-esteem and self-reliance skills by providing sufficient resources to bring to bear towards the healing process.

As detailed above, strengthening the Spleen and Stomach, harmonizing the earth, and addressing any issues of stagnation in the middle are also warranted (e.g., food stagnation, dampness, qi stagnation, etc.). When the Spleen is implicated we often see affliction by dampness and phlegm, and this allows for greater likelihood of phlegm misting the orifices and impacts the clarity of the sensory portals. Ensuring the orifices are clear becomes of paramount importance.

And, lastly, if we have any impact on the reproductive organs, namely the uterus (or the prostate for men), we must look at the connection between the uterus/prostate and the brain via the curious organ relationship. It is not uncommon to see blood stasis in these regions create mental-emotional-psychological symptoms. Another connection comes from the Liver, which regulates blood circulation to these anatomical structures in the pelvis as well as penetrating the brain. Blood stasis can arise here from a multitude of causes, including menstrual irregularities and prostate inflammation from impaired circulation resulting from Heart impairment secondary to trauma, sexual abuse (e.g., rapes, incest, etc.) impacting the reproductive organs, and traumatic physical injuries to the pelvis (e.g., car accidents, falls). As a general strategy in these cases, we would want to purge blood stasis (i.e., Wang Qing-ren's formulas).

A note on the shen and psychological disorders

The Heart, as the Emperor, houses the shen. In this context, when we're talking about the shen we're talking about a collective term for the emotional, mental, and spiritual aspects of our lives. This includes its involvement with learning, intelligence, memory, differentiation of emotions and thoughts, and associations, making all the connections and categorizations, and creating identities. It's also a willingness to engage with something external from oneself. The Heart interacts with all of the emotions; anger can affect and cause Heart fire. Joy and sadness are going to affect the movement of Heart qi. Overthinking is going to affect the Heart by creating Heart blood deficiency; fear and fright affects the communication of the Heart and Kidneys. This is important to be aware of as these interrelationships allow for greater specificity of our treatments.

With personality disorders (zang zao/visceral agitation) we want to prioritize our focus a bit more towards the Kidneys (see the luo vessel chapter for more discussion on personality disorders and the dissemination/irrigation of yuan qi). With confusion disorders (luan/confusion) or with learning difficulties and poor concentration and memory issues where there is difficulty prioritizing or creating context, we tend to focus a little more towards the Spleen and dampness. With dian kuang or bipolar/manic-depressive disorders, look more towards the Stomach (Stomach fire) as well as the Triple Burner mechanism. Behavioral types of psychological issues arise when people lash out and become violent; here we look to a sinew orientation as well as the Liver (hyperactivity), which controls the muscles, sinews, and tendons. And when there is deviant behavior (non-conformist in nature) we address more of the Lung and metal aspects (metal deals with purity and individuation) in our treatment protocols.

If you can't discern some of these distinctions you can always work with the Heart. But the more specific the criteria one can bring towards the treatment strategy only creates better-tailored treatments. In one sense, however, all diseases are diseases of the shen, so formulas and treatments that work on the Heart will always have some value as we always want our treatments to move the patient's spirit. Treatments and herbal formulas for the Heart and shen will be provided in Part II.

From a Daoist perspective on shen disturbances, Jeffrey Yuen speaks about working with the self and self-cultivation as an intrinsic part of treatment. One must have awareness and understanding of what's happening in one's life and the choices and circumstances that have created it. We play a major role in this regard; more than most realize. As the Mother has stated:

> When you have a thought, a well-made mental formation which goes out of you, it becomes an independent entity and continues on its way and it does that for which it was made. It continues to act independently of you.[76]

> One must not admit bad thoughts into oneself under the pretext that they are merely bad thoughts. They are tools of execution. And one should not allow them to exist in oneself if one doesn't want them to do their work of destruction.[77]

And Sri Aurobindo has affirmed:

> Thought is not essential to existence nor its cause, but is an instrument for becoming; I become what I see in myself. All that suggests to me, I can do; all that thought reveals in me, I can become. This should be man's unshakeable faith in himself, because God dwells in him.[78]

One must take responsibility for these aspects as well as for how one perceives one's current situation (even memories, as these too can be colored), as this creates the seeds of one's future. We all have a narrative that runs on a loop day after day, causing us to relive, think, and see things in the same way. This is profoundly so for traumas. Sri Aurobindo notes:

> All it takes is for a group of cells to be struck once by an impression (a fear, a shock, or an illness), and they will begin repeating their fear, their contraction, the particular tendency towards disorder, or the memory of their illness. It is a gregarious, absurd mental process that spreads from one cell to the next, quivering and quivering everywhere, endlessly, forever picking up the same wavelengths, the same decaying suggestions, and forever responding to the same stimuli, like a Pavlovian dog to his bell.[79]

That cycle must be interrupted for healing. The treatments should attempt at reorienting the patient's preoccupation with the negative to something positive, towards self-discovery and acknowledgment of what is good in their life. Again, Sri Aurobindo says:

In fact, the effervescence of Agni is due not so much to a basic cellular incapacity as to the resistance of "our" obscurities. This purifying stillness alone can clear the way and help release Agni's overwhelming Movement without causing the body to quake in unison, to panic and run a fever.[80]

This self-empowerment, making sure we are shifting the responsibility to the individual (rather than them just succumbing to and accepting our external treatments), offering opportunities toward growth, and helping them reclaim their power, is instrumental. Dr. Van Der Kolk, citing his teacher, Elvin Semrad, writes about the importance of patients acknowledging these facts of life: "The greatest sources of our suffering are the lies we tell ourselves."[81] These stories that patients tell are crucial to understanding them and their identification with their suffering. Dr. Hammer states: "Treating…signs and symptoms without reading in them the story of the person is a denial of the role which the patient plays in his or her own disharmony."[82]

There is no magic bullet or easy way out. Western pharmacological medicine has sought these magic pills for years, but as Dr. Van Der Kolk concedes, "psychiatric medications have a serious downside, as they may deflect attention from dealing with the underlying issues. The brain-disease model takes control over people's fate out of their own hands and puts doctors and insurance companies in charge of fixing their problems."[83]

We have to change these things from the inside and not allow ourselves to be judged by external standards. We must take responsibility for our own experiences, shift our thinking, and redirect our shen, as it is the only way to transcend our suffering and move towards healing. True healing allows for patients to change and grow into responsible, self-regulating, and active participants in life. Dr. Van Der Kolk acknowledges that Western medications, while making people (especially children, who are increasingly taking such medications) more manageable and cooperative, "interfere with motivation, play, and curiosity, which are indispensable for maturing into a well-functioning and contributing member of society."[84] And lastly on this topic, he states: "Being a patient, rather than a participant, in one's healing process separates suffering people from their community and alienates them from an inner sense of self."[85] Dr. Hammer further states:

> The medium for new experience and for human growth is the heat, light, and energy of a searing and powerful direct involvement between two members of the human species. In a profound way, each person knows that the experience of being himself can change only when his most hidden selves live again in this intense way with another person, one who will relate to these selves differently from those who bore the original responsibility for labeling his psyche.

Change occurs through new experience with one's hidden self, not through the revolving door of the established circuits of one's inner mind. An outer experience was indispensable for the original inner experience, and a new outer experience is necessary to bring about a new inner experience.[86]

The Nei Jing Su Wen instructs us further:

> The Yellow Emperor asked: "I am told that in ancient times, when a physician treated a disease, he only transferred the patient's thought and spirit to sever the source of the disease. In nowadays, the patient is treated with drugs internally and acupuncture externally. Nevertheless, some of the diseases are cured, but some of them cannot be cured and why is it so?"
>
> Qibo answered: "In ancient times, people lived in the cave of the wilderness surrounded with birds and beasts, they drove away the coldness by the motion of themselves, and evaded the hot summer by living in the shade. They had no burden in heart in admiring the fame and gain, and had no fatigue in the body for seeking a high position, thus, one can hardly be invaded by exogenous evil in this calm and plain environment. So, when one contracted disease, both drugs for curing inside and acupuncture for curing outside were not necessary, but only transferred the patient's emotion and spirit to sever the source of the disease would be enough."[87]

> Yellow Emperor said: "When the body of the patient is declined, his blood and energy are exhausted, why is it that the treating is ineffective?"
>
> Qibo said: "This is because the spirit of the patient can no more play the role it should play."
>
> Yellow Emperor asked: "What do you mean by that?"
>
> Qibo said: "The acupuncture and stone therapy can only conduct the blood and energy, but can do nothing to the spirit and consciousness of the patient. If the spirit and the energy of the patient are disappearing, his will and consciousness are dispersing, the disease can by no means be cured…"
>
> Qibo said: "The patient is the root and the physician is the branch, they must be compatible. Of course, cooperation of the patient is necessary, but only the cooperation of the patient without a good physician is not enough, it is also called incompatible of the root and branch, and the evil cannot be removed either."[88]

Creating this resonance between patient and practitioner is of utmost importance. Skill in creating this intimacy and relationship is a major factor in assisting one's patient to redirect his thoughts and spirit towards healing. Dr. Hammer's treatise *The Patient–Practitioner Relationship in Acupuncture* is instructive in this regard.[89] We must use this relationship to encourage our patients to commit to making the vital changes in their lives in order to move on from (instead of moving in towards) their pain and suffering. Part of this is akin to the physical aspects of invigorating the blood and opening the orifices to help our patients see things from a different perspective. It provides a rite of passage which comes from confronting our fears and pain so that we can leave them behind. This requires the ability to comfort oneself (remember our treatment strategies of nourishing yin and blood) in order to create this change that is so desperately needed. In the words of Dr. Hammer, "The doctor helps, nature cures, and each person is responsible for his relationship to nature and to himself."[90]

PART II

CHANNEL SYSTEM DYNAMICS AND TREATMENTS

———

Acupuncture, Herbal, and
Essential Oil Treatments

In Part I of this text I have created a broad context within which to understand trauma and all the disparate pieces that are required for understanding the scope of Heart Shock. In particular, we looked at the major dynamics implicated in the physiological responses to trauma, the primary and secondary impacts, as well as a host of pathognomonic signs and their most common associated symptoms. Our discussion also included detailed treatment strategies that must be incorporated into successful treatments.

In Part II, I will begin the process of approaching treatment within the context of each individual channel system. In order to accomplish this and make the most out of utilizing these channel systems, for each channel system I will provide a detailed analysis of its energetics and overall uses followed by its relevance in the treatment of Heart Shock and all the myriad pieces within that umbrella diagnosis. In this text, great focus will be given to the collateral channels (sinew, luo, divergent) and 8x meridians as there has been less available instruction in these channels and the perspective provided herein is not generally part of most US schools' curriculums.

Heart Shock has many elements and creates an impact on all of the energetic levels (e.g., wei, ying, yuan) as a systemic diagnosis, and as such, certain channel systems will have a larger impact on specific levels. This knowledge allows one to give a greater focus when symptoms in one level are more heightened, and it also allows for an increasingly varied combination of systems to be utilized simultaneously (either within an individual treatment, or as part of an overall strategy over time).

I will present the channel systems in order from their most superficial aspects (wei qi involvement) to the deepest core aspects (yuan level). But the reader should keep in mind that, while each channel system can be utilized on its own, there are also many interrelationships that allow for tapping into multiple systems concurrently.

Along with the discussion on the primary channels, I will also present the use of specific categories of points not dealt with much in the other channel system discussions, such as the Window of the Sky points and the use of the Heart and Pericardium channel points and the nine palaces/nine Heart pains. Additional treatments that I personally find helpful to many of my patients will also be mentioned, such as Ge Hong's Nine Flower treatment, as well as treatment options and ideas stemming from Dr. Hammer's DRRBF. Lastly in Part II, I will discuss the role of gui/ghosts and gu/parasites in Heart Shock and some of their unique presentations and treatment strategies.

Within each chapter, I will present herbal treatments as well as essential oil recommendations based on the channel system energetics. Some of Dr. Shen's formulas will also be discussed and analyzed from the perspective of multiple channel systems.

CHAPTER 4

Sinew Meridians

Sinew channel introduction

The sinew meridians' domain is that which relates to wei-defensive qi. There are other systems, however, that influence the sinews and wei qi, namely the yuan level and its contribution of yang qi (of which wei qi is a sub-part), as well as the ying level which contributes the raw materials in the creation of wei qi (i.e., the jin-ye from the Stomach). Thus, one should always be mindful of the varied interrelationships affecting the sinew channels and wei qi (production, movement, source). With their relationship to wei qi, the sinew channels will have a major impact on Heart Shock, including management of the portals, the taiyang relationship to the exterior and boundaries, the nervous system functioning (from all the different perspectives discussed in Part I), hypervigilance, armoring, mood regulation, temperature regulation, rate and rhythm and the smooth muscle contractions of the Heart and gut, and fight/flight/freeze responses.

As wei qi covers the entire surface of the body, the sinew channels are very broad channels. Acupuncture channels are commonly depicted with fine lines, since we are generally looking at diagrams of primary channels and their points. The sinew channels, however, are larger and broader as they are more closely related to bands of muscles. Wei qi tends to accumulate in the folds and fleshy areas as well, including the webbings and paddings (e.g., neck, buttocks). They begin at the jing-well point, their only true designated point. All the other points along the channels are considered "ashi," meaning that they are reactive in some way, including being tender, tight, active, painful, swollen, hot, flaccid, weak, cold, etc. The sinew channels are made up of tendons, muscles, connective tissue, and ligaments, and, as mentioned, cover the entire body, even overlapping across other channels. They are the most external part of the body and represent the medium for the circulation and movement of wei qi. The yang sinew channels control the external anatomy, and the yin sinew channels control more of the internal domain, including the smooth muscles of the Heart and the gut (making them responsible for peristaltic activity and regulating cardio-rhythms). Thus, the yin sinews will have a major role in issues such as constipation (from fight/flight/freeze and constant stress reactions), tachycardia, fibrillations, palpitations, etc.

Unlike the luo vessels which we will discuss in the following chapter, the sinew channels exist despite any pathology being present. They are part of one's normal physiology. They have important roles in communicating with the external environment and management of the sensory orifices/portals, which is also a reflection of the health of the zang fu. Each of the zang fu has an associated orifice, and the health of that organ contributes to the clarity of perception of said orifice. This is yet another interrelationship that the sinew channels have with the ying and yuan levels.

The sinew channels also help offer protection from external pathogenic factors. In Part I, I approached the idea of trauma being the result of an external influence assaulting the body and mind. But we all experience a constant bombardment of stimuli (excessive and constant sounds, sights (including the barrage of images from televisions, smart phones, and tablet screens), smells, exposures to wind, cold, damp, pollution, EMFs, etc.) and stresses that endlessly engage our sinew channels. Our sinew meridians are therefore constantly stimulated and highly active, particularly if we are living in a city or fast-paced suburban environment or have experienced any traumas. The sinews are expansive and always acting, as a subset of yang, to protect us while we are awake (yang), and to nourish and strengthen us when inactive and asleep (yin). The sinew meridians don't just work on the exterior; the yin sinew channels go internally. When we have abundant healthy circulation of wei qi, these channels can penetrate into the internal regions of the body and also bring existing pathology back out to the surface of the body to be eliminated.

Distribution of wei qi to the surface is assisted by the movement of Lung qi, which governs wei qi. When the Lungs diffuse, they diffuse wei qi and fluids, bringing them out to the surface to ward off pathogens and maintain the health and integrity of the orifices and the senses. Wei qi is associated with our natural, involuntary, instinctive, reflexive, and spontaneous responses. It prompts us to sweat when we are hot, and shiver when we are cold. And as we don't have to think about removing our hand from a hot flame, we don't have to think about our wei qi responses. Healthy wei qi has its own natural protective mechanism. When wei qi is insufficient or lacking, patients may lack the sensitivity or reflexes to properly respond to external stimuli. One example that we often see occurs in cases of diabetic neuropathy, in which patients are unable to perceive heat, cold, and/or pain, particularly on their extremities. In these cases, patients are vulnerable to burns and other injuries, particularly when using tools like heat lamps and moxibustion, since the wei qi is not being properly activated.

Wei qi also reflects the ways we armor ourselves physically and emotionally, and, usually unconsciously, through our musculature. So, we will often see ashi points in specific areas in people who are tense and tight—that tightness can contribute to vulnerability to external pathogens since wei qi cannot circulate well in this type of terrain. If wei qi does not circulate well it cannot defend well either. Wei qi circulates in the exterior via the Lung's influence (skin and orifices) and Liver (muscles/sinews), as well as the interior (zang organs and also regulating smooth muscle contraction).

Qualities of wei qi

Wei qi is warming in nature. It has its source from Du mai (the yuan level and the birthplace of yang qi). Via the wei qi, the yuan level gets to seek expression. As an example, we can look at the taiyang level and its connection to shaoyin—it allows us to emanate, manifest, and express who we are (Kidney essence) to the world via the Bladder channel. And as part of its warming quality, wei qi helps with its next function, movement.

Wei qi has a significant role in circulation. It homes to the chest at Ren 17, reflecting the energetics of the Lungs, Heart, and Pericardium. This is also an entry point where the yang sinews transition with the yin sinew channels, allowing for wei qi to enter the interior domain at night. Yang sinew meridians move wei qi up to the extremities and into the head (fifth limb), except at night when it moves back into the chest to allow for internalization—sleep and rejuvenation. This internalization allows for the muscles, sinews, and limbs (and head/brain/nervous system) to become quiet and inactive, rest, and recuperate, while internally the organs receive the opportunity to rest, digest, and recharge the batteries. Wei qi internalization is crucial for helping to align sleep patterns with solar and lunar cycles, and an inability to enter the chest and organs is implicated in sleep disorders. This prevents the nervous system and mind from fully relaxing and contributes to its continued hyperactivity. Symptoms such as neck and jaw tension, Temporomandibular Joint Disorder (TMJ), grinding, restless leg syndrome, etc. are further reflections of this inability of wei qi to descend and enter the interior.

Sinew channels and wei qi are very expansive, so the pathways tend to cross over each other, which is one way that pathogens are able to travel and progress into different levels (e.g., taiyang pathogen moving to shaoyang, etc.). This can also happen with musculoskeletal problems wherein pain in one anatomical location and channel begins to move and invade broader areas, and even radiate to other channels (e.g., Triple Burner elbow pain that over time spreads to the Large Intestine or Lung channel). This expansiveness also reflects the diversity of conditions that the sinew channels can treat. In addition to the external invasions that practitioners are accustomed to treating, sinew channels can also be used to effectively address ENT issues (sinus problems, head issues, sore throat, etc.), dermatological problems, musculoskeletal symptoms, neurological problems, metabolic issues, thyroid problems, etc. Sinew channels can also treat insomnia, nocturnal urination (bedwetting), nausea, constipation, and a variety of gastrointestinal problems that manifest with rebellious qi.

Wei qi is protective. Whenever an external pathogen tries to gain access to the body, our instinctual autonomic functions will reflexively occur, such as sweating, fever, nasal secretions, etc., in response. These symptoms reflect wei qi being stimulated, rising to the occasion, and attempting to defend its terrain. Wei qi controls the opening and closing of the pores, which are crucial outlets for external pathogens as well as a way for exteriorizing internal pathogens. From a Classical perspective, we need some type of fluid discharge to effectively release something from the body. As a pathogen tries to move inward (generally at the level of the throat as it attempts to gain access to the chest), fever becomes more pronounced, especially when confronted by the Stomach channel, giving rise to the "four bigs."

And while wei qi is protective, it is not solely defensive. As mentioned earlier, abundant wei qi can reflect a healthy immune system, one that is also offensive and that can penetrate the interior to thrust out retained pathogens. It is also regulatory as the wei qi is responsible for maintaining the health of the heart rate and rhythm as well as peristaltic activity via its dominion over smooth muscle contractions. It circulates to the sensory portals to maintain their health and vitality as well as the purity of its perceptive capacities. All of these features of wei qi should be considered when considering the use of the sinew channel system to address a particular presentation.

Origins of wei qi

Wei qi is derived from food and drink entering the Stomach—the gu qi and the jin-ye; the thin and thick fluids are created here. The thin portion of the jin fluids go to the sensory orifices, and this helps us to clearly perceive what our eyes are seeing and what our ears are hearing. The higher the degree of clarity that our sensory organs can perceive, the greater the benefit to the zang fu organs. As a reciprocal relationship when the zang fu are healthy, the orifices are healthier and more able to perceive without distortions. The thick/turbid aspect of jin fluids goes to the sinews and the skin and helps to produce sweat. This assists wei qi in circulating to the exterior via the fascia and connective tissue.

For the ye, the thin aspect goes to nourish the zang fu and the thick/turbid aspects go to the curious organs (e.g., bones, brain, marrow, vessels, Gall Bladder, uterus, and prostate) and the gao (i.e., gao huang). The gao huang refers to the concept of the membrane (gao reflecting the yin aspect) and the movement in and out of the membrane (huang).

To recap, wei qi is produced from food and drink and circulates between the skin and the sinews and homes into the chest. Yang sinews represent the movement outward, while the yin sinews represent the movement of wei qi as it moves into the chest and interior. Wei qi is also contributed to by the yuan level and yang qi, and can be represented by the shaoyin/taiyang relationship.

Sinew channel sequence

The sinew channels follow a different sequence to the primary meridians which is more reflective of wei qi circulation. It begins with the leg taiyang Bladder with the opening of the eyes (wei qi stimulated by light/sun) and moves through the channel systems in two-hour increments. For the yang sinew channels, the arms and legs do not sequence together like they do in other channel systems. Here, wei qi moves first through the yang leg sinew channels from foot taiyang (Bladder) to foot shaoyang (Gall Bladder), and from there to foot yangming (Stomach). From the Stomach yangming, it travels to the arms and follows the same sequence, arm taiyang to arm shaoyang to arm yangming. Once the yang sinew channel circulation is complete, it moves to the yin sinew channels which reflect the internalization of wei qi. Here the leg and arm channels are paired. From arm yangming, the wei qi circulates to the leg and arm taiyin (Spleen and Lung), then the leg and arm shaoyin (Kidney and Heart), ending with the leg and arm jueyin (Liver/Pericardium). The sequencing of the channels reflects the origin and movement of wei qi, and as such, if we see upper limb symptoms, the presumption is that, barring an injury to the arms, the problem may have originated in the legs and one may need to treat the legs first or concurrently with the arm sinew channels.

The sinew channels have two sequences: one relating to the solar aspects of wei qi, the other, the lunar (discussed infra).

Solar sequence

The solar sequence as listed in the above paragraph is the more common, day-to-day circulation of the sinew channels. And unlike the Chinese clock and the primary channel sequence, with the sinew channels there is no specific time of day associated with any of the channels. As a reflection of wei qi and light, the sequence beginning is dependent on when the individual wakes up, opens the eyes, and registers the influence of yang via the sensory orifices at Bladder 1. From this point, the channels move in a two-hour cycle sequence (Bladder—Gall Bladder—Stomach—Small Intestine—Triple Burner—Large Intestine—Spleen/Lung—Kidney/Heart—Liver/Pericardium).

Wei qi is a subcategory of yang qi. The yang SM moves upward to the head (most yang), then moves inwards to connect to the yin for rejuvenation (yuan source level and yin SM). The yin sinews can internalize and/or help externalize pathogens, its gateway being the chest, where the yin and yang alternate circulation to allow wei qi to go inwards. As wei qi is activated by BL 1 and light, at night it internalizes to allow for sleep and regeneration.

As a result, it can be important to learn when a patient wakes and retires to bed each day. For example, if an insomnia patient wakes up at 3:00am, we can look at the primary meridian and know that time is when qi is moving from the Liver into the Lungs, but if we know when the patient went to sleep we can calculate where this patient is within the wei qi circulatory cycle. If this patient went to sleep at midnight, she would only be a few hours into the yin sinew circulation and that can help to diagnose a potential shaoyin wei qi pathology. Supposing the patient wakes up at 7:00am, she should theoretically begin the process of internalizing wei qi at around 7:00pm. According to this model (which is often not followed by modern

Western cultures), at the end of the yang sinew circulation, ideally she should be home relaxing and winding down from the day rather than heading to the gym and/or socializing. The taiyin sinews (Spleen and Lungs) would begin internalizing as she rests after dinner, the muscles begin to unwind, the breathing can slow down, etc. Then she would be retreating to bed, allowing the wei qi to enter further into the chest and abdomen, which is an important aspect of nourishing the organ systems and "recharging the batteries" so that there is sufficient qi to return to navigate the following day's activities without depletion. Symptoms like insomnia, nighttime urination, and improper digestion can be from the inability of wei qi to internalize at the proper time due to a lifestyle that may force it to remain on the exterior.

Understanding the sequence of wei qi, napping adds a little wrinkle into the picture and impacts the cycle by interrupting the yang sinews and moving wei qi towards the yin sinews. Naps may be very helpful in a number of circumstances, especially for those who are depleted and need to recharge the batteries more often, as well as those whose nervous systems are hyperactive. It is important, however, that wei qi be able to complete its entire circuit to ensure that all the organ systems are getting the benefit of wei qi circulation. If someone is very tired because yang is circulating poorly, a sedentary lifestyle with napping would be counterproductive as one would rather encourage the patient to be more active and allow wei qi to activate the sinews.

For most of our patients, their lifestyles include either an inability or unwillingness to slow down and rest. Artificial light, stimulants, media, technology, and work and life demands encourage us to push past limits and tax the body. This may also disorient wei qi in terms of our biorhythms (both solar and lunar cycles). In the summer, there's more light and people tend to be more active. More fruit is consumed in the warmer weather as it engenders fluids and our bodies try to store those fluids as well as the sugar (glycogen: fat binds sugar) and the yang qi to store back into the Kidney and Dai mai for the winter. With our modern lifestyles, however, these normal evolutionary signals are impacted as it becomes harder to live by and abide by natural rhythms when our environment is artificially controlled. With conveniences like artificial light, heat, and air conditioning we are no longer able to accommodate seasonal changes in the same way. Summer is always here and winter never truly arrives, but our bodies keep storing sugar for energy that it never needs. The more light our bodies perceive, the more it signals yang and wei qi, along with the tendency to think it's summertime. Nowadays, however, we live with light virtually all the time until we flick off the light switch to go to bed at night. The artificial light is also very stimulating to wei qi, promoting the body's natural mechanisms to crave more carbohydrates and sugar and more fruits. It creates a tendency to stay up later, reenergizing us as wei qi remains on the surface, followed by a tendency to feel hungry or crave a snack, creating its own feedback cycle wherein that sugar is stored away as fat and cholesterol for a winter that never comes. This is the cyclical relationship between our eyes, BL 1, wei qi, mood, sleep regulation, and our metabolism, and it leaves us vulnerable to the host of modern diseases like obesity and diabetes, heart disease, and other cardiovascular problems like arteriosclerosis.

When we look at issues related to our nervous systems, metabolism, and sleep, wei qi is very relevant as it must adjust to the different seasons, climate, and natural light exposure. Seasonal affective disorder impacts many, and people tend to become more depressed when there is less sunlight. It is the light that our eyes are picking up via BL 1 that stimulates wei qi, and wei qi is responsible for regulating one's mood.

As such, regulating sleep habits (which determine light exposure) can be a powerful tool to re-establish harmony in the relationship of wei and ying. With any hyperactivity on the wei level, this entire cycle is stimulated, we use and consume our jing-essence faster, and taxation occurs.

Domain of the sinew channels

The sinew channels have domain over all pathologies that are rooted in wei qi. And as we have seen above, wei qi has many functions and regulates activities that impact the entire body, including the ying and yuan levels. Some of the most common areas that one should look to the sinew channels include the following.

External invasions

As all external pathogenic factors (EPFs) will challenge wei qi, we can utilize the sinew channels for the treatment of disorders of external wind, cold, damp, heat, etc. External symptoms such as achiness, runny nose, congestion, fever and chills, sweat, cough, etc. reflect a pathogen on the surface that needs to be expelled via wei-defensive qi.

Pain syndromes

The sinew channels treat all types of pain due to climatic factors (bi-syndromes) as well as qi circulation trapped in the musculature. This can manifest as the varied types of pain (cold/sharp, wind/radiating, damp/heaviness, etc.), as well as stiffness, tightness, tenderness, weakness, numbness, neuropathies, injuries, spasms, etc. The yin sinew channels also address pain as it travels in towards the bone level which reflects the yin of yang. The divergent meridians also exercise domain over this area, and we can often distinguish the use of the yin sinews for more acute pain disorders rather than chronic ones which implicate the divergent meridians.

Allergies (external and internal)

Similar to EPFs, allergies confront wei qi and cause a constant hyperactivity and consequent exterior symptoms such as sniffling, runny nose, sneezing, burning itchy eyes, cough, etc. Internal allergies, however, can also be the result of wei qi hyperactivity as it responds to the irritations in the gut lining. We discussed wei qi's origin as emanating from the Stomach yin, and a relative lack of yin can create irritation and inflammation in the gut as well as also affecting peristaltic activity with the internalization of wei qi.

Dermatology

Wei qi uses the raw materials from the Stomach, and the turbid aspect of the jin fluids circulates in the skin. Wei qi (and Lungs) also regulates the opening and closing of the pores and the ability to discharge pathogens from the skin layer. While there are multiple causes of dermatological issues (i.e., blood heat, toxicity, digestive, Liver, etc.), the sinew channels' domain over wei qi and the exterior makes it an important venue in the treatment of all skin disorders.

Ears, eyes, nose, and throat

As wei qi has a major role in circulating to the sensory orifices and providing nourishment, disorders in these realms are treated by the sinew channels. The ears, eyes, nose, and throat are also areas in which external pathogens gain entry and attempt to internalize in the body, bringing their defense to the realm of wei qi and sinew channels.

Gastrointestinal issues

As mentioned earlier, the gut is the origin of wei qi production and provides the raw materials towards its creation. The wei qi circulates from the Stomach to the Large Intestine and Lung channels to be distributed to the skin and sensory orifices in order to defend our borders and provide proper acuity to our sensory portals. This is done via the yang sinew channels. The yin sinew channels return wei qi back to the interior to nourish the internal terrain. One of the important characteristics of this is that at night one must "rest to digest" and assimilate and nourish our bodies with what we have taken in (food and drink, but also thoughts and experiences). This provides the necessary timing for recharging the batteries and replenishing our reserves. Wei qi is also responsible for the smooth muscle contractions, including peristaltic activity. Disorders such as constipation and diarrhea, irritable bowel syndrome, etc. reflect disharmony of wei qi in the gut. Moreover, as pathogens make their way internally, wei qi travels with the pathogen, still fighting. Wei qi, which is warming, battles with the pathogen in the interior, creating symptoms such as gastritis, inflammatory bowel disease, Crohn's disease, etc. The sinew channels are important channels to tap into to treat such disorders.

Mood disorders

To understand mood disorders, one must differentiate mood, emotions, and temperament. One's mood lacks consciousness of the reason one feels the way one does. Like the wind, a mood can blow in and out without much warning or without one understanding its origin. It is within the realm of wei qi. Emotions have blood and consciousness attached to them. When a person experiences the emotion of anger, he knows why he is angry and the particular circumstances behind it. As such, one creates context and has a particular perception. Similarly, one can also modify that context and perception with different information and/or choice. Emotions are under the auspices of ying qi. Temperament is one's stance in the world and relates more to one's constitution. A metal person tends towards longing and sadness and perceives the world accordingly. It is more hard-wired and is governed by yuan qi energetics. Thus, mood disorders relate to wei qi; they can be automatic unconscious patterned behaviors. People with mood disorders can be highly susceptible to stress and any external influences, including even changes with the weather and barometer. As wei qi also has its root in yang qi, yang qi may also have an influence over this domain as well, but the relationship to, and the utilization of, wei qi in the treatment of mood disorders is crucial.

Nervous system disorders

As mentioned earlier, Dr. Shen's conception of the nervous system is rooted in taiyang energetics and consists of the lightest, fastest-moving energies, i.e., wei qi. In Part I, I detailed all the relationships to this concept of the nervous system, including the taiyang–shaoyin relationship, wei qi–yang qi, Heart and Kidney axis, Liver and sinews/armoring, divergent meridian energetics, etc., but wei qi is the primary manifestation and linkage to all of these dynamics.

Sinew channel pathways

All the sinew channels begin at their respective jing-well points and travel upwards. As the channels ascend, they bind and knot at specific locations along the pathway, mostly the major articulations which relate to the origins or insertion areas of joints, and bony areas like the occiput, face, ankles, hips, etc. And as mentioned above, the only "true" points associated with the sinew channels are the jing-well points. All other points are considered ashi points, as well as the binding areas which have the ability to release the pathogen being held in the channel.

Meeting/convergence points

The sinew channels also contain meeting or convergence points which reflect areas where the trinity of channels meet up. These points have significant import in that they are used to control major areas in which wei qi accumulates. These areas are also commonly needled to prevent transmission of pathology from progressing from one channel into another within the trinity and gaining a stronger foothold. The convergence points are as follows:

Leg Yang Channels (Bladder, Stomach, Gall Bladder): SI 18/ST 3 (cheekbones). The cheekbones are strategically situated in the middle of all the sensory orifices, with the nose medially, the ears laterally, the eyes above, and the mouth below. There is a reciprocal relationship between the senses and motor activity: how one senses the world determines how one moves, and how one moves determines how one senses the world.

Arm Yang Channels (Small Intestine, Large Intestine, Triple Burner): ST 8/GB 13 (forehead). ST 8 moves to Du 23/24, and GB 13 communicates with Du 20.

Leg Yin Channels (Spleen, Kidney, Liver): Ren 3 (pelvis).

Arm Yin Channels (Lung, Heart, Pericardium): GB 22 (axilla/chest)—an important point for relaxing the sinews. GB 22 is a notable point that shares energetics with other channel systems, namely the luo channels and the divergent meridians. The Su Wen names GB 22 as the origin point for the great luo of the Spleen, making this a major area where wei qi meets up with the chest and blood and where wei qi moves into the ying level (and here, as the convergence point of the Lungs, Heart, and Pericardium, this is yet another reflection of that dynamic). The Gall Bladder is in charge of decision-making and to some degree helps determine what we allow into the chest (Pericardium to protect the Heart). Also significant is that GB 22 is a confluent point on the Small Intestine and Heart's divergent meridian. As a region where wei qi internalizes to the chest, one can often find blood stasis here (hence the relationship to the great luo of the Spleen).

Diagnosing the root

Because the sinew channels are broad channels that tend to overlap, an important aspect in using them is to understand the root pathology and sinew meridian involved. When it comes to pain, one must understand the root pathogenic influence is based on the nature of the sinew channel dynamics (i.e., movement), not necessarily the location of pain or presence of ashi points. The presence of pain and/or ashi points still requires local treatment, but the jing-well point to be needled to release the pathogen must be based on the movement diagnosis/nature of pain. The movements and their associated sinew channel correspondences are as follows.

Movement diagnosis

TAIYANG

The taiyang sinew channels are responsible for the extension movements of the limbs (arm/hand/leg/foot). The taiyang channels are implicated with pain initiated by walking, driving (extending foot to press on pedal), extending an arm or lifting an arm or leg, extending the body while standing up from a chair, etc.

SHAOYANG

The shaoyang sinew channels are responsible for rotational movements while the limbs are extended. Pain can be initiated by twisting of the hands, turning of one's head, rotating the legs or any joints (hip, arms, knee, ankle), or any lateral flexion.

YANGMING

The yangming sinew channels manage the bearing of weight when movements are being held in position. Pain initiated by holding weight while extended or while engaging muscles to halt movement implicates the yangming channels. Thus, back pain while standing still, or leg pain that is not felt while running, but rather upon slowing oneself down and stopping movement, is yangming sinew channel pain.

TAIYIN

The taiyin sinew channels are engaged as the body begins to withdraw its energy inwards or when retracting one's muscles. Thus, the taiyin channels would be implicated in pain initiated by bending the arms or legs while trying to move into a seated position, or pain while seated in a retracted position.

SHAOYIN

The shaoyin sinew channels are responsible for rotational movements while the limbs or affected body parts are in a retracted position (shaoyang is when the limbs are extended). Pain experienced while rotating the body while sitting, or rotating the limbs while the elbows/knees are bent, is a shaoyin sinew channel problem.

JUEYIN

The jueyin sinew channels are implicated when any and all movements elicit pain, when there is constant pain, even without movement, and pain and/or limitations with movement (e.g., paralysis). Back pain while lying still in bed, inability to move, and pain with movement in any and all directions warrants a jueyin sinew channel diagnosis.

Thus, when it comes to pain, the movement evaluation is more important than the location of ashi points as it informs about the sinew channel origin. For example, a patient with pain after playing tennis experiences pain while holding a tennis racket and bearing its weight, but the location of pain is found on SJ 14. SJ 14 is needled as the ashi point, but LI 1 must be needled as a reflection of the yangming pathogen via movement diagnosis.

Lunar sequencing: wei qi's monthly cycle

The cycles of wei qi, in addition to following a solar cycle as described above, also have a lunar cycle. The associations of the sinew channels to the monthly cycle describe, much like the Chinese clock, which channels have an abundance of qi (in this case, wei qi) in any given month. The general cycle follows from shaoyang → taiyang → yangming → yangming → taiyang → shaoyang → shaoyin → taiyin → jueyin → jueyin → taiyin → shaoyin → shaoyang and the cycle continues. In our monthly calendar that plays out as follows:

January: Gall Bladder

February: Bladder

March: Stomach

April: Large Intestine

May: Small Intestine

June: Triple Burner

July: Kidney

August: Spleen

September: Liver

October: Pericardium

November: Lung

December: Heart

It is important to note, however, that the Chinese calendar differs a bit from the Western calendar. So, to utilize this information above, we must adjust the information by one month. For example, if a patient comes in for a visit in October complaining of seasonal allergies, we would adjust backwards one month to September and see that the Liver sinew channel would be implicated seasonally. Treatment would be to search the Liver sinew channel for ashi points, releasing areas of tightness and tenderness along the channel and at the binding areas, followed by other ashi areas on the channels based on symptoms. The jing-well point of the Liver, LR 1, would be needled at the end of the treatment, reflecting the lunar root-cause of the allergies.

Our circulation follows a cyclical pattern through the channels, whether it be via the solar cycle with the activation of light, or the lunar cycle as depicted above. This can play out in many ways as our wei-defensive qi has a protective component and can remember and hold onto pathology that recurs at certain times of the year or at "anniversaries" of specific traumas. This is easily seen with seasonal allergies as noted above, but can also occur with physical and/or emotional traumas. With physical traumas, one can see the recurrence of pain in areas that experienced trauma years prior and only becomes symptomatic with flare-ups at the time of anniversary. With emotional traumas, it is not uncommon to see a patient struck by particular moods as the anniversary of a trauma nears, again, even if the trauma was many years before. Utilizing the sinew channels can be a powerful tool for unraveling these traumas and invigorating wei qi to release them.

Sinew channel symptoms

All the sinew channels have their unique characteristics, signs, symptoms, etc. Many of these are summarized below.

Yang sinew channels

The yang sinew channels are focused on stimulating wei qi and the creation of mobility and action.

Leg taiyang Bladder

TRAJECTORY

The leg taiyang Bladder sinew channel is responsible for circulating wei qi throughout the largest muscle channel in the body. It begins at BL 67, the jing-well point, and travels up to BL 60 where it binds. It ascends the posterior aspect of the leg to bind at BL 40, as well as the anterior aspect to bind at GB 34 and BL 39. It travels up the back of the thigh to BL 36 and goes to the back to bind at the sacrum (BL 31–34 and the gluteus). There are multiple branches of the Bladder sinew channel. One goes from the lateral malleolus at BL 60 to the heel and the Achilles and ascends to the back of the knee, from there traveling to BL 36. From the hips and GB 30 area, it travels to the side of the spine and up to the nape of the neck (BL 10) and to the back of the head. From the head it continues to the bridge of the nose and upper eyelid where it binds around the sinuses and continues to the cheekbones. Another branch goes from the shoulder to the cheekbones. A branch from BL 10 goes internal to the root of the tongue. An additional branch is found at BL 16–17, wrapping around the shoulder by SI 11 (its taiyang pair), binding at LI 15 branching to the axillary crease and GB 22, and to ST 12. From ST 12 it moves to the cheekbones (meets SI 18) and another branch goes towards the back of the head at GB 12. And one last branch travels from the BL 13–14 area up to GB 21 where it binds.

BINDING AREAS

> BL 60, 61, 39, 40, 56, 57, 36, 31–34, 1, 2
>
> GB 40, 34, 30, 12, 21, 22
>
> KI 10
>
> SI 11, 12 (scapula), 18
>
> LI 15 (shoulder), 20 (nose)

MOTION

The movement associated with the Bladder sinew is extension.

SYMPTOMS

Common symptoms include pain along the trajectory, taiyang pathogens and wind-cold symptoms and presentations, sinus problems, allergies, rhinitis, back pain, heel pain, joint pain, strained muscles, inability to close the eyes (e.g., Bell's palsy), tongue, throat, and thyroid disorders, axillary lymph swellings, immune deficiency, and asthma.

It's important to note that the gastrocnemius muscle as a major fight/flight/freeze muscle frequently demonstrates tension and sensitivity with Heart Shock and the resulting hypervigilance and armoring. Over time, however, one often finds the calf to be atrophied from long-term adrenaline (Kidney yang) leakage resulting in corresponding symptoms of immune deficiency, asthma, allergies, etc.

Leg shaoyang Gall Bladder

TRAJECTORY

The channel starts at GB 44, binding at GB 40. It travels up the lateral aspect of the leg to bind at GB 34 at the fibula. From there it travels up the lateral thigh to GB 29 and goes to the back to bind at the sacrum (BL 31–34) and gluteus. It continues up to the ribcage to the clavicle and binds at ST 12. There is a branch from GB 22 that goes to the breast and up to ST 12 as well. From there it travels behind the ear, up to the temples and cheekbones, and binds at SI 18. It continues to the nose to meet with LI 20, then up the nose to bind at GB 1. There is a branch from GB 9 which goes to ST 8 and up to Du 20.

BINDING AREAS

> GB 40, 34, 29, 22, 9, 1
>
> ST 32, 12, 8

SI 18

LI 20

Du 20

Sacral Liao points, breasts (via GB 22)

MOTION

The Gall Bladder sinew channels govern the movement of rotation while the limb or body part is extended. (Rotation as a movement is similar to the Gall Bladder's function of decision-making, allowing for choice in movement.)

SYMPTOMS

Pain, spasms, pulling sensations along the trajectory, shaoyang EPFs, bitter taste in the mouth, intercostal pain, nausea, one-sided paralysis, sacral pain, chest pain, breast pain, neck pain, etc.

Leg yangming Stomach

TRAJECTORY

The sinew channel begins at ST 45 and the three middle toes. As it ascends it binds at ST 42, then travels up the tibia to bind at GB 34 (three leg yang meeting point). It continues to the lateral hip to bind at GB 29, goes to GB 25 and LR 13, and then travels to the spine (L2–L4). Another branch goes from ST 42 to ST 35, where it binds. From there it continues up to bind at ST 30, moving to Ren 3 (three leg yin meeting point). It travels up the abdomen to the chest and binds at ST 12 (three leg yang meeting point), then up to ST 5, and splits at the mouth and cheek with a branch going to SI 18 (three leg yang meeting point) and ST 4 to bind. It continues up to the eyes to meet at BL 1. An additional branch from ST 5 goes to the ears.

BINDING AREAS

ST 42, 35, 30, 12, 4

GB 34, 29

Ren 3

MOTION

The Stomach sinew channel is responsible for weight-bearing actions as well as engaging the muscles that slow down or halt movement.

SYMPTOMS

Common symptoms of the Stomach sinew channel include sore throat, throat bi, loss of voice from EPF transforming into heat at the throat (area of internalization), counterflow or rebellious qi, hernia, swellings/distension in inguinal area, abdominal spasms/pain, deviation of the mouth, drooping (and puffy) eyelids which can't open, and urogenital disorders (cystitis, herpes, etc.). The Stomach sinew channel has a major influence on the sense organs and includes such symptoms as tinnitus, ear infections, deafness, eye redness/irritation/styes, mouth ulcers, bleeding gums, etc.

Understanding the relationships between the taiyang, shaoyang, and yangming, one can see that there are adjustments between them in response to pathogenic invasions. When a pathogen exists in taiyang but there is a wei qi deficiency and taiyang is unable to expel it, yangming can come to its aid by providing the thin, jin fluids to bolster wei qi, and that adjustment can cause the typical pattern of the "4 bigs" (fever, sweat, thirst, Rapid pulse). Should the ying level be insufficient, the yuan level may be called upon to convert yuan/yang qi to wei qi; this is done via the shaoyang, wherein the Triple Burner mobilizes Kidney yang to the Heart/chest, often producing symptoms such as chest/ribcage tightness (GB 22) and bitter taste in mouth (Heart fire) to prevent the pathogen from penetrating.

Arm taiyang Small Intestine

TRAJECTORY

The Small Intestine sinew channel begins at SI 1, moves up the arm, and binds at SI 5–6. It then travels up the ulnar side of the forearm to bind at SI 8. From there it continues up to SI 9 where it binds, goes into the scapula, and then the neck, binding at the mastoid covering the area of GB 12, GB 20, and SI 17. From here it circles above and around the ear to bind at ST 5. It then travels to and binds at GB 1, then to GB 13 (three arm yang meeting point). There is a branch from behind the ear that penetrates into the ear.

BINDING AREAS

SI 5, 6, 8, 9, 17

ST 5, ST 8/GB 13

GB 12, 20, 1

MOTION

As a taiyang channel, the Small Intestine sinew is in charge of extension movements such as lifting the arm above the head or extending the elbow outwards. It has a strong connection to the subscapularis (raising arm), rhomboids (connects to scapula and

Du 14), supraspinalis (opens ribcage), and tricep muscles (allows for straightening of elbow).

A couple of important notes on the supraspinalis and the tricep. The supraspinalis helps with opening and extending the arm and ribcage and one can commonly see a jutting forward of the jaw from tightness in these muscles caused by Heart fire. This can be found in patients post trauma as they are constantly searching for threats. The tricep allows for the straightening of the arm and consumes glucose for the arm yang sinew channels much the way the calves do for the leg yang sinews. Like with the calves, one can find flaccidity here in chronic fatigue from constant hypervigilance.

SYMPTOMS

Pain along the scapula and trapezius; inflammation of the axilla; tinnitus (especially difficulty determining pitch); ear pain; pain at the mastoid process; toothache; abnormal contraction of face; twitching eyelids; migraines at temporofrontal area.

The area of SI 12 is where pathogens can find latency and progress to the yin level (and the divergent channels). Cold pathogens, tightness, and armoring are common here and often seen post trauma with hypervigilance.

Arm shaoyang Triple Burner

TRAJECTORY

The Triple Burner sinew channel begins at SJ 1, continues upwards, and binds at SJ 4 and at SJ 10. It ascends the upper arm, shoulder, and neck to connect with ST 5 and from there connects internally to the root of the tongue. From the upper arm, a branch goes to the upper trapezius to meet with the Small Intestine sinew channel. At the region of the mandible (ST 5), the channel travels to the temples. A branch from ST 5 moves to the front of the ear and outer canthus at GB 1. From the eye it ascends the head to ST 8/GB 13.

BINDING AREAS

SJ 4, 5, 10

LI 15

ST 5, 6

Tongue

MOTION

As a shaoyang channel, the Triple Burner manages the rotational movements of the upper limbs (such as opening a jar, turning a doorknob) or trouble with allowing the arms to hang straight. It has a strong area of influence over the deltoid and trapezius muscles.

SYMPTOMS

Pain with rotation of arms/hands, hanging of the arms, turning of the neck, opening the jaw. It can also result from raising the arms (as in taiyang), straightening the arms with tension, headaches near the eyes associated with rotational arm movements, thyroid gland symptoms (e.g., weight issues/fluctuations), swelling, edema around the wrists, muscle pain/tension from tension in the nervous system and/or emotional disturbances or long-term mental stress, or neck, shoulder, abdomen, or knee pain. Because this muscle channel connects with the tongue, it treats curling or contractions with speech disorders (often caused by wind stroke).

Arm yangming Large Intestine

TRAJECTORY

The Large Intestine sinew channel begins at LI 1, moves up the arm, and binds at LI 5. From there it goes up the forearm to bind at LI 11, continuing up to the shoulder to LI 15, up the neck, and in front of the ears, ascending to the ST 8/GB 13 area. From there it travels to Du 20, crossing over the midline to the opposite side of the face at ST 5. One branch goes from the shoulder to the upper spine. Another goes from the neck to ST 5 and binds at LI 20.

BINDING AREAS

LI 5, 11, 15, 20

SI 18

GB 13/ST 8

MOTION

As a yangming sinew channel, its movement is associated with gripping or holding an object in place and bearing its weight.

SYMPTOMS

Common symptoms of the Large Intestine sinew channel include pain with opening the jaw, straightening the arm, and rotating the arms/hands. There is also an inability to turn the neck (inability, not pain—which would be shaoyang), inability to bear weight, fidgeting of the hands/feet (Tourette's) or tension that is difficult to release (Bell's palsy), frozen shoulders, tennis elbow, scapula pain, pain in the upper thoracic spine, and issues of the face, cheeks, mandible (the face is the field of yangming), and the temporofrontal region (opposite side).

The Large Intestine sinew channel has a strong influence over the deltoid muscle and, as such, the dynamics of the chest. Weakness in the deltoid can ultimately cause the chest to collapse, i.e., weak Lungs (asthma, etc.). Over time, the hollowing of the chest will compensate by pushing the shoulders back, causing a barrel chest and emphysema. As the Large Intestine is related to the Metal phase, grief from traumas can impact these muscle groups and become implicated in symptoms of chest pain, shortness of breath, etc.

Yin sinew channels

The yin sinew channels are where wei qi begins to internalize. Here the arm and leg channel pairs converge towards the center of the body (yin regions). Often, here we are confronted with loss of muscle mass and flaccid muscles from lack of tone. Taiyin begins the internalization of yin (thick fluids and blood); shaoyin internalizes for the sake of jing-essence to support the major articulations (e.g., hip, knee, shoulder, elbow) into a state of retraction and ability to rotate the limbs; jueyin signifies the reverting of yin and the movement back out to the Bladder taiyang.

Leg taiyin Spleen

TRAJECTORY

The Spleen sinew channel begins at the SP 1/LR 1 region, ascends, and binds at SP 5 and the medial malleolus. It moves up the medial aspect of the tibia to bind at SP 9, continues up the medial thigh to the groin to bind at SP 12, and then travels to the lower border of the navel where it enters internally. It ascends to the ribcage, wrapping around the ribs to bind near LR 13 and GB 22 where it branches, one branch adhering to the spine, the other homing to the chest.

BINDING AREAS

SP 1/LR 1, SP 5, SP 9, SP 12

LR 13 area

Ren 3, 4, 6, 7 and umbilicus

GB 22 area

MOTION

The Spleen sinew meridian allows for the retraction of the lower body, the ability to move into a sitting position, and the retraction of joints of the lower limbs.

SYMPTOMS

The cardinal symptoms of the Spleen sinew channel are related to its areas of influence. It has an impact on the genitalia region at SP 12 (cold pain/hernia, prostatitis, discharges, swellings, herpes); it connects to the umbilicus (hernia, dampness, or spasms in the abdomen); wei qi is internalized and there are smooth muscle contractions (abdominal pain, diaphragmatic spasms, chest and Heart symptoms); and there are channel pathway symptoms (chest pain, rib pain, spine pain, bunion pain, pain during sitting (prolonged sitting damages the Spleen), tension or flaccidity in lower intercostals/oblique muscles (Gall Bladder channel area), weak knees, ankles, and back pain referring to the abdomen).

The Spleen sinew channel has an influence over the adductor muscles which are essential for maintaining the pelvic structure. Flaccidity here can be found with infertility, hormonal changes during menopause, hot flashes, etc. Stiff shoulders can result from adductors being flaccid, thus creating flaccid intercostals/Dai mai. Similarly, tension in these muscles can create significant stagnation as the Spleen sinew attempts to astringe this leakage. This can create symptoms such as cysts, fibroids, and other tumors and inflammatory processes in the pelvic region. As a sequelae to sexual traumas, these muscles can frequently become tense, hypervigilantly protecting oneself, leading to the host of stagnations listed above. Additionally, certain repetitive exercises that utilize these muscles excessively can likewise create this problem, even specific lineages of taijiquan, such as the Yang style, which prioritizes a closing/tightening of the kua (hips and inguinal area). It is not uncommon for men who engage in these practices to develop prostate issues. The sartorius muscle (GB 27/GB 28/SP 12 to SP 9 area) is also under the Spleen sinew channel and allows things to move in a rotational aspect, giving birth to shaoyin's movement. Problems with this muscle may cause weak, heavy knees or cracking and knocking from sinking Spleen qi.

Arm taiyin Lungs

TRAJECTORY

The Lung sinew channel originates at LU 11, and travels up the arm to bind at the thenar eminence at the LU 10–9 area. It ascends the radial aspect of the wrist and forearm, binding at the elbow and LU 5. It travels up along the Lung channel to the deltoid muscle and shoulder at LI 15, then to the lower border of the clavicle at ST 12. From the collarbone, it descends to the chest and diaphragm.

BINDING AREAS

LU 10–9 area

ST 12

LI 15

MOTION

The motion of the Lung sinew allows for retraction. These muscles allow for bending the arms, chest, and ribcage. The Spleen allows for the sitting position in relation to the lower body, i.e., retraction of the ankles, knees, and pelvis. The Lungs allow for compression and retraction of the ribcage, without which bending would be difficult.

SYMPTOMS

The symptoms of the Lung sinew channel include insomnia from a difficulty falling asleep due to the chest being unable to sink/allow wei qi to descend as well as its relationship to the Heart. One sees symptoms along the trajectory such as rib pain/tension, hypochondriac pain, fibrocystic breasts, hiatal hernia, etc. Counterflow qi, coughing, hiccups, hemoptysis, etc. are also common. The LU 10 area of the thenar eminence is an analogous reflection of the sacrum. When flaccid, one will often find lesions on the sacrum which must be released before resolving long-term Lung issues. The movement of the thenar eminence can relax the chest, elbow, and knees and allow for the Kidneys to grasp Lung qi. The area of LU 2 can also show nodules and gumminess here, often related to metal toxicity and toxicity in lymph from poor elimination. The thenar eminence area should once again be utilized to release this toxicity, as well as releasing the sacrum.

Leg shaoyin Kidney

TRAJECTORY

The Kidney sinew channel begins at the little toe and crosses under the foot, communicating with KI 1, emerging along the navicular bone around KI 2 where it binds around the Achilles tendon at the KI 3, 4, 6 area. From here it ascends the leg to bind at KI 10, BL 40, and BL 39. It continues up the thigh into the genitalia and moves from the pelvis into the spine (connecting to the psoas/iliopsoas), and up to the occipital region to meet with the Bladder sinew channel and to bind at the occiput. Another branch ascends the abdomen and enters into the chest.

BINDING AREAS

KI 2, 3, 4, 6, 10

BL 40, 39, 10

MOTION

As a shaoyin channel the Kidney sinew manages rotational movement while the body is in a retracted position.

SYMPTOMS

The Kidney sinew channel establishes lots of connections which are associated with its primary symptoms. One connection is to the head and brain. The Kidney sinew channel can be used for floating yang with wind such as seizures and epilepsy, convulsions, and occipital headaches. As it deals with rotation, neck and head pain is a Kidney sinew problem. Moving the head up and down implicates taiyang, and while shaoyang doesn't have a large impact on occipital pain, it should be ruled out as the channel will traverse the GB 20 area. Lower back pain while the person sits and rotates, or while lying down and attempting to move, reflects the Kidney sinew channel.

Chronic dermatological conditions can implicate the Kidneys as well in their relationship to the Lungs and taiyin's role of internalizing wei qi. Where that wei qi cannot internalize, we can see skin disorders, especially if the Kidneys are unable to detoxify via the fluids. One may also see cramping/pain, allergies, asthma, etc.

The knees are also traversed by the Kidney sinew channel. Pain above the knee reflects the Kidneys (where pain at the patella is the Stomach channel, and pain below the knee is typically Spleen related). Needling KI 1 is excellent for relaxing the knees and providing suppleness.

A role of the Kidneys is to move fluids, and this includes the sexual fluids. From the perspective of wei qi movement into the sexual organs, the Spleen brings fluids and blood to the flesh (e.g., elongation of the sexual organs and stimulation), the Kidneys are responsible for the movement of the sexual fluids in the uterus/vagina/penis, and the Liver manages the release of those fluids. Symptoms such as vaginal dryness or irritation with sexual activity can implicate the Kidney sinew channel and stagnation of wei qi. Traumas involving sexual activity, rapes, incest, etc. can cause sinew channel issues of the pelvis.

Like all of the sinew channels, the Kidneys deal with pain along their pathway. This includes low back pain, spine pain, leg pain, hamstring and calf pain, bone spurs, plantar fasciitis, heel spurs, pain at the nape of the neck, bone degeneration and pain in the joints, arthritis, pain in the legs while rotating from a seated position, and difficulty bending the chin upwards and downwards. (Whiplash tends to be a Kidney sinew problem as it is often caused by being struck from behind in car accidents, i.e., while sitting. The pelvis contracts in anticipation of (or responding to) the impact (and fear is often involved with the preparation of impact); this can be released by working on the heel at KI 3 and KI 4, as well as the pad of the little toe.)

The Kidneys also deal with fear and can displace fear into the muscles of the pelvis, legs, spine, etc. The Kidney sinew is also related to the adrenals and Du mai and tends to be very sensitive with allergies (relationship to taiyang) and asthma (Lung/Kidney relationship). When there is an external expression of chronic issues, one can treat the Bladder and Kidney sinew meridians together.

As the Kidney sinew channel reflects Du mai energetics and its relationship to the Bladder sinew channel, it has a big impact on posture. Where someone walks hunched forwards (with a cane and/or buffalo hump), often it is because the back has become flaccid, implicating a weak Kidney sinew channel.

Arm shaoyin Heart

TRAJECTORY

The Heart sinew begins at HT 9 and ascends to HT 7 where it binds. It travels up to and binds at HT 3, then goes up the axillary region to HT 1 (goes to the armpit connecting with GB 22) and spreads, wraps, and embraces across the chest in a horizontal axis. From there it descends to the umbilicus via the midline.

BINDING AREAS

HT 9, 7, 3, 1

GB 22

Umbilicus

MOTION

The Heart sinew channel manages rotational movements towards the midline of the body.

SYMPTOMS

The symptoms of the Heart sinew include pain with bending the arm at the shoulder towards the midline, implicating the pectoralis major muscle. This muscle has a relationship to the brain via its connection to the Heart channel and the sternum. Ren 15 at the tail of this bone is the source point of yin and has a direct impact on the brain. Excess stress or prolonged concentration can make Ren 15 very tight and sensitive to touch. Flaccidity here can suggest a weak Heart or that mental concentration is poor. This also creates a connection to yangming seen with ulcers caused by excessive worry. This can be treated by releasing the binding areas of the Heart sinew meridian (i.e., minor eminence, HT 7, HT 3, GB 22, Ren 15) and palpating the intercostals for lumps and releasing those. This can treat Stomach fire, angina, mental stress, etc.

Based on its location, the Heart sinew channel also treats chest and breast symptoms, including mastitis, fibrocystic breasts, hiccups, belching, esophagitis (passes through the diaphragm), fainting, shock, anxiety, and running piglet qi (connection to the umbilicus, lower dantian, and yuan qi).

Arm jueyin Pericardium

TRAJECTORY

The Pericardium sinew channel begins at tip of the fourth and middle fingers and travels to the palm to PC 8, continuing to the wrist and binding at PC 7. From there it travels up to the elbow and binds at PC 3, and follows up the arm to the axillary region where it binds. From here it descends to the lower ribs and also binds at the diaphragm (Ren 17/15 area).

BINDING AREAS

PC 7, 3

Ren 17–15 area

Axillary region

Diaphragm

MOTION

As a jueyin channel, the Pericardium sinew manages pain with all or no movements, including the inability to move (paralysis).

SYMPTOMS

Pericardium sinew channel symptoms include the inability to move the tongue (including post stroke), difficulty moving the upper part of the body, chronic stiff neck, loss of ability to speak or swallow, spasms along the trajectory, fatty qi (Liver accumulations felt under the right side of the ribcage), symptoms related to the pectoralis muscle, including floaters and dizziness (impact on eyes from Liver toxicity), chest pain, stuffiness in the chest, chronic headaches, and xi fen syndrome (Lung qi stagnation due to phlegm and heat accumulation, with symptoms such as a mass below the hypochondrium, pleurisy with chills, fever, cough, vomiting, and harsh and painful breathing).

Leg jueyin Liver

TRAJECTORY

The Liver sinew begins at the lateral side of the big toe at the corner of the nail and travels in front of the medial malleolus where it knots at LR 4. From here it ascends along the medial aspect of the tibia to the medial aspect of the knee and knots. It then moves to the medial aspect of the thigh to the external genitalia where it knots.

BINDING AREAS

LR 1, 4, 8

Ren 3

MOTION

Like the Pericardium, its jueyin pair, the Liver sinew manages pain with all or no movements, including the inability to move (paralysis).

Symptoms

The Liver sinew treats stiffness, spasms, pulling sensations of the big toe, pain in the medial ankle, knee, or thigh area, symptoms of the external genitalia, including impotence from excess sexual indulgence, damp-heat congestion, or cold invading the Liver channel, orgasmic dysfunctions and inability to reach climax (common with sexual abuse), spasms from internal or external cold or damp cold (hernias, shan), and pain or abnormal discharge from external or internal heat.

Sinew channel pulses

As the sinew channels reflect wei qi dynamics, and wei qi has its greatest influence in the exterior, pulses for the sinew channels are mapped superficially on the skin (yang sinew channels) as well as the contour of the radial artery (yin sinew channels). As we have already discussed, wei qi has its roots in the Stomach (ying level) as well as the Kidneys (yuan level), so the presence of wei qi and sinew activity does not negate a root elsewhere. A full pulse diagnosis should always include an evaluation of the ying and yuan as well as all the channel systems to determine root causes and other relevant diagnoses.

When looking at the pulses from a Classical perspective we orient towards the patient's wrist with his palm facing upwards. The area from the skin down to the bone is separated into five general components (classically based on beans of pressure), each equidistant from the next. Each gradation of pressure should be equal to the last, so there are five equal depths from the skin (3 beans) to the bones (15 beans). The area that we will be most focused on for the sinew meridians is the 3 beans (yang sinew channels) and 6 beans (yin sinew channels) of pressure. Pressure is applied to the radial artery equally with the practitioner's three fingers on the cun, guan, and chi positions simultaneously, moving as one unit (see Figure 4.1).

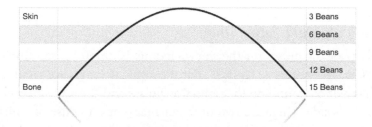

Figure 4.1: Pulse depths

- Wei level is 3 beans of pressure: skin and yang sinews

- 6 beans: yin sinews and luo

- Ying level is 9 beans of pressure: vessels

- 12 beans: flesh (embodiment of all the organs)

- Yuan level is 15 beans of pressure: bone

- Even deeper: marrow

Wei qi is reflected on the exterior portions of the pulse. At 3 beans of pressure one establishes connection to the yang sinew channels. At 6 beans of pressure one sees an adjustment between the wei and ying level. As such, 6 beans can reveal the presence of yin sinew meridian activity, or activity in the longitudinal luo (see Chapter 5 for criteria to determine if the 6 beans are reflecting luo vessel activity). Thus, 6 beans are still reflecting wei qi activity, but they are going inwards (or externalizing: see below for how to differentiate). The 6 beans are still technically the wei qi and floating level. The 9 beans of pressure are reflecting the ying level, 12 beans are where the ying and yuan are accommodating each other, and 15 beans are the yuan level.

In general, pulses that signify a sinew meridian problem are ones that are suggestive of stagnation and/or a pathogenic factor being retained on the exterior wei level. This will manifest with a Floating pulse (in this context, meaning the 3 or 6 beans of pressure[91]) combined with some other quality to suggest wei qi being held or in conflict with a pathogen. Some typical associations include:

Floating and Tight: wind-cold or taiyang pathogen.

Floating and Wiry: more severe restriction, where yang can't ascend. This tends to show up with pain and typically in the lower body and the yin sinew channels.

Floating and Rapid: wind-heat or yangming pathogen.

Floating and Slippery: wind-damp or shaoyang pathogen.

Basic sinew channel reflexology

The reflexology of the pulses for the sinew channel is different from the reflexology of the pulses for the primary channels that most practitioners are taught. Here, the leg sinew channels are found on the right-side pulses and the arm sinew channels are found on the left side. There are two different mappings, the use of which depends on whether or not the pathogen is internalizing from the wei level to the interior, or whether or not the pathogen is being externalized to the wei level.

When a pathogen is found on the exterior and is confronting the body and wei qi, one palpates the principal impulse more laterally. In this scenario, the taiyang Bladder sinew channel is found on the cun/distal position, the shaoyang Gall Bladder sinew channel on the guan/middle position, and the yangming Stomach sinew channel on the chi/proximal position. As one presses from 3 beans to 6 beans, one finds the associated leg yin sinew channel. Thus, the shaoyin Kidney sinew channel is found on the cun/distal position, the jueyin Liver sinew channel on the guan/middle position, and the taiyin Spleen sinew channel on the chi/proximal position.

The left-side pulses reflect the arm sinew channels as follows: the taiyang Small Intestine sinew channel is found on the cun/distal position, the shaoyang Triple Burner sinew channel on the guan/middle position, and the yangming Large Intestine sinew channel on the chi/proximal position. As one presses from 3 beans to 6 beans, one finds the associated arm yin sinew channel. Thus, the shaoyin Heart sinew channel is found on the cun/distal position, the jueyin Pericardium sinew channel on the guan/middle position, and the taiyin Lung sinew channel on the chi/proximal position.

When an interior pathogen is being released to the wei level, one palpates the principal impulse more medially. Here, the yin level at 6 beans is moving pathology to the wei level at 3 beans to be expelled from the body. In this scenario, on the right wrist at 6 beans one finds the jueyin Liver sinew channel in the cun/distal position, which reverts and communicates with the taiyang Bladder sinew at 3 beans. In the guan/middle position at 6 beans, the taiyin Spleen sinew communicates to the yangming Stomach sinew at 3 beans. In the chi/proximal position at 6 beans, the shaoyin Kidney sinew communicates with the shaoyang Gall Bladder sinew channel at 3 beans.

On the left wrist at 6 beans, one finds the jueyin Pericardium sinew channel in the cun/distal position, which reverts and communicates with the taiyang Small Intestine sinew at 3 beans. In the guan/middle position at 6 beans, the taiyin Lung sinew communicates to the yangming Large Intestine sinew at 3 beans. In the chi/proximal position at 6 beans, the shaoyin Heart sinew communicates with the shaoyang Triple Burner sinew channel at 3 beans.

These mappings are depicted below.

Pathology internalizing	Pathology externalizing
3 beans → 6 beans	6 beans → 3 beans
Taiyang → Shaoyin	Jueyin → Taiyang
Shaoyang → Jueyin	Taiyin → Yangming
Yangming → Taiyin	Shaoyin → Shaoyang

When an EPF enters, it generally confronts taiyang first due to its responsibility for defending the exterior and being the largest sinew channel, thus containing the most yang qi. If the wei qi is deficient/insufficient, it will then confront either the shaoyang or yangming. A Floating pulse in any of these positions is a sign that something on the wei level cannot be released. When Tight we are confronted by cold, but one should apply a broad understanding in that it can reflect other representations of cold, namely obstructed movement and pain. Thus, a Floating pulse can indicate tightness or tension in its respective areas, e.g., Floating and Tight at the left cun/distal reflecting the Small Intestine sinew channel with pain and tension around the scapula, cheek, etc.

If we understand that sinew channel pulses are assessing wei qi and its ability to perform its varied functions as discussed above, we can see that it requires that wei qi be unobstructed and its sources of nourishment be sufficient and communication open. Thus, in addition to evaluating the particular sinew channels and their six channel differentiations, we also want to assess (1) Kidney yang; (2) Stomach fluids; (3) patency/free flow of Liver qi; and (4) Lung qi diffusion (to make sure that wei qi can circulate to the exterior, release pathogens, and nourish the portals).

One method of determining the diffusion of Lung qi is to place all three fingers on the 9 beans of pressure and pump down on the chi position, pump down on the guan position, and lift up on the cun position to determine if something pushes your finger back up to the wei level. If so, the Lungs are diffusing wei qi appropriately.

Sinew pulses and the nervous system

Within the Shen-Hammer lineage, there are also pulses that help us to consider the impact of wei qi and the sinew channels. The depths of pressure found in the Shen-Hammer system are analogous to that of the Classical pulse, with the difference that in Shen-Hammer we orient the wrist with the radial bone and thumb upwards and the little finger and ulnar side resting down on the table. The proportions of the depths remain the same as in the Classical pulse, though due to the impact of gravity, the pressure required is slightly different, usually requiring finding the qi depth and utilizing a bit more pressure than finding the 6 beans. Figure 4.2 depicts the Shen-Hammer pulse depths.

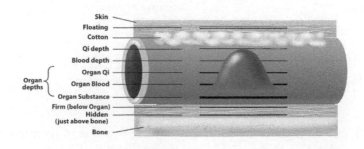

Figure 4.2: Shen-Hammer depths
Reproduced with permission from Eastland Press

Thus, the area from the skin to the qi depth is considered the "above qi depth" and in general (there are a number of exceptions) determines more superficial, wei level, and acute presentations. Then we find the qi depth (akin to the 6 beans), the blood depth (analogous to the 9 beans), and the organ depth (which reflects the "qi of organ depth" and is similar to the 12 beans), and find with a bit more pressure the "blood of organ depth" and "organ/substance of organ depth" (which corresponds to the 12–15 beans).

Findings on the above qi depth and the qi depth relate to issues of the nervous system. When one finds Tense or Tight (more severe) pulses uniformly at the qi depth or above, one can diagnose a "nervous system tense" condition. Where there is also weakness below, especially in the Kidneys (Deep, Reduced Substance, Feeble, Absent, or Empty pulses), it signifies a "nervous system weak" condition. Assessing the left distal position and the Heart as well as the left middle position and the Liver is also helpful in determining more complexity with these diagnoses. Should a Hesitant pulse wave also be present, it is further evidence of Heart and nervous system involvement.

From a Classical perspective, when the Tight pulses are uniform on all three positions (Long pulse) on the 3 beans of pressure, one can diagnose a Du mai pulse. When that pulse is also vibrating (Rough Vibration), it signifies current pathology in the Du mai from the Classical perspective. From the Shen-Hammer lineage, we would understand this to relate to shock and trauma and their impact on the nervous system. More information will be provided on this in the chapter on the 8 extraordinary meridians.

Sinew channel treatment

Treating Heart Shock with the sinew channels requires a multi-pronged approach which involves distinguishing root from branch, including the nature of the pathogen, its associated movement, knowledge of transmission, needling techniques, and sinew releases. Each of these topics is considered below.

Evaluating root and branch

Determining the root of a sinew channel problem relies on understanding its origination in terms of its climatic influence (e.g., wind, cold, damp, etc.) and how that manifests in its symptomatology, whether it be the nature of pain (e.g., sharp, stabbing, heavy, radiating, etc.), its restricted movement, and/or other external presentations. One must be clear to not mistake the branch (i.e., destination, ashi points, etc.) for the root cause, taking into consideration the solar as well as lunar cycles of wei qi, and a proper evaluation of the pulse.

Transmission and confluent points

Understanding root and branch relies on an awareness of how sinew channel issues progress and move to implicate additional sinew channels. The confluent points are important treatment areas to prevent such transmission as well as address symptoms in multiple channels. Often these confluent points can be reduced/dispersed to prevent pathogens from internalizing and spreading. This can be done via needling (described below) or even plum blossoming and/or gua sha. These points can also be tonified if there is underlying wei qi deficiency to bolster wei qi in the area to prevent the pathogen from progressing. The confluent points exist on the head (ST 8/GB 13) and face (SI 18/ST 3), as well as the chest (GB 22) and lower abdomen (Ren 3).

Needle technique

The needling technique for the sinew channels and to affect wei qi involves needle rotation/circular needling or the chiseling technique (particularly good for fatty tissues, nodules, gummy areas). With rotational needling one is circling the needle in a tornado-like fashion to create a spiraling of qi. When there is blockage or a pathogen to be released, one needles from small tight circles to larger broader ones to create a movement upwards and outwards as well as to create a sweat. When deficiency exists, the reverse is done to draw qi into the point. The needling speed is faster to release a pathogen, and slower to bring wei qi inwards.

The chiseling technique is where the needle is repeatedly re-angled into the ashi point superficially looking for release of the tissue/muscle layer. When releasing a pathogen, the jing-well point should be needling down the channel and towards the exterior. A fire needle is often used as well. When trying to tonify wei qi in the channel, it is needled upwards and moxa can be added. Needling is generally done shallowly and superficially to access the wei qi. If the patient is weak, supplemental needling can be done wherein multiple needles are placed in a point to reinforce it.

One can also use the round needle or do gua sha or cupping to release a pathogen to/from the surface. And moxa can and should be used if there is evidence of cold or damp or flaccidity.

The nature of the EPF helps determine the needling techniques used when pain or bi-syndrome is the main presentation. When wind is the major pathogenic factor with wandering bi (radiating pain), one needles from the destination of pain back to the origin with no needle retention. The needling technique is circular in order to lift the wind out. With damp fixed bi, one needles with indirect moxa on top of the needle. Cold painful bi is needled after causing friction in the area, followed by indirect moxa. With heat, one bleeds to bring out the heat and uses more needles in order to reduce. The jing-well points are used to finish the treatment.

Interconnected channels

Along with the sinew channels, additional channels can be added into a sinew treatment. Earlier I discussed the interrelationships between the wei level and the ying and yuan, as wei qi relies on both of these levels for its own functioning. To protect the ying level from pathogens moving internally, the luo meridian can be needled obliquely to promote movement outwards towards the wei. This is particularly helpful when the Lungs are unable to diffuse its qi to the exterior or there are other emotional causes at the root of the pathology (see the luo vessels chapter). It can also be needled transversely to put a pathogen into latency at the yuan level.

Wei also goes to the yuan via the divergent channels, which attempts to put the pathogen into latency, often in the joints and bony cavities. As many of the divergent meridian areas are located in proximity to sinew channel binding areas, they also utilize wei qi to maintain the latency along with yin. Once pathogens enter the yuan level, Kidney yin (yang retreats back to yin) becomes damaged, presenting symptoms such as steaming bone syndrome, lymphomas/leukemia, damage to the marrow, etc. Needling the divergent channels and releasing to the sinews is a common strategy which helps to bring out the acute process, the aggressive aspect of the unchecked heat that cannot be fully vented.

From the primary channel perspective, he-sea points affect the divergent channels and this layer because they regulate the bowels and wei qi controls the smooth muscles of the gut. Shu-stream points can also be needled as well if the patient is weak and/or vulnerable with insufficient qi on the wei level. As the shu-stream point energetically relates to where pathogens enter deeper in the primary channels, it should be needled distally towards the jing-well point. Xi-cleft points can also be helpful where the wei level begins to affect the ying level, creating qi and blood stagnation. Here we may see an inability to discern the nature of the pathogen (i.e., wind-cold, wind-heat) or what elicits the pain as blood stagnation is now more primary. Xi-cleft points are powerful analgesics and for this purpose should be needled using a dispersing technique. Additionally, points on the Lung and Liver channels can be added in to sinew channel treatments. From a primary channel perspective the Lungs deal with the amount of wei qi and the Liver deals with its movement (muscles, sinews).

Du mai can also be incorporated into a sinew channel treatment, especially when a nervous system tense condition is present or there are roots on the yuan level. It should be cautioned, however, that the yuan level should not be used simply to release an EPF. To do so would be to compromise the yuan-yang qi where there are other safer options as outlined above.

Sinew releases

Utilizing sinew releases is a powerful tool in the treatment of wei qi disorders. First, releasing any obstructions in the movement of wei qi at its source (yang and Du mai) is essential for freeing up the wei qi to expel pathogens trapped in the exterior.

Thus, one of the first steps in treating the sinew channels is to release yang and wei qi if there are any obstructions in the lower back (Du 4) and upper back (Du 14). Once wei qi is freed, there is more wei qi available for a successful sinew channel treatment.

The premise of how one releases the sinews is a bit different from other types of therapies that use bodywork and resistance. The idea of the sinew release is to mimic a complete state of tension (yang) in order to bring it into a state of relaxation (yin). Thus, to accomplish this, the practitioner will assist the person in consciously contracting the area to be released, which would presumably take one towards a future state of increased pathology or lack of movement, while the practitioner assists the patient in bringing it back to a state of full mobility. This is very different than physical therapy which attempts to force movement in the direction of increased mobility. With sinew releases, the patient attempts to move towards future pathology in order to get to the past with diminished pathology. Releasing areas of the body that involves the patient in exercises empowers them and brings consciousness to something they were previously unaware of.

This is done as follows.

Du 4 release

Diagnosing an obstruction in taiyang, shaoyang, or yangming:

Have the patient lie on their back, bending one leg with the sole of the foot placed on the table at the level of the other leg's knee, shoulder width apart.

Have the patient drop her bent knee outward laterally. If there are no restrictions, the patient's lateral leg should touch the table.

If she cannot, this suggests a taiyang obstruction.

Next have the patient drop her bent knee inwards towards her extended leg. No obstructions would allow her leg to touch the other thigh.

**If she cannot reach the straightened leg, this
would suggest a shaoyang obstruction.**

**If she cannot hold the leg in place at the extreme of her
movement, it suggests a yangming obstruction.**

To release the yang aspect:

Cradle the patient's leg/knee and instruct the patient to push against your resistance in the direction of increased restriction of movement (i.e., future). For example, if the patient shows a taiyang restriction and cannot drop her leg laterally onto the table, she should be trying to engage her adductor muscles to move her leg/thigh medially towards the other leg (i.e., worsening mobility). The patient's hands should be placed on her abdomen to prevent anchoring or compensation/cheating by using muscles in addition to the leg.

The practitioner should be providing resistance only to the patient's movement.

The patient is to use all of her force to push and, every few seconds, should be directed to move the leg a few inches in the opposite direction (the past) while still maintaining intention on pushing towards her other leg. The practitioner allows the movement back towards the table and very subtly back towards the original direction of the patient's force (the other leg), creating a slight rocking motion. This should be done repeatedly until the patient's leg reaches the table or there is no additional progress.

At the end of the release the patient should completely relax and let her leg go limp while the practitioner moves it back and forth throughout its full range of allowed movement.

The release should be performed in both directions and both sides to release any taiyang, shaoyang, and yangming restrictions bilaterally.

It should be noted that these releases ask the patient to utilize significant effort and can be difficult for them both physically and mentally. Often patients will experience an emotional release during the procedure or shortly afterwards.

After the release, the patient should be questioned on the location of any ashi points that were felt while doing the release. These are holding areas that should be needled and released with the next phase of the sinew channel acupuncture treatment.

Du 14 release

> With the patient lying on his back have him place one hand on his forehead and one hand cradling his occipital region.
>
> **The practitioner should hold the patient's elbow and hand on the forehead.**
>
> Making sure the patient's arm is horizontal, the practitioner should rock the neck/head back and forth to create relaxation of the cervical and Du 14 area. This rocking motion should be gently performed, and once it is felt that the patient is sufficiently relaxed for a while, abruptly turn the patient's head to its full range of motion. This should be repeated a few times on both sides.
>
> **Needle any ashi points on the neck and upper back after the release.**

Sinew releases can be performed on most muscle groups and should follow the basic tenet as set forth above: bring the patient to a state of complete tension moving towards the future, and gently guiding the patient towards the past. The releases above are tremendously useful in any sinew channel protocol, but are also profound in the treatment of Heart Shock and nervous system disorders. Freeing up yang qi in the Du mai (freeze response), and making that yang qi available to nourish the back-shu points (Triple Burner dissemination) as well as accommodate wei qi circulation (nervous system tension and armoring), satisfies a number of Heart Shock treatment strategies. And as sinew releases can be used on any muscle group, they will be particularly helpful for our purposes on the taiyang Bladder channel, which is directly implicated in the fight/flight/freeze responses detailed earlier. Below is a good release for the calf which is often tight in Heart Shock cases.

Taiyang Bladder channel sinew release for the calf muscle

> Have the patient lie on his back and bring his toes up as far as he can while stretching the gastrocnemius muscle to test his range of motion. Hold the patient's foot and have the patient push downwards as you eventually guide the toes up to a full range of motion of the calf muscle.
>
> Next, have the patient roll his toes outward towards the table and try to keep/move them towards the lateral table while you resist and guide them back medially to the center of the table.
>
> For both of these make sure to support/stabilize the knee so that there is no compensation with other muscles.
>
> Do this in both directions to get their toes to point up and inwards.

Qigong

Muscle/tendon-changing qigong is very consistent with the above, and instruction within this style would be a wonderful lifestyle practice to incorporate for patients. This also goes for marrow-washing qigong as a further development (and associated to the 8x meridians), and warranted to treat the yuan level. While this topic is vast and outside the scope of this text, further exploration is suggested.

Synopsis of sinew channel treatment

Proper treatment comes from evaluating the root sinew meridian implicated, which informs about the proper jing-well point that must be released. Knowledge of the nature of the pathogen informs us about the needling technique (e.g., a cold pathogen requires moxibustion and blowing on it to disperse the cold, a damp pathogen should be needled with moxa on the needle, and a heat pathogen can be reduced and bled or dispersed via gua sha). One must also be aware of and address any underlying deficiencies and/or stagnations (e.g., wei or yang qi, Lung and Kidney qi, Stomach fluids, Lung diffusion, Liver qi stagnation). Where more than one channel is implicated, the confluent points should be treated as well, and the most interior sinew channel is treated first as one works his way back to treat the more superficial channels. The channels should be palpated, areas of tension/tightness should be released, and areas of weakness/flaccidity should be tonified.

Sinew channel strategies

1. Evaluate root sinew meridian:
   a. Pulse diagnosis
   b. Movement diagnosis.
2. Diagnose nature of the pathogen (wind, cold, damp, etc.):
   a. Pulse diagnosis
   b. Symptoms and other signs.
3. Address underlying deficiencies.
4. Address blockages/stagnations.
5. Treat the most interior channel first and work backwards.
6. Release wei qi via sinew releases (Du 4 and Du 14).
7. Palpate areas of tension/tightness and release (acupuncture, moxa, tuina, gua sha (using blood to disperse wind), sinew releases to affected areas, etc.).
8. Palpate areas of weakness/flaccidity and tonify (acupuncture, moxa, etc.).
9. Address other relevant channel systems.

10. Needle jing-well point of root sinew meridian (e.g., Bladder 67 taiyang wind-cold, Gall Bladder 44 shaoyang wind-damp, Stomach 45 yangming wind-heat, etc.).

Additional concepts related to the sinew channels

PROGRESSION

Unresolved EPFs often lead to rebellious qi (e.g., coughing, nausea and vomiting, flatulence, borborygmus, etc.) as it moves to the yin level of the chest. As it moves into the yin level, it is presumed that the yang (head) is involved, too. To address this, one should palpate the head and release the affected zone (e.g., taiyang, shaoyang, yangming). Once in the chest, the pathogen has either entered shaoyang or yangming. It becomes important to needle Du 20 and SI 18, which assists in allowing for the exit of the pathogen.

THROAT

The throat is an important thoroughfare for the entry/exit of pathogens, even with ENT conditions. Use of the Window of the Sky (WOS) points, which impact the sensory orifices, becomes important. Choosing the proper WOS points is based on the related yang channels as below:

Wind-heat/yangming: ST 9, LI 18

Wind-cold/taiyang: BL 10, SI 16

Wind-damp/shaoyang: SJ 16, SI 17 (used to be Gall Bladder point)

TERRAIN

Chronic conditions typically have a wei qi deficiency and are also related to yangming as it provides the entryway to the interior domain. As such, releasing the sinuses is a common strategy employed when addressing an interior chronic problem. Wei qi homes to the chest (Heart and Pericardium) and expresses the self through the tongue and speech. Working on the throat assists in opening Ren 17 (below) and the sinus region (above). In chronic conditions, one might also need to release the major articulations such as BL 40, GB 29, LI 15, nape of the neck, the SCM area, diaphragm, and chest. As these areas release, one may experience a healing crisis as yang becomes aroused in the exterior. Symptoms such as sinus infections, conjunctivitis, skin outbreaks, upper respiratory conditions, etc. may present.

ADDITIONAL CORRESPONDENCES

Wind tends to manifest in the portals and sensory orifices, heat and chronic inflammation often implicate yangming and the throat, cold enters through the chest, and damp enters via the chest and head. Internally, wind manifests with signs of distension; dampness with fullness/heaviness; heat with pain and inflammation, shen disturbances, and signs of fluid depletion/discharge; and cold with severe pain and, when in the abdomen, accompanying constipation.

IMPORTANT ANATOMICAL AREAS

The SCM is the bridge between the cranial and thoracic cavities and helps mediate the internalization/externalization of wei qi. Many of the WOS points are located nearby as well, making it an area that impacts the portals. The abdominal rectus is the bridge between the thoracic and pelvic cavities on the anterior body, and the paravertebrals support the spine and the connection between the pelvis and abdominal rectus on the posterior. These, along with the diaphragm and the psoas muscle, become common holding areas for wei qi pathology and traumas. Interestingly, there are other disciplines using sinew release techniques for the psoas muscle to address the impact of trauma.[92]

SENSORY ORIFICES/PORTALS

The sensory orifices as mentioned earlier are a crucial component of the Heart Shock treatment strategies. Knowledge and understanding of these anatomical areas are important to obtaining a proper release. Below in table form are some of the major points that help to release the portals.

Eyes		
	BL 67	Pain/inflammation in the eyes (also opens up the sinuses)
	GB 44	Affects the eyes (pain, difficulty in focusing, constant blinking, visual dizziness)
	LI 1	Acute optic neuritis, blindness from inflammation, beginning stage of MS, optic neuritis from heat causing wei atrophy or acute sudden blindness
	PC 9 LR 1	Treat inflammation of the eyes, swollen eyes from heat pathogen, or facial edema from heat stagnation
Sinuses		
	BL 67	Clear watery discharge
	ST 45	Thick yellow nasal congestion
	LI 1	Nosebleeds from heat
	SI 1	Nosebleeds (also impacts the tongue)
	KI 1	Nosebleeds
	LU 11	Persistent nosebleeds

cont.

Ears		
	GB 44	Tinnitus, dampness blocking the ears causing loss of hearing, fluid in the ear
	LI 1	High-pitched ringing in the ears
Tongue		
	SI 1	Curled tongue; difficulty expressing self; can affect speech and throat (sore throat)
	SJ 1	Stiffness of the tongue, difficulty in articulating one's voice
	KI 1	Throat bi, pain, inability to use voice (Divergent meridian symptoms)
Head		
	BL 67	Occipital and vertex
	SI 1	Treats all headaches and more effective than Bladder 67 for occipital. Excellent for sinus headaches
	GB 44	One-sided headaches
	ST 45	Facial swellings, Bell's palsy, deviated mouth and eyes
	SJ 1	Sinus headaches
	KI 1	Headache with vertigo/dizziness upon standing
Restore yang	ST 45 HT 9 PC 9 LR 1 KI 1	Moxa on these points can resuscitate yang; bleed Liver 1 and Pericardium 9 to open the portals; can bleed, then moxa to open portals and return yang (e.g., stroke, hemiplegia)

Sinew channel treatments for Heart Shock

Each of the sinew channels has its role and importance in the potential treatment of Heart Shock depending on the patient's presentation. There are a multitude of potential applications; however, this discussion will focus on the ones most commonly seen within my practice and clinical experience. It should also be kept in mind that the ideas set forth below utilizing the sinew channels can also be further adapted and incorporated into treatments with other sinew channels as well as other channel systems. This can be done within any given treatment or staged over time in longer-term strategies.

Bladder sinew

The Bladder is the largest of the sinew channels and traverses through the muscle groups responsible for the fight/flight/freeze response. As a taiyang channel it is where yang is first mobilized into action. With trauma, this channel is triggered, and in those with a strong enough nervous system, the fight/flight/freeze muscles become activated and often remain hyperactive, creating a nervous system tense condition. Where the nervous system is inadequate, one can see the freeze response as yang qi becomes unable to rise to the occasion. This tension in the Bladder sinews creates pain and stiffness and lack of mobility (calf, hamstring, lower back, neck, occiput, etc.). Both of the above scenarios prevent the dissemination of yang qi via the Triple Burner, and this stagnant yang weakens the Kidneys over time. One common presentation of this is depression. This tends to be an endogenous-type depression as Dr. Hammer states in *Dragon Rises, Red Bird Flies* (DRRBF). And, as a mood disorder, patients are mostly unaware of its onset or reason and it seems as if a dark cloud follows them. The fear generated by the trauma, and responsible for the freezing of yang, creates an inability to emanate and move in the world, resulting in a sense of impotency. Releasing the wei qi stagnation from the Bladder sinew via ashi points, binding areas, and the jing-well is instrumental in managing and correcting this. Also warranted is to nourish back the Kidney yang with appropriate points as well as moxa. Gua sha as well as cupping should be performed if there is tension in the nervous system. This allows wei qi to disseminate, but also yang qi to anchor itself in the Kidneys. Freeing up this qi obstruction and nourishing back the Kidneys is instrumental in helping a patient move past traumas.

The Bladder sinew channel also expresses to the head, eyes, and nose. Nervous system tense disorders resulting from traumas typically have the impact of clouding the sensory orifices, creating either a lack of acuity, or a hyperactivity of wei qi. This is seen clearly with allergic rhinitis and the constant sinus irritation that results. Additionally, as we discussed in Chapter 1, the eyes are a major portal implicated in hypervigilance and the constant need to scan our environment and search out potential threats. Typically, there will be tension around the eyes, tearing and straining, irritation, etc. Releasing the Bladder sinew is a method for addressing these symptoms of hypervigilance.

Additionally, the Bladder sinew channel makes connections to the Heart via GB 22 as well as its internal pathway to the root of the tongue. GB 22 is a meeting point of the three yin of the arms (Heart, Pericardium, Lungs) and as such has a strong influence over the dynamics of the chest. It is also an opening point to the great luo of the Spleen (see Chapter 5), managing blood stasis that has entered into the chest, diaphragm, and, to some degree, systemically. As a luo point, it has an influence over one's psychological status and can quell heat from stagnation in the chest and Heart with such symptoms as anxiety, panic, insomnia, etc. In this case, it can be needled to release tension and knotting, as well as cupped, bled, or released via gua sha to engage blood in supporting wei qi. GB 22 has additional dynamics that make it important in Heart Shock, namely being a confluent point of the Heart divergent channel (more to be discussed on this in Chapter 7), which assists in bringing wei qi into the chest and, specifically, the Heart itself. The other confluent point of the

Heart divergent channel also lies on the Bladder sinew channel, namely BL 1. This creates a further relationship to the eyes, hypervigilance, distortion of perceptions, allergies based on wei qi hyperactivity (which the Heart divergent channel treats), etc. Combining Bladder sinew treatments with Heart divergent treatments is a common strategy I use in my clinic for the sequelae of Heart Shock.

Creating a relationship to the tongue is also instructive. While going to the root of the tongue (Kidney association) and not the tip (Heart association), the tongue as a whole is related to the Heart in its governance over speech and the ability to articulate in general. To speak from one's Heart, open the chest, and release pain, hurt, grief, etc. plays an important role in overcoming trauma. Utilizing the Bladder sinew to release stagnation in the chest (Heart) and its connection to the tongue (Heart and speech) assists in the transformation of traumatic experiences and allows healing to ensue.

Gall Bladder sinew

The Gall Bladder sinew covers some territory similar to the Bladder sinew in that it spreads across the GB 22 area and the chest as well as traversing to the eyes. In addition to the chest dynamics, however, the relationship of the eyes is slightly different as GB 1, while helping to open the portals, also allows for peripheral vision, hence the ability to see things from different angles. Using GB 1 can allow a patient to begin to view differing perspectives on their trauma and hence create a modified narrative. The Gall Bladder deals with decision-making and rotation. Here we are provided with the capacity to rotate our perspective and make new decisions. Healthy decision-making comes from an internal knowing of what is right and true for each of us as individuals. It is based on the clarity of our perceptions, on the pureness of our Heart, and the rooting of our Heart's communication with the Kidneys. GB 22 (and 34) create a dynamic to the chest and Heart, and the Gall Bladder sinew traverses and knots in the lower back connecting to Kidney energetics. The Gall Bladder sinew also traverses the ears, allowing for connection to a second portal (governed by the Kidneys) and for one to hear one's true voice. Releasing obstructions in these areas assists with opening the portals, proper perceptions, and the ability to see multiple points of view, change one's narrative, hear one's inner voice, and move past the trauma.

Stomach sinew

With the Stomach sinew we begin to see a pathogen transitioning to heat as it enters yangming. At this point, from a Heart Shock perspective, we can see patients exhibiting anxiety and manic behavior. Treating this with releasing the entryway to the interior, the throat, can be helpful in addressing this behavior. In addition, one can gua sha the area called the "ring around the collar" (this will be discussed more in Chapter 7), which includes such points as ST 9, ST 12, LI 15, GB 21, and Du 14.

This releases the heat back out to the exterior with the help of the interior/ying layer mobilizing blood to externalize the internalizing wei qi.

Other symptomatic manifestations of this attempted internalization of wei qi include the various possibilities of rebellious qi. As the Stomach sinew channel represents yangming and wind-heat symptomatology, it is instructive to note that the psychological presentation of wind-heat personality includes irritability and frustration and eventual manic behavior. Often patients who have experienced trauma are in a constant state of irritability and frustration as the nervous system maintains its hyervigilance and hypersensitivity from the heat which manifests as a result of the chronic stagnant qi. Eventually, this heat damages yin, creating more nervous system irritation which can also manifest internally with such symptoms as food allergies, a nervous stomach, and IBS-type presentations. Eventually, one might begin to see dysbiosis take place with candida, SIBO, etc. as internalized wei qi stagnation breeds heat, inflammation, and the response of distorted yin (dampness) to accommodate it. These are the branches one can see with a root of Heart Shock that has impacted the sinew channels and internalized via yangming to the gut.

As heat internalizes at the throat, attempting to gain access to the chest and abdomen, it is not uncommon to see inflammation and heat in the thyroid. Of course, the thyroid has a strong relationship to the Stomach channel as it traverses this area, and the thyroid regulates temperature dynamics and a host of other wei qi autonomic functions. Symptoms related to the hyperthyroid such as tachycardia, arrhythmias, irritability, etc. can be common with this presentation. Here we see the Stomach fire contributing to Heart fire and impacting the Emperor. Treating the Stomach sinew channel can rectify such problems without having to needle Heart channel points. Stomach sinew channel ashi points, binding areas, ST 9, and local points to the throat and chest can be used with ST 45 to release this presentation.

Like the two preceding channels, the Stomach sinew visits the portals, and in this case creates a connection to all of the sensory orifices (e.g., the eyes at ST 1 and BL 1, the ears with a branch from ST 5, the mouth at ST 4 and 5, and the sinuses at SI 18). With a further connection to the eyes, ears, and sinuses, now the Stomach reaches the mouth, a main portal for taking in that which is external to us and transforming it into something useful and nourishing. No longer is one simply being exposed to external stimuli, but here one has the opportunity to chew it, process and assimilate it, and decide to swallow it.

Connections are also made with the Stomach sinew channel to the lower back (GB 25, lumbar 2–4), lower abdomen (ST 30, Ren 4), and chest (pectoralis). This creates further dynamics to help in regulating the Kidneys (adrenaline surges and hyperactivity responses) and the Heart. Again, symptoms such as tachycardia, insomnia, anxiety, mania, etc. are very common with Heart Shock, and the Stomach sinew channel can play an important role in treating these dynamics.

Small Intestine sinew

The Small Intestine sinew channel as part of the taiyang is the first defense in regulating the musculature most directly associated with the fight/flight/freeze response. As part of the channel's armoring from nervous system tension, one typically sees a chronic neck and shoulder tension that is resistant to short-term treatments. When it has its root in Heart Shock, the nervous system tension becomes hard-wired as if the individual's new baseline is to maintain a hypervigilant stance in the world, requiring constant surveillance and readiness in one's muscles. Over time, these areas burn out, creating weakness and flaccidity, eventually impacting the shoulder. Treating the pain and tension or the weakness and atrophy of the shoulder requires the use of the Small Intestine sinew to open up areas of obstruction and allow wei qi to re-enter and strengthen the tissues. As one releases the shoulder and scapula area, a secondary impact is that it reduces tension in the Heart and calms the spirit. As mentioned earlier, the supraspinalis assists with opening of the ribcage and has an impact on the chest. Tension here creates heat, which can harass the spirit and create symptoms of Heart fire. Reciprocally, Heart fire can create tension in the shoulder blade, tighten these muscle groups, and create a forward jutting of the jaw and neck. This is a common stance, with hypervigilant patients post trauma always trying to have their heads precede their bodies in order to be on the lookout and spot danger. This constant worry can create tightness in these muscle groups, and releasing this sinew channel can relax the nervous system while simultaneously treating the Heart fire pattern.

Tightness in these muscles can also represent the repetitive thinking and recurrent narrative that takes place after trauma. Also commonly present in these circumstances is a Hesitant pulse wave. When the area has become fatigued and flaccid, often the impact on the mind is that one has difficulty learning and retaining information. It is not uncommon for patients with Heart Shock to be spacey and have difficulty processing (the Small Intestine is in charge of sorting and separating pure from turbid) and assimilating information. In my experience, a majority of the patients I have seen or have known to develop dementia and Alzheimer's had significant traumas in their past, and one impact of this was the loss of memory capacity and the proper sorting of information (blood stasis is another significant contributing factor).

Triple Burner sinew

The connections to the sensory orifices are furthered by the arm yang channels, the Triple Burner going to the eyes and ears and contributing to reducing inflammation and clearing the portals of consciousness. Additionally, this sinew channel, as a fire element, impacts temperature regulation and autonomic functions related to the thyroid gland. Hyperthyroid symptoms such as tachycardia, palpitations, insomnia, restlessness, etc. (Heart fire symptoms) can be addressed due to its connection to the Heart. It has a large impact on the throat as well as the tongue (the channel connects from ST 5 to the root of the tongue), enabling speech (often patients who have experienced traumas have a difficult time speaking up for themselves) and the articulation of one's voice and Heart.

Two additional areas in which the Triple Burner binds are commonly needled in my practice with Heart Shock patients: SJ 10 at the elbow I use often to relax the Heart and bring qi from the Triple Burner to anchor back to and pacify the shen; and GB 21 and GB 13 (ben shen) are powerful points for calming the spirit and relaxing the sinews.

Large Intestine sinew

The Large Intestine sinew channel also addresses the portals, communicating with the ears and nose. Its circulation on the deltoid muscle can be seen in this muscle's impact on the chest (chest hollowing from weak deltoids), asthma, and grief, sadness, and loss from traumas. Fidgety hands (a constant need to touch and receive stimulation) are part of this presentation as a yangming channel mediating heat in the nervous system (see also the following chapter on the luo vessels in which its metal pair, the Lung luo, has a similar presentation).

The Large Intestine sinew channel has the unique characteristic of creating polarity as it connects to Du 20 and the brain, then crosses over the midline to the opposite side of the face at ST 5. Another trajectory moves to the upper spine, creating further connection to the Du mai, the spine, brain, and nervous system functioning. As a yangming channel, releasing the Large Intestine sinew can clear heat from and prevent further pathology from entering the Du mai, brain, and nervous system.

Spleen sinew

The taiyin sinew channels represent the internalization of wei qi into the chest and abdomen. The Spleen has a major influence over the pelvis and adductor muscles and, as mentioned earlier, can be associated with pelvic floor obstructions like fibroids and cysts (wei qi stagnation), as well as hormonal dysregulation and flaccidity (wei qi deficiency). A common occurrence in patients who have been sexually molested or assaulted is a significant guarding of the abdomen and pelvis and contracted adductor muscles. The stagnation over time develops into toxic heat accumulations with obstructions in the reproductive organs as well as inflammatory conditions like pelvic inflammatory disease, herpes, HPV, prostatitis, infertility caused by blood, yin, and qi stagnation, etc. Deficiency manifests over time and can be a primary factor in infertility as well. The connection to the umbilicus further substantiates the relationship to the lower abdomen, but also to source qi.

As wei qi creates the smooth muscle contractions of the gut, and the Spleen has influence over the abdomen, the Spleen sinew can be used for poor motility (constipation) or hypermotility from nervous system inflammation and irritation causing frequent bowel movements. In the context of the Shen-Hammer lineage this constitutes the nervous system tense condition overacting on the digestive system. As it also circulates to the muscles of the intercostal spaces, the chest dynamic can be impacted, causing Heart symptoms such as palpitations, diaphragmatic spasms, and tachycardia. The channel binds at the area of GB 22, which is the original luo point for the great luo of the Spleen (see Chapter 5), and as such can be implicated in many of the psycho-emotional disturbances related to shock and trauma.

Lung sinew

The Lung sinew is most useful in Heart Shock in terms of its relationship to the chest. Trauma often causes stagnant wei qi throughout this entire area, including the intercostal muscles and diaphragm. Dr. Shen's Heart Closed pattern is a common scenario, as is finding a Diaphragm pulse, representing trapped qi in the diaphragm, with suppressed emotions, anger, shortness of breath, asthma, and insomnia as common symptoms.

The Lung sinew also has a role in circulation through the breast, and one can often find symptoms such as fibrocystic breasts as well as fibroid tumors, cysts, and even breast cancer develop from long-term stagnation here post trauma. With breast issues there are two signature pulses that I find. The first is in the Special Lung Position which is a branch off the radial artery, the superficial palmar artery (roughly found between LU 9 and PC 7). This pulse generally extends the length of the artery. When this pulse is Restricted (a quality wherein the sensation is cut off and only felt along a portion of the artery) it signifies an obstruction in the chest, usually due to some physical blockage such as a tumor. Typically, this pulse will also be Muffled (see Figure 4.3) and possibly also Choppy[93] (see Figure 4.4) or Rough.[94] When the left middle position reflecting the Liver is also Empty, I always correlate a breast pathology. And significant to the Liver findings is that often there is suppressed or repressed anger/frustration/irritability at the root of the pathology, often intertwined with grief and sadness. The Lung sinew can help rectify trapped wei qi throughout this area.

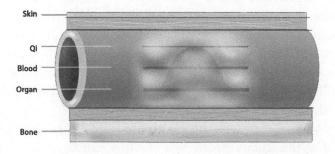

Figure 4.3: Muffled pulse
Reproduced with permission from Eastland Press

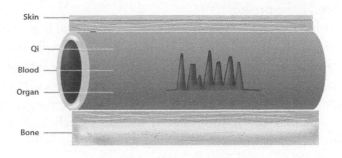

Figure 4.4: Choppy pulse
Reproduced with permission from Eastland Press

The relationship of the thenar eminence to the sacrum and lower back has been discussed earlier. By releasing obstructions along the Lung sinew, one can help establish the proper dynamic of Lungs descending to Kidney as well as the grasping of qi in order to root yang qi as well as address symptoms such as rapid breathing and hyperventilation which can be common with anxiety and nervousness post trauma.

Kidney sinew

The Kidneys and Heart share an intimate connection, both paired as shaoyin channels. Heart and Kidney communication and the fire–water balance is the fulcrum that all other systems rely upon for stability. The Kidney sinew channel relies on this relationship as it circulates wei qi along its pathway to the lower abdomen, lower back and spine, chest, and even the brain, solidifying its impact on the Heart, mind, and nervous system. As we discussed earlier, Heart Shock creates a destabilization systemically, one reason being that the Heart–Kidney axis becomes obstructed. Using the shaoyin sinew channels, one can restore communication.

Due to its connection to the spine, stagnation here can prevent yang from anchoring, creating symptoms of floating yang with wind such as seizures and epilepsy, convulsions, and occipital headaches. And, of course, whiplash, lower back pain from traumatic injuries, especially while the person is sitting and rotates, or while lying down and attempting to move, as well as any locations along the pathway (or implicated by movement diagnosis), can be addressed with the Kidney sinew channel.

As touched on earlier, the Kidneys have a role in circulating sexual fluids in the reproductive organs. Stagnation secondary to sexual abuse and traumas often impact this movement, resulting in vaginal dryness or irritation, pain with sexual activity, frigidity or lack of interest, and diminished libido. The Kidney sinew channel can play an important role in releasing this stagnation, assisting in restoring function back to the reproductive organs.

The Kidneys have a primary relationship to the emotion of fear, and this emotion can be displaced into the musculature post trauma, particularly the lower back, spine, pelvis, and psoas muscles. Sinew releases of Du 14 and 4 can be extremely effective in releasing the trapped wei qi and repressed fear, a necessary process to overcome one's trauma. Fear can create hypoactivity and paralysis from frozen yang. Hypersensitivity in the nervous system resulting from trauma is equally likely and creates excessive adrenal activity, wei qi hyperactivity, and allergic responses which are effectively addressed with the Kidney and Bladder sinew channels.

As the Kidneys have an impact on the back, spine, abdomen, and chest, this channel can be effectively utilized to treat postural imbalances, especially when grief or guilt weaken the qi of the chest and muscles of the upper back causing hollowness in the front, with a hunching forward, eventually resulting in hypothyroid conditions and the buffalo hump.

Heart sinew

The Heart sinew strengthens the communication of Heart and Kidney via its channel pathway. Following the trajectory of the Heart primary meridian, the sinew channel covers the same terrain, but additionally binds throughout the chest, breast, and muscles of the pectoralis and intercostals (binding at GB 22, the three arm sinew meeting point as well as a Heart divergent confluent point). As such, one of its main uses is for stuffiness/stickiness and oppression in the chest. This can manifest with shortness of breath, anxiety, insomnia, palpitations, claustrophobia, etc., all common in the sequelae of traumatic experiences. An associated finding with chest oppression is a Tense and Sticky[95] pulse in the left distal position. With a major impact on the circulation of wei qi throughout the chest, one often finds that the stress post trauma can create chest and breast symptoms, including mastitis and fibrocystic breasts (and eventual breast cancer from long-term heat creating toxic heat). Earlier, I described the pectoralis and brain connection with the Heart sinew channel symptomatology including poor concentration/spaciness when flaccid, and nervous system tension with anxiety (heat that develops from stagnation) when tight. The pectoralis attaches to the sternum and with prolonged stress Ren 15 can present with exquisite tenderness after traumas. As the heat from stagnation at Ren 15 is directly above the stomach, nervous system tension and worry can create inflammation in the gut with canker sores, reflux, esophagitis, belching, and other signs of Stomach fire.

A unique feature of the Heart sinew channel is that it binds down the midline of the abdomen (covering the Ren mai and Kidney channel) and directly connects and binds to the umbilicus, creating a strong connection to yuan qi. As Heart and Kidney communication is a primary disconnect with Heart Shock, the Heart sinew can release obstructions preventing proper communication and allowing rooting of yang qi in the lower dantian. Symptoms such as anxiety and panic disorder (running piglet qi), tachycardia, arrhythmias, fibrillations, etc. can be effectively treated with this sinew channel.

When treating the Heart sinew channel, typically the chest is extremely knotted when symptoms such as the above are present. Palpating the intercostal spaces should be done with a side-to-side pressure as the Heart sinew manages rotational movements. Needling is typically done on a horizontal lateral-medial plane between the rib spaces, and caution should be used with the depth of needling. As we are addressing wei qi and the sinews, typically needling can be rather superficial. Due to the large territory this channel covers on the chest and breast, multiple needles may be necessary to release enough of the restrictions to be successful. Typically, I find the most sensitivity around the areas that would correlate with the Kidney, Spleen, and Stomach primary trajectories, along with the area of GB 22. If there are restrictions on the Kidney channel of the chest and abdomen, palpating the lower trajectory should also be included, and if knots and tenderness are found, KI 1 should be added to the treatment.

Because of the direct connections of GB 22 to the Heart sinew as well as divergent channel, the Heart divergent channel can be, and is often, included in a broader treatment plan. BL 1 is the upper confluent point of the Heart divergent channel (which plays a major role in allergies) ,and combining this with the Bladder sinew is extremely effective for treating allergic responses from hypersensitivity of wei qi. Combining the taiyang–shaoyin relationship, the Kidney sinew can be needled as well.

One of the findings I commonly discover with Heart Shock is a Knotted or Spinning Bean pulse in the left distal position. Always reflective of significant stagnation, a Knotted/Bean pulse that presents in the more superficial aspects of the left distal position (especially within the 3–9 beans) warrants the use of the Heart sinew channel. Often a treatment (or short series of a few treatments) will completely eliminate this finding and the associated restriction of wei qi within the chest.

Pericardium sinew

The Pericardium sinew channel, like the Lung, Large Intestine, and Heart sinew, has a major impact on the circulation of wei qi in the chest and can be used to treat all the chest and breast symptoms mentioned above. As the Heart Protector, and a jueyin channel, it assists in mediating the relationship between the Liver and Heart (and hence, diaphragm), and qi's role in blood circulation. It is particularly helpful when traumatic experiences cause a closing of the Heart as a protective measure to insulate one from emotional pain. Like the Heart sinew, the Pericardium also binds in the axillary region and maintains some role in lymph congestion in this area (lymph circulation also homes to the chest and thoracic duct). Thus, stickiness and oppression in the chest, along with anxiety, panic, rapid heartbeat, arrhythmias, etc., can be treated effectively with the Pericardium sinew.

As it relates to the Heart sinew, and the mind and nervous system, often the Pericardium sinew can present with a chronic stiff neck. This symptom reflects the attempt to block heat and wind from chronic nervous system tension reaching to the brain, which would result in seizures, epilepsy, stroke, etc. It is an ecological response and an adaptive measure.

It should be noted that many believe the jing-well point of the Pericardium to be the tip of the middle finger, not the 0.1 cun proximal to the corner of the nail. In my experience, I have needled both depending on the sensitivity of the patient (tip of finger being much more sensitive for most) with equal results.

Liver sinew

The Liver sinew's influence only extends as high as the lower abdomen and the sexual organs, but in this regard can have a major impact over traumas of a sexual nature and betrayals of intimacy. The Liver's role over wei qi is responsible for the release of sexual fluids, and traumas to this region can prevent the ability to relax during sexual activity (often with pain and discomfort) and not being able to reach orgasm. Additionally, as qi is responsible for moving the fluids, often the Liver channel is utilized where stagnant fluids have created cysts, HPV, damp-heat in the Bladder, etc. Another common and related Classical diagnosis is cold invading the Liver channel; this can result in pain, discomfort, cramping, frigidity, etc. When needling the Liver channel for pelvic symptoms, after releasing knots and ashi points along the channel of the leg, one can needle tender ashi and tight points on the lower abdomen obliquely towards the pubic bone, manipulating the needle to achieve a sensation traveling to the reproductive organs.

Additional treatments with the sinew channels

In addition to the specific characteristics of how each of the above channels relate to treating Heart Shock, many of the channels can be combined or used to treat specific concepts within a Heart Shock framework. For example, some of our strategies within the sinew channels that relate to Heart Shock include nervous system tension, pain, opening the portals, etc. Below is a short list in table form reviewing which point categories and sinew channels are most commonly utilized for some of these topics.

Topic	Categories/Channels	Comments
Phlegm misting the orifices	Window of the Sky points	Each of these points have a powerful impact on the sensory orifices
	Confluent points	SI 18: all orifices of the face ST 8/GB 13: connects to Du mai and brain
	Jing-well points	Releases portal of associated channels

Pain	All sinew channels depending on location treat pain within its own trajectory	All pain can impact the Heart and spirit, and the Heart channel can always be utilized in conjunction with other channels
Nervous system tense	Tension in the nervous system can be directly treated with multiple sinew channels and can correspond to tension along the channel trajectory. Can also relate to specific energetic concepts. For example:	
	• Fight/flight/freeze response	Bladder/Small Intestine (taiyang)
	• Eyes	Gall Bladder shaoyang for peripheral vision and ability to see options; Stomach and Large Intestine for heat and inflammation; Bladder for relationship to light and wei qi activation, taiyang, and tearing/wind sensitivity
	• Throat	Stomach, Triple Burner, Small Intestine
	• Chest	Large Intestine, Lung, Heart, Pericardium, Stomach, Spleen, Kidney
	• Nervous system tense overacting on digestive system	Spleen, Stomach
	• Nervous system impacting circulatory system and reproductive functioning	Liver, Kidney
	• Brain	3 yang leg channels, Large Intestine
	• Jaw	All yang channels
Insomnia	Wei qi internalizing: yangming and taiyin communication Nervous system tense: relaxing sinews as above Chest stagnation: Lung, Large Intestine, Pericardium, Heart Abdominal stagnation: Spleen, Stomach	Area of the jaw (grinding, clenching signs of wei qi trapped): SI 18, ST 5, ST 9
Anxiety	Hyperactivity of nervous system: as above Chest stagnation: Large Intestine, Lung, Heart, Pericardium Running piglet qi: Heart and Kidney sinew channel	
Depression	Bladder, Kidney: endogenous type Heart/Pericardium: betrayal, cyclothymic Large Intestine, Lung: traumatic loss, grief	
Anniversaries	Lunar cycle	

cont.

Topic	Categories/Channels	Comments
Dreams/ Nightmares	Taiyin (Lung/Spleen)	First returns back here as the breathing gets deeper and relaxes: "relaxation/concentration"
		Time to reflect on yourself, your life. Need to let go of the day, e.g., turn off TV, emails
	Shaoyin (Heart/Kidney)	Communication with above/below; opening access with Heart/Kidney
		Sinew wraps the chest and draws down to the Kidney. The Kidney connects with the sternum
		When person begins to fall asleep, so nightmares come here and person wakes up; lucid dreaming also occurs here
	Jueyin (Pericardium/Liver)	Body releases unresolved issues: comes in images. The body is trying to release to the Pericardium
		Body attempts to help person to find resolution, so there is an opportunity here to do so
		Liver: Where your dreams are prophesies—Hun and Liver projects out. Time is already written, future is there, and you only have to pick up on it (vibrations) to see the future
		Deep relaxation occurs if you have no issues to resolve

Treatment and clinical management

As the sinew meridians and wei level are unconscious, the more treatments a patient receives, the greater the impact. After treatments, as wei qi has been aroused, some patients may experience adverse reactions such as dizziness (wei qi is coming up), insomnia (wei qi not entering the chest), flushing, sweating, tremors/spasms, etc. These are expected effects and not considered pathological as they represent wei qi's adjustments to the treatment. As wei qi homes to the chest, we must assist with its movement internally for these symptoms to subside. One can teach patients how to massage certain acupuncture points to encourage this internalization of wei qi back into the chest. Points such as PC 6 and 7 can be effective in buffering the treatment if patients experience symptoms post treatment.

Sinew meridian formulas: Releasing the exterior, calming the nervous system, treating pain

Herbal strategies

Herbal strategies utilizing the energetics of the sinew channels rely on the activation of wei qi. To impact wei qi, one looks to herbs that are spicy and aromatic, that release the exterior, as well as having affinities to the Lungs and Liver, the two zang fu with a wei qi association. As wei qi is warming, initially herbs with a warming–hot nature are preferred. As a pathogen moves inward, heat is produced as the pathogen becomes embroiled with wei qi in the interior and as yang qi mobilizes to defend its terrain. In that case, herbs that are cooling can be used; however, aromatic herbs are still prioritized. As the heat progresses it can begin to tax and deplete the wei qi and eventually qi and yang of the body. Typically, a pre-existing wei qi deficiency is present to allow the pathogen to internalize, the heat being created further weakening it, requiring the inclusion of qi tonics in the formula.

From this general perspective and understanding of wei qi, strong heat-clearing herbs (e.g., Yin Qiao San) should not be commonly utilized and they can damage the body's innate ability to defend itself. If cold herbs are to be used, aromatic ones are chosen such as Shi Gao (Gypsum) and other warming herbs are combined into the formula. Not so dissimilar from antibiotics, they can create cold and damp in the interior, leading to further stagnation, qi deficiency, and eventual dysbiosis as long-term stagnation breeds damp-heat.

Zonal herbs

Herbs that resonate with the zonal areas of the body should be utilized when trying to focus the impact of a formula. The zonal herbs and their correspondences are as follows:

Taiyang: For the taiyang, Gui Zhi, Wei Ling Xian, Qiang Huo, and Ma Huang are the most relevant, though Ma Huang is less frequently used nowadays.

Gui Zhi: sweet, warm, acrid; Lung/Bladder/Heart affinities.

Wei Ling Xian: salty, warm, acrid; Bladder affinity.

Qiang Huo: bitter, acrid, warm, aromatic; Kidney/Bladder affinities.

Ma Huang: warm, acrid, slightly bitter; Lung/Bladder affinities.

Shaoyang: For the shaoyang, Qin Jiao, Fang Feng, and Chuan Xiong are most commonly used. As temperature can swing in either direction with shaoyang pathologies, having herbs that are slightly cooling or warming to neutral is most helpful.

Qin Jiao: bitter, acrid, slightly cold; Liver/Gall Bladder/Stomach affinities.

Fang Feng: slightly warm, sweet, acrid; Bladder/Liver/Spleen affinities.

Chuan Xiong: acrid, warm; Pericardium/Liver/Gall Bladder affinities.

Yangming: For yangming, Bai Zhi is the most important zonal herb. The heat here is not pathological. It is generated to prevent the pathogen from going to the interior, into the organ system (starts at yangming pair). If it goes to the LI then we follow the movement, try to cool it off, and get it out of the body.

Bai Zhi: acrid, warm; Lung/Stomach affinities.

Taiyin: For taiyin, the representative herb is Hou Po, though Cang Zhu and Huo Xiang can also be used.

Hou Po: bitter, spicy, warm; Lung/Large Intestine/Spleen/Stomach affinities. (Stimulates yang qi to exteriorize wei qi to surface.)

Cang Zhu: bitter, acrid, warm, aromatic; Spleen/Stomach affinities.

Huo Xiang: slightly warm, acrid; Spleen/Stomach/Lung affinities.

Shaoyin: The shaoyin representative herb is Rou Gui.

Rou Gui: sweet, hot, acrid; Liver/Spleen/Kidney/Heart affinities.

Jueyin: Jueyin's representative herb is Wu Zhu Yu (often used with Huang Lian to balance temperature).

Wu Zhu Yu: bitter, acrid, hot, slightly toxic; Liver/Kidney/Spleen/Stomach affinities.

Additionally, as a strategy utilizing the sinew channels, it is recommended to choose herbs that support wei qi with yang qi. These include:

Du Huo: bitter, acrid, warm; Kidney/Bladder affinities.

Qiang Huo: bitter, acrid, warm, aromatic; Kidney/Bladder affinities.

With chronicity, yang will affect its yin pair, and may go internally and affect the blood. Bitter herbs are needed to clear the blood level. Once in the blood level, one may have intermittent symptoms as the blood holds on to the pathology (yin stagnating either blood or phlegm). (If there is a phlegm complication then one should treat the sacrum or thenar eminence with bleeding or cupping as mentioned earlier in the Lung sinew discussion.) Once the pathogen moves towards the chest, yin begins to bind the qi and one sees the signs of phlegm and/or blood stasis. Herbs that are effective in treating wei qi stagnation in the chest mixed with damp and phlegm include Gua Lou Ren/Gua Lou Pi (very commonly used in Shen-Hammer formulas for Heart Shock) and Tian Hua Fen. To regulate wei qi in the chest, especially with Liver and Lung affinities, Chai Hu, Qing Pi, and Chen Pi can be utilized. Where blood and phlegm are both stagnating, Si Gua Lou is an effective herb (also commonly used in Dr. Shen's formulas).

Sinew channel herbal protocol

1. Identify affected zone/sinew channel, e.g., yangming, shaoyang, taiyang, etc.

2. Severity:
   a. A more severe diagnosis warrants an increase in the herbal formula dosing. For example, 30g of Gui Zhi can be decocted and boiled down to 3 cups of liquid to be drunk every three hours for tightness in the occiput and paravertebrals.

3. Chronic issues:
   a. Support wei qi with yang qi, e.g., Qiang Huo/Du Huo.
   b. If the chronic issue impacts the blood or phlegm, the use of Gua Lou/Tian Hua Fen and/or Si Gua Lou is warranted.
   c. If yangming is the prevailing issue and is a chronic problem, one has to protect its elemental pair, taiyin (Lung/Spleen). To do so, the use of spicy bitter herbs to exteriorize the pathogen is warranted.
      i. Hou Po treats the Lung/Large Intestine/Spleen/Stomach.
      ii. Cang Zhu treats the Spleen/Stomach only.
      iii. Huo Xiang treats the Lungs and Spleen/Stomach where the patient feels achy, heavy, sluggish, etc.

4. When the root is Heart Shock, add appropriate herbs to satisfy other treatment strategies from Part I.

Treatment example

A patient comes in with a chief complaint of chronic lower back pain that resulted from a traumatic injury. From the movement diagnosis, there is pain when walking, signifying a Bladder sinew channel problem. The nature of the pain is tight, worse with cold, and radiating from BL 25–40, confirming a taiyang (wind and cold) pathogen. Palpating the sinew channels reveals dryness along the trajectory and flaccidity suggesting a movement towards deficiency, e.g., Kidney yang and/or Stomach yin. To treat, the focus is on creating resonance to the taiyang zone and Bladder sinew channel with warming and aromatic herbs due to the cold pathogen, e.g., Gui Zhi and/or Wei Ling Xian. Next, addressing the location of radiation, one can choose herbs that have an association with the legs, e.g., Che Qian Zi and/or Niu Xi. The deficiency present (dryness and flaccidity) warrants utilizing herbs to address yang qi and its support of wei qi, e.g., Du Huo and Qiang Huo, as well as Stomach yin and muscle tone, e.g., Xi Yang Shen, Shi Hu, Tian Men Dong, Mai Men Dong, or Sha Shen. If any discoloration exists or the pain is intermittent, one can add Mu Dan Pi, which also has a descending action. A representative formula would consist of:

Gui Zhi
Wei Ling Xian
Chuan Niu Xi
Du Huo
Qiang Huo
Xi Yang Shen
Mai Men Dong
Mu Dan Pi
Zhi Gan Cao

The last focus is to accommodate any of the diagnoses present from our Heart Shock strategies. Thus, we must assess Heart yin deficiency, Heart qi deficiency, blood stagnation, Kidney yang deficiency, nervous system tension, stagnation in the chest, opening the portals, and strengthening the Spleen/Stomach if any such diagnoses exist. The above herbs already accommodate some of these potential diagnoses. Xi Yang Shen and Mai Men Dong strongly nourish Heart yin and make up two of the most commonly used herbs in Shen-Hammer formulas for Heart Shock. Gui Zhi strengthens Heart qi and promotes circulation in the chest. Du Huo activates and stimulates Kidney yang via its connection to Du mai. Qiang Huo helps to open the chest as it wraps from the Bladder channel to the front of the body and opens the taiyang and Du mai (having some capacity to open the portals). Mu Dan Pi assists in moving the blood. These last few herbs open the spine, regulate the Bladder sinew, and relax the Liver, accomplishing the function of calming the nervous system. Xi Yang Shen and Mai Men Dong strengthen the Stomach, and Mai Men Dong also clears any heat irritating the Heart and shen. If necessary, an additional herb to open the portals can be added. With the addition of Zhi Gan Cao, one further strengthens the earth as well as nourishes Heart qi, strengthening the formula's ability to move qi and blood without compromising the Heart, and calms the spirit. Dosing should be consistent with which particular aspects of the diagnoses one wants to highlight.

Gui Zhi Tang (Cinnamon Twig Decoction)

Gui Zhi	9g
Bai Shao	9g
Sheng Jiang	9g
Da Zao	4pcs
Zhi Gan Cao	6g

Gui Zhi Tang is perhaps one of the most famous Classical formulas for the exterior, and no discussion of wei qi and the sinew channels would be complete without at least mentioning it. The formula represents a beautiful adjustment to the dynamics of wei qi, and its production and relationship with ying qi. The formula is most often used with a wei qi deficiency where stronger medicinals would create further taxation. Thus, Gui Zhi, a taiyang zone herb, is being used to warm the channels and disperse cold, Sheng Jiang and Bai Shao for adjusting ying and wei, and Da Zao and Zhi Gan Cao for strengthening the middle, nourishing blood, and harmonizing. As Bai Shao strengthens Stomach yin, and Stomach yin is the main post-natal mechanism for producing wei qi, Bai Shao's presence serves two functions: producing enough yin-fluids to boost wei qi as well as to create enough sweat to thrust out the pathogen.

As a Heart Shock formula, Gui Zhi Tang should be modified to accommodate other strategies. It is not uncommon for a Heart Shock patient, while in the midst of treatment, to be struck with a wind-cold invasion requiring treatment to prevent internalization of the pathogen and further taxation to the system. Simple modifications of the formula can allow for tailoring of Gui Zhi Tang to make it appropriate without compromising the other treatment strategies. For example, one can strengthen the Heart yin component (Bai Shao already nourishes the yin to some degree) with the addition of Xi Yang Shen or Mai Men Dong; Heart and Kidney qi can be further nourished (Gui Zhi already strengthens Heart qi) with Ren Shen, Rou Gui, or Fu Zi; the chest can be further opened (Gui Zhi opens circulation in the chest) with Qiang Huo, which will also further strengthen the taiyang release and relax the nervous system; blood can be moved more strongly (Gui Zhi promotes circulation) with the addition of Rou Gui as above; and the portals can be impacted with Xi Xin and Yuan Zhi (which will also calm the shen). Thus, the new formula can address the taiyang wind-cold invasion, protect the interior, nourish the earth, and address the Heart Shock strategies simultaneously. Once the wind-cold invasion is resolved, a more specific Heart Shock formula can be utilized.

Gui Zhi Tang Modified (Modified Cinnamon Twig Decoction)

Gui Zhi	9g
Bai Shao	9g
Sheng Jiang	9g
Da Zao	4pcs
Zhi Gan Cao	6g
Rou Gui	9g
Ren Shen or Xi Yang Shen	9g
Fu Zi	9g
Qiang Huo	6g
Xi Xin	3g
Yuan Zhi	6g

Xiao Chai Hu Tang (Minor Bupleurum Decoction)

Chai Hu	24g
Huang Qin	9g
Ban Xia	24g
Sheng Jiang	9g
Ren Shen	9g
Zhi Gan Cao	9g
Da Zao	12pcs

Xiao Chai Hu Tang treats the shaoyang level with alternating fever and chills, bitter (or sour) taste, hypochondriac pain, fullness in chest, dizziness, nausea, etc. While an extremely versatile formula, its best use as a Heart Shock treatment comes with modifications, one famous formula being Chai Hu Jia Long Gu Mu Li Tang, below.

Chai Hu Jia Long Gu Mu Li Tang (Bupleurum plus Dragon Bone and Oyster Shell Decoction)

Chai Hu	12g
Huang Qin	4.5g
Gui Zhi	4.5g
Da Huang	6g
Long Gu	4.5g
Mu Li	4.5g
Qian Dan (or Dai Zhe Shi/ Hu Po, etc.)	4.5g
Ren Shen	4.5g
Fu Ling	4.5g
Ban Xia	6g
Sheng Jiang	4.5g
Da Zao	6pcs

A variation of Xiao Chai Hu Tang, Chai Hu Jia Long Gu Mu Li Tang is used for a pathogen in all three yang stages with fullness in the chest, irritability, palpitations, heaviness in the body, irregular heartbeat, etc. With the additions of Long Gu, Mu Li, and Dai Zhe Shi, this formula is more suitable in Heart Shock with significant disturbance to the shen, and heat signs, especially with the inclusion of Da Huang. Da Huang assists with moving the blood, which will be assisted by Gui Zhi, and Chai Hu's rectification of qi in the chest, diaphragm, and hypochondria. Should Hu Po be used over Dai Zhe Shi, this will increase the blood invigoration aspect, so as to further calm and settle the shen, treating palpitations and an irregular heartbeat.

Heart yin should be protected with Xi Yang Shen, with Ren Shen retained as it will strengthen and protect the Kidney yang. The earth is protected with Ren Shen, Fu Ling, Sheng Jiang, and Da Zao, and Ban Xia will treat phlegm, and hence the clouding of the spirit. The nervous system is relaxed with Chai Hu, Da Huang, Long Gu, and Mu Li.

Shao Yao Gan Cao Tang (Peony and Licorice Decoction)

Bai Shao	12g
Zhi Gan Cao	12g

While not a Heart Shock formula, Shao Yao Gan Cao Tang can become a foundation for formulas that can impact and relax the nervous system. It treats irritability, spasms, abdominal pain, etc. and can be modified to further include the Heart Shock strategies easily on a case-by-case basis.

E Jiao Ji Zi Huang Tang (Ass Hide Gelatin and Egg Yolk Decoction)

E Jiao	6g
Ji Zi Huang	2 yolks
Sheng Di Huang	12g
Bai Shao	9g
Zhi Gan Cao	1.8g
Gou Teng	6g
Shi Jue Ming	15g
Mu Li	12g
Fu Shen	12g
Luo Shi Teng	9g

E Jiao Ji Zi Huang Tang utilizes the Bai Shao/Zhi Gan Cao combination as mentioned above. Best for a chronic condition where yin has been compromised from long-term nervous system tension and heat, this formula strongly calms the sinews and nervous system (and wind) with Bai Shao, Gou Teng, Shi Jue Ming, Mu Li, Fu Shen, and Luo Shi Teng. It nourishes Heart yin (E Jiao, Ji Zi Huang, Sheng Di Huang), anchors to the Kidneys (Sheng Di Huang, Shi Jue Ming, Mu Li, Fu Shen), calms the shen (Sheng Di Huang, Mu Li, Fu Shen), treats bi-syndrome and unblocks the collaterals (Luo Shi Teng), opens the portals (Shi Jue Ming), and protects the earth (Fu Shen).

Dr. Shen's formulas

Dr. Shen's nervous system tense formula

Chuan Xiong	Rz. Ligustici Chuanxiong	5g
Yu Jin	Rx. Curcumae	6g
Lu Lu Tong	Fr. Liquidambaris	12g
Jing Jie	Hb. Schizonepetae	12g
Bai Shao	Rx. Paeoniae Alba	6g
Yin Chai Hu	Rx. Stellariae Dichotomae	3g
Xiang Fu	Rz. Cyperi	2g
Yan Hu Suo	Rz. Corydalis	10g
Huang Qin	Rz. Scutellariae	2g

Dr. Shen's nervous system tense formula, while not treating Heart Shock per se, can be very useful in treating the tension, hypervigilance, and armoring that is seen with trauma. This formula is primarily focused on relaxing the Liver, from a zang fu perspective, moving qi and blood, and regulating the sinews. The Liver lies between the shaoyin and the taiyang from a Five Elemental perspective as a wood element and mediates between water and fire. This formula releases the stagnation at the level of the Liver and nervous system to allow for proper communication between the Heart and Kidneys. Chuan Xiong and Yu Jin move qi and blood (Lung's relationship). Lu Lu Tong opens the diaphragm and blockages between the upper, middle, and lower jiaos to ensure proper communication. Xiang Fu strengthens the movement and communication between the three burners and regulates Liver qi. Jing Jie as a surface medicinal opens the orifices and the pores and releases the skin and muscle layer. It helps to prevent the vulnerability to, and contraction of, additional external influences as one is relaxing the exterior terrain. Bai Shao helps to nourish the blood and soften the Liver to regulate qi, and Huang Qin clears any residual heat created by the stagnation. Yin Chai Hu assists with clearing heat that may have damaged the yin, and Bai Shao helps to nourish it back and soften the sinews. Yu Jin also serves to open the portals of consciousness, while Xiang Fu and Bai Shao help to regulate mood.

Dr. Shen's alternate nervous system tense formula

Shi Chang Pu	2.4g	Heart nerves
Chuan Xiong	4.5g	Relax nerves
Jing Jie	3g	Relax skin nerves

Bai Shao	6g	Relax "inside" nerves
Xiang Fu	4.5g	Relax organ nerves
Ge Gen	4.5g	Relax muscle nerves
Yu Jin	6g	Relax organ nerves
Gua Lou Pi	9g	Relax organ nerves

Over time, Dr. Shen modified or created alternate formulas based on the systems theory concepts. The alternate nervous system tense formula above demonstrates a few important concepts. The first is Dr. Shen's associations of herbs with the nerves, and specifically which class of nerves each herb impacts (see the formula above). Shi Chang Pu relaxes the Heart nerves, Chuan Xiong the nerves in general, Jing Jie the skin nerves, Bai Shao relaxes the "inside" nerves, Xiang Fu, Yu Jin, and Gua Lou Pi the organ nerves, and Ge Gen relaxes the muscle nerves. Potentially, Dr. Shen may have conceived this formula for someone with nervous system tension that has begun to impact the nerves in the yin sinews as well with the "pathogen" having entered the interior. Also notable is the addition of Shi Chang Pu, which strengthens the impact of Yu Jin on opening the portals and can be used where there are additional distortions to one's perceptions after trauma. Lastly, this alternate formula demonstrates a stronger influence over the dynamics of the chest (which becomes impacted as the pathogen moves to the interior), in particular phlegm and stickiness/heaviness in the chest, with the inclusion of Gua Lou Pi. Ge Gen and Bai Shao may also treat the dryness and flaccidity that can result from long-term stagnation impacting the muscles and sinews.

Dr. Shen's circulatory system formula

Qiang Huo	Rz. Se Rx. Notopterygii	6g
Si Gua Luo	Fasc. Fasc. Luffae	6g
Dan Shen	Rx. Salvae Miltiorrhizae	6g
Sang Ji Sheng	Ram. Sangjisheng	12g
Yuan Zhi	Rx. Polygalae Tenuifoliae	6g
Da Zao	Fr. Ziziphi Jujubae	10g
Dang Gui	Rx. Angelicae Sinensis	6g
Mu Gua	Fr. Chaenomelis	12g
Fang Feng	Rx. Ledbouriellae Divaricate	6g

Dr. Shen associated the circulatory system with shaoyang energetics. The focus with this formula is to unblock stagnation in the channels and the chest in order to restore Heart and circulatory function. One of the first things to notice with the above formula is the inclusion of two of the zonal herbs from the wai ke/external medicine tradition, Qiang Huo (taiyang) and Fang Feng (shaoyang), which comprise the major focus on the sinews. Second is the use of herbs to address phlegm in the chest and to open the orifices (Yuan Zhi and Si Gua Lou). Si Gua Lou and Dan Shen also open the chest, as does Qiang Huo, which is related to Du mai and the taiyang channels. Thus, it has a strong influence over the upper back and is said to wrap around the front of the body as well to the area of Ren 17–15. Si Gua Luo, Sang Ji Sheng, Mu Gua, and Fang Feng deal with the shaoyang aspects, move qi, relax the sinews, and dispel wind-damp. Dan Shen, Dang Gui, and, to a lesser extent, Si Gua Luo also move blood, with Dang Gui nourishing it as well. Mu Gua, Fang Feng, Sang Ji Sheng, and Qiang Huo assist with moving the damp stagnation from the muscles, and Dang Gui with Da Zao helps to ameliorate the drying aspects of the zonal and damp/phlegm-clearing herbs.

While not specifically a Heart Shock formula, many of the herbs satisfy strategies consistent with Heart Shock, such as calming the nervous system (Qiang Huo, Dan Shen, Sang Ji Sheng, Yuan Zhi, Mu Gua, Fang Feng), opening the chest (Qiang Huo, Si Gua Lou, Dan Shen, Yuan Zhi), activating Kidney yang and Du mai energetics (Qiang Huo), strengthening Heart qi (Dang Gui, Da Zao), invigorating blood (Dan Shen, Si Gua Lou), opening the portals (Yuan Zhi), calming the shen (Yuan Zhi), and strengthening the Kidneys (Sang Ji Sheng). Tweaking this formula with herbs to strengthen Heart yin and anchor Heart Yang, further nourish and anchor Kidney yang, etc. can easily be accomplished.

Sinew meridians and essential oils

The use of essential oils can be very powerful in the treatment of Heart Shock and there are many ways one can specifically address sinew channel energetics with this modality. As essential oils are substance and energetic medicines which are topically applied to the acupuncture points and channels, they can serve as multiple modalities (acupuncture energetics as well as herbal). With an understanding of the acupuncture energetics as well as the functions and uses of essential oils, the combinations and possibilities for using oils on the sinew channels are diverse. Below are some suggestions, many of which have come from Jeffrey Yuen's teachings and have been utilized by myself (and others) over the years.

With essential oils we want to create signatures that resonate with the level of wei qi, and that place an emphasis on top note oils. There are a number of methods for using the oils to impact the sinew channels, which include taking baths (trying to sweat and stimulate wei qi), creating liniments (for musculoskeletal injuries), inhalation/diffusion (to impact mood and psyche, as well as respiratory conditions), and creating blends to apply on the acupuncture points. For this latter function, oils can be tailored to meet the energetics of the point categories, functions, channels, etc.

Additionally, as essential oils are aromatic, most have the ability to open the sensory orifices in some capacity, making them particularly effective in the treatment of Heart Shock. Rosalina is one notable oil that clears the sensory orifices; it is particularly good for acute allergic responses as well as clearing internal heat (yangming) back out to the surface. Another, eucalyptus radiata, is known to open the portals and is very safe to use, an important consideration when treating children. A third commonly used oil is camphor, which happens to be a good oil for resuscitation as it treats sudden shock, fainting, and dampness and turbidity in the upper burner and head, and has a dilating effect on the vessels as well as the portals. As part of the cinnamon family, it also strengthens Heart qi.

Some of the more commonly used oils, and their zonal associations, are listed below.

Zonal essential oils

YANG SINEWS

Taiyang: basil, spruce, cinnamon twig

Shaoyang: rosemary, celery, lemon

Yangming: rosalina, bitter orange, petitgrain, peppermint

YIN SINEWS

When the pathogen is in the level, one has to break up the yin stagnation (dampness) in order to exteriorize the pathogen.

Taiyin: damp/phlegm preventing diffusion of wei qi: eucalyptus oils, especially eucalyptus polybractea.

Shaoyin: cold phlegm obstructing the chest, preventing descension of qi into the Kidney (e.g., Kidneys not grasping Lung qi): eucalyptus polybractea, benzoin, sage.

Jueyin: hot phlegm trapping wei qi, potentially occurring with blood heat: myrrh (blood stasis and hot phlegm stasis), German chamomile, clary sage.

Essential oils can be very effective in the treatment of traumatic injuries and their associated pain. In this regard, one should choose oils that are top note and quick-acting oils that impact the level of wei qi. These signature oils include grapefruit, mint, wintergreen, birch, eucalyptus, etc. Next, one should look to the source of wei qi, yang qi, to gain support, including oils that can impact Du mai, such as cinnamon bark, ho leaf, and clove. As with all our treatment strategies thus far, opening the sensory portals with oils such as eucalyptus, rosalina, camphor, etc. should be included. Next, one must address the nature of the condition (e.g., wind-cold, wind-damp, etc.). Litsea, for example, treats pain from wind, damp, and cold. Additionally, oils which can regulate the circulation of qi and reduce pain such as birch and/or wintergreen can be added to the oil blend. If the condition is caused by hot bi-syndrome with damage to the nerves and tissues, one must add oils to promote tissue growth by nourishing yin (e.g., geranium, clary sage, fennel), and if there is weakness and flaccidity, one should add oils to tonify qi (oils containing linalools can accomplish this, e.g., basil, thyme, etc.). Lastly, oils to address any of the Heart Shock strategies not accounted for above should be included. For example, geranium, clary sage, and fennel already address strengthening of Heart yin and qi as well as Kidney yang, camphor or eucalyptus address the portals, oils for regulating qi and reducing pain often invigorate the blood, etc.

Treatment protocol for pain with essential oils

1. Choose top note signature oils to impact wei qi.
2. Choose oil with an impact on yang qi to support wei qi, including resonance to the spine.
3. Choose oil to open the sensory orifices.
4. Choose oil based on the nature of the pain.
5. Choose oil to regulate qi and reduce pain.
6. If hot bi is present with damage to the nerves/tissues, choose oil to rebuild tissue and nourish yin.
7. If there is flaccidity, choose oil to tonify qi.
8. Address other Heart Shock strategies if present.

There are a host of essential oils that can satisfy many of the above strategies. Below is a short list of oils for the underlying climatic issues involved with pain.

Essential oils for wind: radiating pain, limited motion, spasms, cramping, numbness, etc.

Spruce

Celery

Spikenard

Essential oils for damp: swelling, heaviness, achiness, soreness, etc.

> Cinnamon
>
> Hyssop
>
> Benzoin
>
> Parsley
>
> Birch
>
> Wintergreen

Essential oils for cold: severe pain, no inflammation, tightness

> Styrax (Lu Lu Tong)
>
> Litsea
>
> Lemongrass
>
> Basil
>
> Clove
>
> Fennel

Essential oils for heat: redness, pain, swelling, inflammation, atrophy

> Cajeput
>
> Fir
>
> Galbanum
>
> Sweet marjoram
>
> Lovage
>
> Yarrow
>
> Chamomile
>
> Sandalwood

Pain from traumatic injuries requires understanding the phases of healing to properly choose the appropriate oils. There are three phases: the acute phase, intermediate phase, and late stage. Below is a list of oils and strategies for the treatment of each of these phases. Each of these oils and strategies should be added to the understanding as set forth above and included within the overall Heart Shock paradigm.

ACUTE PHASE

The area presents with swelling, pain, and inflammation.

Treatment principle: invigorate blood, relieve pain, promote circulation, reduce inflammation, disperse swelling.

Method: alcohol liniment is the best method of administration.

Oils: litsea, ginger, ho leaf, peppermint, lavender, eucalyptus, spruce, orange/lemon peel, cinnamon.

INTERMEDIATE PHASE

After the acute phase, lasting up to three weeks. Generally, the affected area will appear deep red and purplish in color.

Treatment principle: relax sinews, disperse stasis, invigorate blood, break up congestion.

Method: steams, soaks, compresses.

Oils: ginger, cinnamon leaf, clove, bay laurel.

LATE STAGE

Residual pain lingers with certain movements, minor signs of stasis, and persistent achiness and stiffness.

Treatment principle: regulate and invigorate area, dispel damp or cold stasis, relax sinews, strengthen bones.

Method: steams, soaks, compresses, plasters, liniments.

Oils: lemongrass, fennel, clove, cinnamon.

Essential oils for depression, anxiety, nervousness, etc.

Using oils to help manage and treat mood disorders and nervous system tension can be a very effective treatment, either on its own or in conjunction with other modalities. Below is a list of oils that have been shown to be effective for a variety of wei qi and psychological profiles. As a general rule, top notes can be used for acute issues, and base notes for chronic issues.

Stress management and nervous system tension

Chamomile

Orange, and all citrus, including tangerine and lemon/lime

Lavender (calms the nervous system, disperses wind,
    moves the Liver qi, opens the diaphragm)

Melissa

Neroli

Petitgrain

Rose (clears Liver fire and anchors Heart and
    Kidneys, promoting communication)

Sandalwood (opens chest/Heart)

Valerian (clears Heart fire)

Anxiety (tranquilizing)

Chamomile

Fir (warming)

Orange

Petitgrain

Rose

Geranium

Marjoram

Juniper

Nutmeg (warming)

Nervousness

Cedarwood (especially Himalayan, which gives a sense of
    protection; clears Lung heat/judgment/inadequacy)

Roman chamomile (increases white blood cells, hence a sense of protection)

Palmarosa (for someone prone to being infected by others' thoughts and feelings; good for allergies and those sensitive to their environment; good for pestilent factors and clears wind-heat and infections)

IRRITABILITY/AGITATION

Sandalwood

Roman chamomile

Cistus

Melissa

RESTLESSNESS

Vetiver (antispasmodic, good for restless legs)

Lavender

Lemon (antispasmodic)

Clary sage (Liver wind, tremors, spasms)

Carrot seed (nourishes Liver blood)

Sweet marjoram (treats Liver fire and high blood pressure, breaks hot phlegm)

FEAR/NIGHTMARES

Citronella (especially for kids who hear voices or see things at night)

Rosemary (secures wei qi, protective against ghosts/gui)

Mandarin/orange (clear Heart fire and agitation)

Neroli

Angelica archangel (calming, anti-parasitic, wards off negative spirits, attracts angelic beings)

Creating the essential oil blend

Generally, when using essential oils topically, it is done as a blend or formula consisting of a number of oils, just like with herbal medicine. With a sinew meridian formula, a 6–10 percent dilution is common, especially with an acute injury. To create a dilution, one mixes a specific number of drops of essential oils per specific volume of carrier oil. An 8 percent dilution is 80–96 drops of essential oils per 1oz. of carrier oil, or other carrier, such as rice wine, vinegar, grain alcohol, etc., depending on the desired impact of the formula. For sinew formulas, I most often use either safflower oil, as it can invigorate the blood, or rice wine or grain alcohol for the invigorating blood effect as well as the impact on the spirit. Very commonly, when creating more of a liniment to treat pain, I will combine carriers, using 50 percent alcohol and 50 percent safflower oil, as it creates a better consistency to be massaged into the affected area. For use specifically on the acupuncture points, I most commonly use safflower oil alone.

CHAPTER 5

Luo Vessels

Introduction to luo vessels

The luo vessels reside in the domain of ying qi and blood and include the longitudinal luo pathway (which becomes visible with a trapped pathogen), and the transverse luo (which mediates the interrelationships of internal pathways and connections between the yin-yang paired systems). Visibility in the longitudinal luo is often revealed by spider veins, varicose veins, nodules/gummies and discolorations. One may also find temperature changes and different textures to the skin, such as dryness, rashes, hot sensations, etc. As the realm is ying qi and blood/fluids, luo vessels are impacted from internal influences such as the emotions, diet, lifestyle etc., but also from external factors bypassing the sinew channels and gaining entry into the interior. The experience of trauma is one such cause and can be thought of as both an internal pathogen which stems from one's perceptions and relationship to the experience (e.g., internally generated fear, fright, worry, grief, guilt, etc.), as well as an external pathogen assaulting the nervous system and body as described in the sinew meridians chapter. The luo vessels' role in latency is that they have the capacity (using its resource of blood and fluids) to create the space/environment (ying relationship to Earth phase) to hold and contain pathogens that seek to come in and move internally and invade the primary meridians, or translocate internally generated pathology outwards.

The luo channels also help us understand and reflect on where a person is stuck in their lives from a psycho-social developmental aspect. We can know if they are trapped in particular emotional states of development and assess their ability to adapt. This is particularly useful in the management of Heart Shock. Ying qi deals with our internal relationship and environment as well as to some degree our conscious awareness, but as we see with the concept of latency, it's also a place where we can suppress pathology (both emotional and physical). When we're looking at the luo we're relating to ying qi, we're relating to the blood and the jin-ye, and we know that it has a major influence over, and impact on, the shen/spirit and also on the hormonal components (endocrine and exocrine functioning). Thus, the jin-ye can also be seen as a measure of our emotional health.

Luo vessel applications

There are a few different areas that the luo vessels are most commonly used for. They include:

1. Internal heat: One instance is where an internal condition is beginning to produce heat, and that heat is moving in to invade the blood and/ or the organs. It can be very helpful in many types of inflammatory processes. With Heart Shock, we often find inflammation from nervous system tension and hypervigilance as well as the hyperactivity of the adrenals. In our culture, inflammation and stress are ubiquitous. With stress outweighing our collective abilities to discharge it, we see a constant internalization and suppression of pathology moving into the blood. From the Shen-Hammer perspective we might see Blood Heat (see Figure 5.1) on the pulse, or some type of retained pathogens reflected in the blood itself. We may see fluids being compromised as heat starts to generate and burn off the yin of the body. The body then begins to leach calcium from the bones to quell the heat, kicking off a vicious cycle that consumes the body.

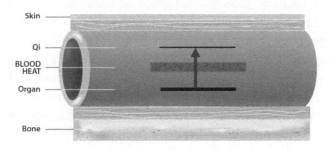

Figure 5.1: Blood Heat pulse
Reproduced with permission from Eastland Press

2. Rebellious qi: We look at the luo vessels when we see rebellious qi and when we are trying to clear pathology. We discussed rebellious qi as one of the impacts of Heart Shock and fright earlier, in Part I.

3. Blood pathology: The involvement of blood in any capacity is important, whether we're trying to move blood, invigorate blood, or break blood stasis. (Moving blood uses the energetics of the Lung qi; invigorating blood uses Heart qi; and breaking blood or cracking blood uses the capacity of Kidney yang supporting Heart yang.)

4. Pain: Another instance when you want to use the luo vessels would be in musculoskeletal conditions, more specifically pain along channel pathways, and often this is done in conjunction with sinew treatments. It is important to note, however, that the luo vessels don't penetrate the "great" articulations, so they have more to do with the minor articulations: the elbows, knees, ankles, wrists.

5. Shen disturbances: The luo channels are also used to treat emotional issues and shen disturbances.

6. Heart pathology: When talking about blood we have to always think about the Heart. The luo can assist treatment of any type of Heart pathology. The luo do not go to their zang fu-associated organs, except the Heart and Pericardium.

Luo channel energetics

From a Classical perspective, we know that the luo channels originate from their respective luo point and then go to their yin-yang pair's source point (some commentators believe it goes to the luo point of the yin-yang pair) and use this source qi to displace the pathogenic factor that has moved inwards: this is often referred to as the Transverse Luo theory. The luo point can also create collaterals off the primary meridian to displace pathogens to the surface by trapping them within the blood. At this point the pathogen becomes "visible" with varicosities, broken blood vessels, discolorations, or nodules: this is referred to as the Longitudinal Luo theory.

The Nei Jing discusses 16 luo meridians: 12 representing the primary channels plus the Ren and Du (Nan Jing says Qiao mai) and the great luos of the Stomach and Spleen. There are two competing or conflicting sequences mentioned in the classics, but we can use whichever one is most appropriate in any given circumstance. The Ling Shu discussed the movement from the Lung to the Heart to the Pericardium (which are the Yin channels of the arm) moving to the Yang channels of the arm, which are the Large Intestine, Small Intestine, and Triple Burner; and then the Bladder, Gall Bladder, Stomach, Spleen, Kidney, Liver, Ren, Du, and then the great luo. This sequence was applied by Wang Qing-ren in terms of his cardiovascular model. The other model follows the same sequencing as the primary meridians and adds in the great luo of the Spleen and the Ren and then the Du.

The physiology of the luo vessels is that they are trying to translocate an external or internal pathogen which the body was insufficiently strong to expel, whether it didn't have enough resources or was unable or unwilling to direct its attention to deal with it. Unable to resolve it, it lingers in a state of latency as a protective measure. Pathogens can make an entry via the channel systems, e.g., the sinews, as it internalizes, or the primary channel via the shu-stream point. The luo will use the blood and the fluids to trap the pathogen and attempt to exteriorize it via longitudinal channels to protect it from going towards the source qi and the interior. Should the pathogen travel to the he-sea point we know it gets to the bowels and the organ systems. The luo moves the pathology to prevent it from going deeper. This concept will be discussed again with the divergent channels, which push the pathogen out to the joints to prevent internalization. If we can't rid the pathogen, it can become trapped and symptoms such as bi obstruction are experienced (a Classical symptom of the luo channels).

The luo utilize ying qi and blood to contain pathogens and make them latent. They do not treat or get rid of the pathogen—the practitioner does via bleeding. The luo vessels themselves are simply channels of containment which use the blood and fluids as their resource.

The longitudinal luo have concepts of fullness and emptiness. In response to a pathogen, blood and jin-ye are mobilized to create a holding space (e.g., spider veins) to contain the pathogenic factor and the luo become visible. This is called fullness of the longitudinal luo. When fullness reaches its max, the pathology begins to empty back into the primary meridians, giving potential access to the zang fu. This is called emptiness and is a progression of fullness where the longitudinal luo has failed in its capacity to sequester the pathogen and it returns back to the primary channels, with access to the constitution (source/luo relationship and transverse luo theory). Emptiness often reveals itself with nodules or swellings often only found via palpation. To protect the source, the body mobilizes its jin-ye to more densely trap the pathogen (e.g., nodulations). As/if that becomes insufficient, one begins to see transverse luo symptomatology which essentially are heat signs and inflammation in the organ systems. Of course, we know that heat consumes qi and blood causing the body to search for another holding place (i.e., yin-yang pair's source point). Treating the transverse luo requires venting this heat back toward the longitudinal luo so it can be released towards the exterior (and bled).

The luo channels have unique trajectories, and knowledge of them is important for utilizing these channel systems in the varied treatments of Heart Shock (and for other diagnoses). For convenience, I will present them in the order of the primary channel sequence (not the Ling Shu sequence as utilized by Wang Qing-ren and the cardiovascular model).

Lungs: LU 7 down to LU 10 to PC 8. This trajectory is trying to release pathology from the chest.

Large Intestine: LI 6 to LI 11, LI 15, ST 5 (branches to ST 4/teeth and SI 19/SJ 17 at the ears).

Stomach: ST 40 to ST 13, Du 20, crossing over the midline of the body to ST 9 (area of thyroid) on the opposite side. For the luo, it is the first channel that establishes polarity.

Spleen: SP 4 to the intestines and into the Stomach (area of Ren 12).

Heart: HT 5 to HT 1, LU 2, ST 11, BL 1 (branches from HT 1 to Heart organ and from ST 1 through ST 5 to ST 11; Su Wen says to Ren 17, 14, 23). The Heart channel goes from HT 5 to HT 1 and wraps around to LU 2, ST 11, and BL 1 where it branches from HT 1 to the Heart organ and from ST 1 through ST 5 to ST 11. Su Wen has a few other points in there as well (Ren 17, 14, 23).

Small Intestine: SI 7 up the arm to LI 15.

Bladder: BL 58 down to KI 4, then follows the Kidney luo to Du 4.

Kidneys: KI 4 to KI 21, Ren 14, Du 4. KI 4, goes up to KI 21, to Ren 14, and then wraps internally and goes down to Du 4.

Pericardium: PC 6 to HT 1, PC 1, Heart organ, and the three jiaos. The Pericardium luo vessel goes to HT 1, PC 1, and then into the Heart organ itself and then communicates with all three jiaos.

Triple Burner: SJ 5 to LI 15, LU 2 and 1, Ren 15, then to the three jiaos (Su Wen says to LI 15 or GB 21, ST 17, Ren 17; later Ren 12 being added). From SJ 5 it goes up to LI 15, wraps with LU 2 and 1, then to Ren 15, and then also to the three jiaos.

Gall Bladder: GB 37 to ST 42. GB 37 will go straight down to ST 42. It then follows the Liver channel.

Liver: From LR 5 it travels to Ren 2 and the genitalia.

Ren: From Ren 15 the channel spreads and fans out over the abdomen.

Du: From Du 1 the channel splits into two branches to follow both sides of the spine (Hua Tou Jia Ji); at BL 10 it splits again and one branch goes over the head to BL 1 and the other goes into the paravertebral muscles down the Bladder sinew meridian.

Great luo of Spleen: From SP 21 it spreads and wraps around the front and back covering the axilla, breast, and ribs. (Classically, GB 22 was the luo point.)

Great luo of Stomach: The channel begins in the Stomach, enters the diaphragm and makes its way under the left breast to where the heartbeat is felt.

Signs and symptoms of the longitudinal luo

The psycho-social perspective of the longitudinal luo maps out one's emotional development. Different stresses and/or traumas (all relative to the individual of course) can impact this unfolding by stunting or blocking its progression or causing underlying insufficiencies at one or more levels of development. This creates the various dysfunctions congruent with luo vessel symptoms. The various levels of development are discussed in detail in the following section. And while they are applicable to a myriad of potential diagnoses, looking at it from the lens of a Heart Shock diagnosis is helpful in understanding where any given patient has become stunted as a result of a traumatic experience.

Lung luo

The Lung luo starts when a child is born and now has the opportunity to sense and perceive the world around him. The function of the Lungs is how we inhale, take things in, and are inspired by our environment. From the physiological level, we associate with the skin and a need for contact. The quality of our bonding with caregivers at an early stage of development impacts the Lung luo vessel, and insufficient bonding creates a heightened desire for contact with the outside world to satisfy those needs. With fullness of the Lung luo the individual cannot get enough bonding and/or stimulation. The Classical symptom is hot palms, which can be reinterpreted as someone who is constantly needing to touch, feel, and experience different stimuli with excessive wei qi activity. The fidgeting is a need for more stimulation. One can see this with ADD and ADHD types of presentations and a desire for contact and bonding. This can also reflect heat from stagnation in the chest which results from the internalizing of a pathogen.

Emptiness of the Lung luo is demonstrated with a need to retreat from stimulation. The person is bored, with little interest in life. There is no desire for stimulation, motivation declines, and the person is uninspired, sad, and tends to live a more depressive type of life.

Rebellious qi in the Lung luo is frequent yawning (a symptom of trying to rid a pathogen from the chest) and frequent urination (additional attempt at ridding the pathogen from the Lungs, via its connection to the Bladder). The diffusing of the Lungs helps with the upward movement to expel, but also descension and the release of both the Large Intestine and the Bladder itself (e.g., taiyang pathogens and the use of Gui Zhi Tang or Wu Ling San).

In response to trauma, we often see patients presenting with Lung luo symptoms, including fullness, emptiness, and rebellious qi.

Large Intestine luo

The Large Intestine luo is where the child begins to develop processing and differentiation of the varied stimuli. We see this played out with the teething process, where the child is not simply accepting and swallowing, but chewing and processing via repetitive movements of the jaw which allows for time to think and experience on a more active level. When stimulation is excessive (e.g., over-feeding, exposure to bright colors and visual stimuli, noises from toys and games, etc.), it can overwhelm the senses.

With excessive stimulation or stimulation that is too early developmentally, especially if there has been insufficient bonding from the prior stage in the Lung, it can produce the fullness of the Large Intestine luo which is a chronic need for repetition in an attempt to fully process the information. There may be a constant need to repeat phrases over and over again, rocking motions, or the constant stimming commonly seen in autism. One may see toothaches, acute deafness and other ear disorders, bleeding gums, TMJ (and grinding teeth) from an inability to process the excess wei qi activity and descend it to the chest, etc.

All of the overstimulation can create a shutting down of response, leading to emptiness of the Large Intestine luo with such symptoms as the inability to process or assimilate and discern sensations. Fullness is trying to repeat to assimilate; emptiness is an inability to discern resulting from the overload. A Classical symptom of this is coldness of teeth (inability to chew more or engage in the process of assimilation) as well as diaphragmatic numbness, representing an inability to animate our feelings.

Rebellious qi manifests as toothaches (rebelling against the demands of trying to assimilate) and acute deafness (channel goes to mouth/teeth and then to ears).

Metal: Lung and Large Intestine luo symptoms
LU

- Full: hot burning palms, constant need for contact, stimulation, desires, lack of concentration, can't sit still, restless legs, excess wei qi activity.

- Empty: shortness of breath, enuresis, lack of interest, indifference, numb to stimulation, sighing, boredom.

- Rebellious qi: yawning, frequent urination.

LI

- Full: toothache, gum disease, deafness, ear disorders, bleeding gums when brushing teeth, jaw tension, TMJ, constantly trying to assimilate information.

- Empty: cold teeth pain, stifling sensation in chest/diaphragm, diaphragmatic numbness (inability to anchor the qi to KI), hard time making links and assimilating info (feel flabbergasted), hard time chewing, autism and inability to separate from the stimulation, i.e., repetition because they can't assimilate/process, poor self-control.

- Rebellious qi: toothaches, deafness.

Stomach luo

From the prior levels of psycho-social development, one can chew, process, and assimilate stimuli/food, etc. and make it one's own. Now a person starts to make discernments of whether or not he likes or dislikes something which becomes the beginning of the emotional response (i.e., gut feelings, not intellectualized). These feelings can be quite strong (consider a young child and tantrums…). When feelings tend to become denied regularly, or not valued or suppressed, the emotions can overwhelm the mind and rationality.

Classical symptoms of the Stomach luo include hysteria (dian kuang), but can be thought of as intense feelings (arousing actions) such as temper tantrums and impulsive reactions. We can see mania, schizophrenia, epilepsy, insomnia, irritability, and restlessness. The Stomach luo channel goes into the head and the brain (to Du 20 and crosses the midline). It also goes to the throat and tongue. Strong vocalized expressions of one's internal feelings often result in this luo where the heart is stronger than the head.

With emptiness of the Stomach luo one sees weakness of the lower limbs, reflecting the person's inability to animate or create strong feelings or have a sense of where or how one wants to move one's qi. There's a lack of will and a feeling of being lost. The Stomach helps maintain tonicity in the flesh and muscles as it creates wei qi from its yin. Here the Stomach luo creates flaccidity and weakness from its failure to mobilize its yin.

Rebellious qi in the Stomach luo presents with obstruction of the throat, goiters, swellings around the throat, sudden hoarseness of the voice, and aphasia/loss of speech from an inability to vocalize one's feelings.

The Stomach luo also contains another trajectory which is shared with the Kidney luo which runs up the Kidney channel from the abdomen to the chest. Symptoms associated with this trajectory include severe panic attacks, even what may be termed temporary insanity, where the Stomach and the intense emotions created become overwhelmed by fear and can result in either uncontrolled actions or paralysis. Remember from Part I that fear can create the fight/flight/freeze response, but also paralysis and tonic immobility.

Spleen luo

The Spleen manages the blood and provides context to our emotional experiences, emotional intelligence, and how to think about our feelings and emotions. Too much thinking about our emotions creates a fullness of the Spleen luo with obsessive thinking and behavior, extreme habituation, and an inability to create closure on our thoughts. Repetitive behaviors, an inability to let go, and a constant retelling of the same story and internal narrative ensue. Physically one experiences sharp pains in the intestines, abdominal distension and fullness from not being able to process, assimilate, and move the digestate, and the full range of eating disorders.

Emptiness of the Spleen luo shows up with addictions, drum-like swellings of the abdomen and intestines (e.g., gu syndrome and parasites), childhood nutritional impairment, and autistic qualities such as repetitive thought and difficulties creating context.

Rebellious qi symptoms include acute vomiting and diarrhea, severe abdominal pain, and dehydration symptoms.

Earth: Stomach and Spleen luo symptoms

ST

- Full: mental disorders, dian kuang, schizophrenia, manic-depression, insanity, epilepsy, insomnia, unable to sort out emotions (mania), like everything or dislike everything, irritability, restlessness, strong emotions, panic attacks and temporary insanity (second trajectory shared with KI), feeling sabotaged.

- Empty: atrophy, weakness, flaccidity of muscles of leg/feet, especially shin area, inability to feel satisfaction, negativity, disengage and retreat from stimulation, limbic obstruction, not being able to bring their blood to what they're attracted to, can't bring enthusiasm.

- Rebellious qi: obstruction of throat, goiters, swellings around throat, sudden hoarseness and aphasia/loss of speech.

SP

- Full: colic pain of ST and intestines, sharp pains, lack of stability, abdominal fullness, drum distension, eating disorders.

- Empty: drum distension, ascites and intestinal swellings, childhood nutritional impairment, flatulence, abdominal fullness and distension, never satisfied with where they are, eating disorders, addictions, autism, repetitive thoughts/feelings/contact, habituation, weak intelligence, weak memory.

- Rebellious qi: acute vomiting, diarrhea, severe abdominal pain, dehydration (like acute attack of cholera), gu syndrome.

Heart luo

The Heart governs relationships, maintaining contact and engagement with the outside world. To do so effectively, it must be open and animated, able to set goals, and articulate its thoughts and feelings well. When our goals are not met, or we find ourselves betrayed, then the Heart luo suffers a broken heart. Fullness of the Heart luo is heart pain, being stuck in painful emotions, and not able to fully express oneself, impacting the throat and creating a suffocating feeling in the chest. Dr. Shen called this "Heart Closed."

Emptiness of the Heart luo is the loss of one's voice (which also includes one's inner voice). The individual is heavy hearted, feels betrayed, and can't bring oneself to speak about it. This loss of verbalization can also manifest in an inability to articulate, dyslexia, Tourette's, and a host of different types of language issues (e.g., stuttering, stammering).

Small Intestine luo

The Small Intestine is responsible for separating the pure and the impure. As that breaks down in the luo, there becomes a need for feedback; to constantly gauge one's thoughts, feelings, and opinions with those of others. Fullness is where the individual is preoccupied with whether or not they are on the right path: thinking, eating, doing the right things, and distilling and assimilating the essence of those things into one's life. There is a constant need for approval due to the insecure internal dialogue, and a looking for self-recognition through feedback from others. When they cannot receive it, they become jealous, aggressive, fanatical, and violent. Physical symptoms include stiffness of elbows (inability to articulate movement and rotation) but can also be thought of as the inability to see things from different perspectives. In some ways, the Small Intestine fullness is obsessiveness about being comfortable with who one is, because of an inability to separate the pure from the impure.

Emptiness is the constant need for affirmation and inability to receive criticism and see things from different perspectives. Physically it manifests in pebbly stools, looseness/instability of the elbows and joints, and small itchy and flaky swellings and scabs (e.g., flat warts, dermatitis, fungal infections, psoriasis).

While both the Small Intestine and Spleen luo deal with habituation and obsession, it is only the Small Intestine which seeks to weigh opinions; the Spleen is just stuck in the same way of thinking/seeing.

Fire: Heart and Small Intestine luo symptoms

HT

- Full: distension and fullness in the chest and diaphragm, stickiness in chest, weight, oppression of chest, feeling of disappointment and betrayal and being cheated.

- Empty: aphasia/loss of speech, disorders of the vocal cords, inability to vocalize one's pains and discontents, loss of spirit.

SI

- Full: instability and weakness of joints, weakness and paralysis of elbow and arm, sensitivity to criticism (react with rebuttal), stiff elbows.

- Empty: flat warts, small itchy swellings that scab, dermatitis, eczema (when scratched, fluids come out, maybe even blood), pebbly stools, nausea, bloating, flatulence, burping, fatty deposits, jealousy, sorting out morality (deciding about whether to be a good or bad person), surveying of opinions to hear what you want, want others to say it for you, manipulation.

Bladder luo

A role of the Bladder is helping to establish boundaries between ourselves and the external environment (taiyang). When there is too much external feedback and outside influences, a fullness of the luo begins, wherein the individual's alarm system starts to get triggered. The person feels threatened all the time and can experience panic attacks. This inability to shut down and reset the alarm causes symptoms akin to post-traumatic stress disorder (PTSD). The Bladder luo travels down from BL 58 to KI 4 and then follows the Kidney channel. An aspect of the Kidney channel reflects the ability to contain oneself. As the Bladder luo is unable to handle the external assault, it seeks solace in the Kidneys. The Bladder luo is about reactivity and hypervigilance, always ready for a crisis, mobilizing for a fight/flight/freeze response. Physical symptoms include nasal congestion, allergies, sinusitis, headache, low back pain, PTSD, and a startle reflex.

Emptiness manifests when a person loses the ability to know her limits. The alarm is always sounding, feedback systems break down, and the person becomes unsure of boundaries and limits and cannot defend themselves. Toxic activities are engaged in, addictive behavior increases, there are eating disorders and binging to the point of exceeding boundaries, as well as vomiting, and there is an overall inability to say "no." These individuals have a constant need of feeling loved, engage in compulsive sex, or feel extremely vulnerable or lack emotion. Physically, the symptoms also include clear nasal discharge and nosebleeds. PTSD can manifest with Bladder luo emptiness as well as fullness.

Kidney luo

The Kidneys govern the will and self-direction, and when misdirected or unable to be controlled, it can lead to obsession. Fullness is an extension of the Bladder's alarm, an inability to reprogram the alarm system causing obsessive-compulsive behavior and risk taking, sado-masochism, etc. Physical symptoms include blockage of the two lower yin orifices, where the person is not able to urinate or defecate, reflecting the inability to let go of attachments, fears, etc.

Emptiness is when paranoia sets in. The person now becomes afraid of themselves, afraid of loss, and afraid of being left alone. They can experience intense depression, darkness, and despair. The distinguishing factor between Kidney luo and the PTSD of the Bladder is that there's no triggering event with the Kidneys or reliving any particular trauma. It emanates from an adrenal exhaustion and, in *Dragon Rises, Red Bird Flies* (Chapter 13), Dr. Hammer distinguishes it as the endogenous deep depressions and phobias. From a physical standpoint, we see pain in the lumbar region, compulsiveness, and self-harm (cutting, etc.).

Water: Bladder and Kidney luo symptoms

BL

- Full: nasal obstruction, clear nasal discharge, headache, back pain, alarm system, over-exceeding limits, panic attack, PTSD, can't turn off alarm, overwhelmed by fear.

- Empty: nosebleeds, chronic clear nasal discharge, sinusitis, deep-seated polyps, second level of addiction (not knowing when enough is enough), can't desensitize self, fetishes.

KI

- Full: lumbar pain, auto intoxication, blockage of lower orifices (constipation, urination), too caught up in their own ego, can't take criticism, obsessive-compulsive, sadist, masochist.

- Empty: restlessness, anxiety, fear, depression, stuffiness of chest and epigastrium, low back pain, genital pain (also dysmenorrheal), paranoia, catatonia, fear of being discovered, impending doom (projection into future).

Pericardium luo

The Pericardium is the Heart protector; it provides intellectual control over our emotions and is responsible for our adaptive/coping mechanisms. The Pericardium provides solutions and prioritizes options (directs our qi in ways that fulfill the Heart) to address the problems that we are experiencing. It helps us to manage stress and assists in generating empathy. As Jeffrey Yuen says, while the Heart offers hope, the Pericardium offers help; help is always available, hope less so. The Pericardium is problem management, biding its time until the Heart can be restored and hope reignited.

Where there are constant failures and disappointments, inability to achieve one's goals, or betrayals (first experienced in the Heart luo), it can affect the Pericardium luo. Fullness manifests with an inability to control one's emotions, prioritize solutions, or call on higher-level adaptive responses, creating hopelessness. As such, people seek quick solutions; they lie and have little remorse. Physically, they experience chest pains, angina, palpitations, and anxiety.

Emptiness presents physically as a stiff neck, and pain in the neck and head. This can be seen as an ecological response, preventing the pathology from rising up to the brain. People with Pericardium luo emptiness often become reclusive and can no longer interact with others or see/perceive from points of view other than their own. They have a difficult time controlling their emotions and can become sociopathic.

Triple Burner luo

The Triple Burner controls one's temperament and temperature. It helps us work out and handle certain situations by allowing us to see through different lenses and use our ingenuity and intuition (fire tapping into water). It provides resources (Triple Burner dissemination) for our problem solving.

If our intuitive creativity becomes blocked, disregarded, or discouraged by others or our own failures, the Triple Burner luo can become full, with symptoms such as rigidity (physical and mental) and stubborn fixed attitudes—people who live for the sake of survival with a hardened attitude and austere personality with unwavering opinions. Physically, we may find dark spots on the Liver channel, rigid elbows, spasms, cramping, and dislocations.

With emptiness of the Triple Burner luo, we see physical symptoms of weakness and loss of tone of the elbows, and pain and difficulty bending the elbow or when bearing weight. Emotionally, the person becomes indifferent, numb, and unwilling to react or take sides/express opinions on anything. They have become a shell, hardened on the outside and hollow within. This indifference is distinguishable from the Stomach luo where the person cannot take on any more feelings (the ability has been compromised). With the Triple Burner the person has been hurt with past experiences and has become depressed, uninterested, and ultimately suicidal.

Fire: Pericardium and Triple Burner luo symptoms
PC

- Full: cardiac pain, angina, chest pain, person cannot control their emotions.

- Empty: restlessness, irritability, rigidity and pain in neck and head (not realizing they have options), lack of social skills, doesn't know how to interact.

SJ

- Full: spasms of the elbow joint, bi obstruction, elbows stiff and dislocated, RA, person rigid in how they handle things, stubborn, hard character.

- Empty: flaccid muscles of the arm, difficulty flexing/bending elbow, hard to rotate, indifference, ostracized.

Gall Bladder luo

The Gall Bladder is responsible for decision making and a vision for seeing new possibilities, providing access to the portals of vision to see and perceive the world differently in order to initiate healing. GB 37 goes to ST 42 where the pure yang of the Stomach rises to irrigate the sensory orifices to allow for proper, clearer perceptions. As a curious organ, the Gall Bladder also connects to the constitution, and has the ability to mutate/morph and change when confronted with stress.

Fullness of the Gall Bladder luo manifests with cold legs and feet and potentially collapse from an underlying yang deficiency. The person with this condition has lost the ability to move/decide/change and sees no options other than living the same unfulfilling hopeless existence. They become introverted and lack the courage to face new challenges or adversities in their lives. Frustration ensues from this dead-end path, and many begin to hurt themselves or allow themselves to be hurt by others.

Emptiness comes with paralysis or weakness/flaccidity of the lower limbs, inability to stand up or rise from the sitting position, feelings of loneliness, isolation, lethargy, emotional inertia, and despair. They have given up on life, and become a hermit or a "wandering corpse."

Liver luo

The Liver regulates the qi dynamic, generates creativity (association to genitals and ability to create/reproduce life), and drives us to achieve our goals and interests. The Liver mobilizes the jing-essence and ensures that our lives continue, whether it be from our accomplishments (psychologically) or through having children (internally).

Fullness manifests with a disinterest in achievement and one's current reality. Some additional symptoms include frequent or abnormal sexual arousal, hearing voices, talking to oneself and hallucinations, development of multiple personalities (creating new reality as stunted in current one), and schizophrenia. Daydreaming is a mild variation where the mind is always off in some other direction breaking from the reality of the present moment.

With emptiness the multiple personalities are more destructive and shift more frequently. The Classical symptom is a persistent cruel and unbearable itch through the genitalia (inability to create what one desires) which can include STDs, herpes, etc.

The rebellious qi aspect is the swelling and pain of the ovaries, testicles, and scrotum representing the frustration, creating stagnation and inability to move the jing-essence which becomes trapped internally.

Wood: Gall Bladder and Liver luo symptoms

GB

- Full: cold sensations of feet and lower limbs.

- Empty: weakness, flaccidity of muscles of the foot, causing difficulty standing, paralysis of lower extremities, lethargy, lassitude, emotional inertia, isolation, loneliness, barrenness, infertility.

LR

- Full: abnormal erection, multiple personalities, schizophrenia (creating own realities).

- Empty: unbearable itching of external genitalia (herpes, syphilis, gonorrhea, HPV, eczema, candida, vulvitis, etc.), constant shifting from one personality to another.

- Rebellious qi: swelling and pain of testicles and scrotum, hernia.

Great luo of the Spleen

The great luo of the Spleen controls all of the sinews of the body, and eventually all pathology of all the luo comes to the Spleen's great luo. Fullness manifests as pain all over the body (the idea that life is suffering and that unfinished business and desire breeds another incarnation), chronic fatigue, and fibromyalgia. Blood is now occluded into the Heart, and our awareness is that of continuous suffering.

Emptiness manifests with looseness of joints, muscular atrophy (wei syndrome), and flaccidity. The Spleen deals with contextualizing our feelings, and here suffering is habituated into the mind. The body feels weak (chronic fatigue syndrome), and there is a lack of will to live. The suicidal components of these last luo channels have led to a lack of integrity of structure breaking down the bones/joints/muscles/flesh.

Great luo of the Stomach

The great luo of the Stomach is located in the diaphragmatic area just below the Heart. It manages the heartbeat, the qi that drives the blood, and has an association to the Chong mai. Fullness manifests with irregular breathing, rapid breathing, chest congestion, and things like congestive heart failures.

Emptiness produces suffocating sensation in the chest, asthmatic breathing, palpitations, fibrillations, and tachycardia.

Great luo of the Stomach and Spleen symptoms

GREAT LUO OF ST

- Full: rapid breathing, irregular breathing, dyspnea, chest congestion, palpitations.

- Empty: suffocating sensation in chest, asthmatic breathing, cough, angina, heart attack.

GREAT LUO OF SP

- Full: whole body pain, multiple site arthritis, bi-syndrome.
- Empty: muscular atrophy and flaccidity, weakness/looseness of the joints, weakness of whole body.

Ren and Du luo

The Ren and Du provide a last ditch effort to alter the perceptions of our suffering into something productive in the present moment. If we are unable, it will create the blueprint for the next incarnation via the Chong mai.

The Ren luo encompasses all the suffering of the yin luos. Fullness is abdominal pain. Emptiness is nodules and abdominal itching.

The Du luo encompasses all the suffering of the yang luos. Fullness is represented by a stiff spine, scoliosis, spinal stenosis, etc. (rigidity and inability to change one's yang dissemination). Emptiness manifests with nodules of the spine, and a heavy head with shaking (i.e., wind and Parkinson's-like symptoms).

Ren and Du luo symptoms

REN

- Full: pain of skin of abdomen.
- Empty: itching of skin of abdomen.

DU

- Full: rigidity and stiffness of spine, scoliosis, stenosis.
- Empty: heavy sensation of head, dizziness, vertigo, shaking forward.

Other diagnostics of the luo

The psychological and symptom profiles as described in the preceding pages constitute sufficient evidence to diagnose luo vessel pathology and proceed into treatments. Treatments for the luo vessels will be described shortly, but first, there are other ways of diagnosing luo vessel activity—namely looking, and palpation (channels as well as pulse).

Looking and palpating the channels

Earlier I mentioned that one of the main characteristics of identifying luo issues is via the concept of visibility. As one scans the channels, visually we may identify broken blood vessels, spider veins, discolorations, raised or protruding areas, varicosities, etc.; touching, we may notice swellings, sponginess, bumps, and/or nodules. All of these signs are indicative of luo vessel pathology and can orient one towards treating the luo vessels. There are other factors to consider, however, when deciding on how to treat the luo vessels. Namely, the status of the blood, contributing factors such as whether or not the Liver is able to store blood, the Spleen to manage blood, the Lungs to move blood, the Heart to invigorate blood, the Kidneys to crack/break blood stasis, the status of the jin-ye, the amount of fluids in the blood (e.g., Blood Thick[96] via Shen-Hammer pulse lineage; see Figure 5.2), whether the Spleen is ascending to the chest to allow for more blood production, etc. This information can be gleaned from the pulse to round out one's treatment strategies and prevent any negative consequences from a bleeding treatment.

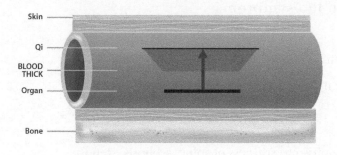

Figure 5.2: Blood Thick pulse
Reproduced with permission from Eastland Press

Pulse diagnosis for the luo vessels

Looking to the pulse can be very helpful as often patients are not willing to share their deepest emotional and psychological issues, especially not early on in the relationship. Being able to palpate the pulse and diagnose a specific luo vessel pathology (or multiple ones) can open up valuable dialogue with a patient and drive treatment strategies and treatments that otherwise may not be considered. The pulse can help direct specific questions that reveal the roots of many problems. It also assists in confirming other signs and symptoms that may have been revealed in other aspects of the diagnostic process.

When looking at the pulses from this Classical perspective we orient towards the patient's wrist with his palm facing upwards. The area from the skin down to the bone is separated into five general components (classically based on beans of pressure) each equidistant from the next. Each gradation of pressure should be equal to the last, so there are five equal depths from the skin (3 beans) to the bones (15 beans). The area that we will be most focused on for the luo vessels is between 3 beans (wei level) and 9 beans (ying level) of pressure. To assess the luo we will be looking at how the ying level is communicating and interrelating with, and adjusting to, the wei level. Pressure is applied to the radial artery equally with the practitioner's three fingers on the cun, guan, and chi positions simultaneously, moving as one unit:

- Wei level is 3 beans of pressure: skin and yang sinews

- 6 beans: yin sinews and luo

- Ying level is 9 beans of pressure: vessels

- 12 beans: flesh (embodiment of all the organs)

- Yuan level is 15 beans of pressure: bone

- Even deeper: marrow.

There are four criteria on the pulse to determine a luo vessel issue. The first is that the cun positions (primarily the right cun) are Floating and Empty (or Weak). A Floating pulse exists when we have qualities present on the 3 beans of pressure (just resting on the skin). With slight pressure towards 6 beans, if nothing pushes back against our finger we can say that it is an Empty or Weak pulse. This reflects an insufficiency of either wei/yang qi or ying qi to maintain the integrity of the wei level.

The second criterion is a Flooding pulse. This is created when the wei level mobilizes ying and qi to bring it to the surface to deal with something that it's not able to deal with on its own. As the body pushes blood to the surface it becomes more Floating and Full and strong. This reflects ying transforming into wei, and the wei qi becomes stronger and more rapid. This Floating Full and Rapid pulse becomes a signature of luo vessel pathology. One might present with heat signs and blood coming to the surface (e.g., nosebleeds, coughing blood, bloodshot eyes, etc.).

The third criterion is a Rough and/or Choppy pulse on the wei level. Flooding is basically tension that is squeezing the ying and bringing it up to the wei level. Over time this creates a Rough pulse. It hits the finger more at a point and feels a little sharper. If it gets to a point where it exhausts the ying, and the blood becomes very deficient, it becomes more Choppy and fine.

The fourth criterion is either the Lung not diffusing the wei qi and/or the Spleen not ascending to the Lung. One method for assessing this is to place all three fingers on the 9 beans of pressure and pump down on the chi position, pump down on the guan position, and lift up on the cun position to determine if something pushes your finger back up to the wei level. If so, the Lungs are diffusing wei qi appropriately.

Go back to that 9 beans of pressure, push down on the cun a little deeper, push on the guan position, and then slowly lift up the cun to assess if there is a pushing up of that finger representing the Spleen ascending to the Lung. Lung diffusion is a sign that it can release pathogens without support from the ying/luo level. The Spleen's ascension demonstrates the normal support of ying to wei. If the Lungs are not diffusing it requires blood to come and support it to get rid of the pathogen. Sweat is the fluid of the Heart (which controls the blood), so blood and the luo will be utilized to assist wei; as sweat is insufficient, blood will be required to release the pathogen.

If one of these four criteria is satisfied, the pulse confirms an active luo issue wherein ying is moving out to the wei. The sinew channels are reflected at 3 (yang sinews) and 6 (yin sinews) beans of pressure. The luo is reflected at 6 beans of pressure as one moves down from 3 to 6 beans and up from 9 to 6 beans. The yin sinews are differentiated from the luo based on the four criteria set forth above. If one is present, our lens switches from the sinew channel to the luo channel. What we're looking for are qualities associated with stagnation as the luo vessels are channels of holding/containment, preventing pathogens from moving to deeper layers. This is what creates the fullness of the longitudinal luo.

From a practical process-oriented approach, we press from 3 beans down to 6 beans and note the quality of the pulse (e.g., perhaps it is Tight or Tense reflecting stagnation, Choppy reflecting blood stasis, or Slippery showing stagnation of jin-ye) and we also go to 9 beans and lift up back to 6 beans noting that quality. If the pulse is Tight moving from 3 to 6, that implicates a yang luo channel. The reflexology follows that of the primary channels, so assuming the right-side cun gets Tight from 3 to 6, it's reflecting a Large Intestine luo vessel problem. If it's Tight coming up from 9 to 6, then it's the yin luo (Lung luo). If we feel a pulse of restriction/stagnation going down from 3 to 6 as well as up from 9 to 6, the implication is that both yin and yang luo are impacted and is suggestive of a transverse luo pathology (see below for transverse luo symptoms).

If the pulse is Thin and Tight or Thin and Weak, this will indicate an emptiness of the luo rather than a fullness. As we will see soon, this requires that, after bleeding, moxibustion will be warranted.

Luo pulses and the great luo/Da Bao

An additional pulse configuration that presents itself commonly (especially in those with Heart Shock) is where the entire 6 beans of pressure become a Long pulse, generally Tight or Tense as one presses from 3 beans down to 6. This quality is a reflection of activity in all of the yang luo channels. When this is felt, treating the great luo of the Spleen along with the Da Bao/Bao mai/Dai mai is warranted (see below for instruction on this treatment).

Luo vessel treatments

Treating the luo vessels primarily involves bloodletting. According to Jeffrey Yuen, bleeding makes the pathology obvious, brings it to one's consciousness, and allows for the condition to change. The lance needle (or lancet) is used to take out a few drops of blood. One can also pinch the skin and lance it to release the blood (and hence the pathogen). As the blood has been stagnant, often it will come out dark, and the area should be expressed until the blood turns a fresher color; it's not necessary to release a lot of blood, often just a few drops is all that is required.

One can also do plum blossoming (7 star hammer) or even gua sha over the affected point/area/channel. When there is constitutional or blood deficiency underlying, this can stimulate wei qi to provoke a response (the area turns red) without the loss of blood. Additionally, if one uses the luo and expresses some blood in a blood-deficient patient, it is advised to harmonize the blood by needling one point proximal to the he-sea point to prevent dizziness or fatigue. One can also needle points related to blood such as BL 17, BL 15, BL 20, BL 11, LR 8, SP 6, etc. to help harmonize the blood. If there is an emptiness of the luo, one should also moxa the luo point to vitalize yang qi to assist in releasing the pathology. The yang qi from the moxa pulls the pathogen back into the longitudinal luo where it can be bled out and fully released. One can also surround and needle directly into the nodules. Ganglion cysts and nodules are found oftentimes along luo point areas.

Classically, the luo is treated every other day to release its pathology, stopping when the condition has resolved. The course of treatment for the blood level is approximately six weeks, then reevaluated, being mindful that acute conditions may resolve more quickly than chronic ones. As it is unrealistic for most patients to receive treatments on this schedule, either for time or financial reasons, an essential oil blend can be created and the patient taught how it can be massaged into the luo points/channels on the days they are not able to come in.

It should be noted that with luo treatments (like all treatments) one may notice that patients experience releases, both emotionally and/or physically as energetics move from the ying to the wei level.

Longitudinal luo vessel treatment protocol

Fullness and emptiness of the luo are treated as follows.

FULLNESS

- Bleed the luo point.

- Address visibility and stagnations along the channel by bleeding, needling, and/or gua sha.

- Harmonize the blood (needle point one point proximal to the he-sea).

- Can needle source point of yin/yang pair to protect the source.

EMPTINESS

- Bleed the luo point and perform moxibustion on it.

- Address stagnations and/or modules along the channel by bleeding, moxa and/or gu shua.

- Harmonize the blood (needle point one point proximal to the he-sea).

- Can needle source point of yin/yang pair to protect the source.

Treat every other day (can use essential oils on the points if the patient cannot come in on that schedule: see below for discussion on essential oils).

Additional aspects of the longitudinal luo channels

The longitudinal luo channels also have associated symptoms of rebellious qi. As they don't require significant elaboration, I will simply list them for one's reference.

Rebellious qi symptoms

Channel	Symptoms	Shen-Hammer Pulse Possible Findings
Lungs	Frequent yawning; frequent urination	Diaphragm pulse, Tense Robust Pounding in Right distal position
Large Intestine	Frequent bowel movements; gas (trapped gas pains, flatulence)	Tense Robust Pounding in LI complementary position
Stomach	Nausea and vomiting	Distal portion of Right middle position and/or Esophagus pulse Inflated and Slippery
Spleen	Intestinal pain, bloating, borborygmus	Right middle position Tight, possible Tense and Inflated
Heart	Palpitations, rapid heart beat, irregular beats (e.g., PVCs)	Robust Pounding in Left distal position

Small Intestine	Reflux, GERD	Esophagus Inflated Pounding Tight
Bladder	Urinary retention and decreased output	Right proximal position Tight or Tense at Qi depth
Kidney	Shortness of breath, wheezing	Tight Right proximal position
Pericardium	Palpitations, anxiety	Positive Pericardium complementary position that is Tense to Tight Pounding
Triple Burner	Alternating symptoms (e.g., fever and chills)	Disparity between upper, middle and lower burner pulses
Gall Bladder	Alternating symptoms (e.g., nausea, diarrhea, sudden turmoil	Gall Bladder complementary position Tense Robust Pounding Slippery
Liver	Dizziness, headaches, frequent outbursts	Left middle position Tight or Tense and Robust Pounding at Qi depth

Transverse luo

The transverse luo channels also have their associated symptomatology. These reflect pathology that has moved deeper into the interior towards the organs and reflect the beginning of heat signs and inflammation.

Transverse luo symptoms

Channel	Symptoms	Shen-Hammer Pulse Possible Findings
Lungs	Shortness of breath, cough and asthma, hot palms	Right distal Tense Pounding, possible Inflated. Diaphragm pulse Inflated on right
Large Intestine	Dry lips, mouth and throat	Right distal Thin Tight, possible Robust to Reduced Pounding
Stomach	Fever and sweat, stomach distention, phlegm, pain along pathway	Right middle position Tense to Tight, Slippery Robust Pounding at Qi depth

cont.

Channel	Symptoms	Shen-Hammer Pulse Possible Findings
Spleen	Heart and/or tongue pain, stiff body, frequent bowel movements	Right middle position Tense to Tight, Slippery Robust Pounding at Blood to Organ depth
Heart	Yellow eyes, pain along pathway	Left distal Tight, possible Flooding
Small Intestine	Tinnitus, deafness, swellings along jawline	Left distal superficially Tight, possible Flooding and Rapid
Bladder	Yellow or watery eyes, headaches and neck pain, hemorrhoids	Tense to Tight Pounding at Right proximal position Qi depth
Kidney	Cold and numb legs, diarrhea (especially cock's crow), depression, lack of interest in life, running piglet qi	Deep Tight at Right proximal with possible Reduced Substance moving towards Empty or Feeble
Pericardium	Heart pain, depression, hot palms or poor circulation	Pericardium complementary position Inflated Tight
Triple Burner	Sweating and pain along pathway	Entire Right side Tight Pounding
Gall Bladder	Sweating and aching of joints	Gall Bladder complementary position Tight Pounding
Liver	Nausea and vomiting, loss of appetite, tension around diaphragm, loose stools, incontinence or anuria	Left middle position Tight to Tense Slippery; Ulnar Liver engorgement complementary position Tight and Inflated, Diaphragm pulse on Left

The treatment strategy of addressing transverse luo pathology consists of attempting to clear internal heat. As yangming is where heat internalizes, one can always begin by clearing heat in the Stomach. Thus, bleeding ST 40 is our entry way to the internalized heat condition. One can then tonify the associated paired channel's source point, SP 3, to protect against transmission and have the support of the Spleen.

At this point, one looks to the affected transverse luo channel implicated in the inflammatory process (e.g., if the patient's symptoms are tinnitus and deafness, the Small Intestine luo is treated) and that luo point is bled while needling its associated yin-yang pair to prevent transmission.

Using other channel systems with luo treatments

To assist with luo treatments, other channel systems can be added in such as the primary channels, divergents, sinew, and 8 extraordinary. The idea is that one uses points that resonate with the strategies one is trying to implement, e.g., using 8x points when addressing yuan qi with transverse luo treatments or using sinew channels to address the wei qi when working on pushing a pathogen out. Regardless of whatever channel system one is utilizing, if the patient is experiencing strong emotional symptoms or shen disturbances, luo treatments can be very helpful. This can be accomplished within the same session or one can alternate treatments. Sinew channels, of course, can be used if one is addressing body pain or armoring in addition to other luo vessel symptoms. In addition, from a strategic point of view, a main goal of using the luo vessels is to bring one's sensations, moods, and involuntary reflexive-type behaviors and patterns (wei level and sinew channels) to one's consciousness so that they can be understood and assimilated. This relationship of the ying and wei is mediated by the longitudinal luo, giving us an excellent opportunity to adjust to these psycho-emotional issues. As Peter Levine states:

> [I]t is the dynamic balance between the most primitive and the most evolved/refined parts of the brain that allows trauma to be resolved and difficult emotions to be integrated and transformed.
>
> The key to this delicate undertaking is being able to safely sense both intense and subtle body sensations and feelings… Together, insula and cingulate help us make sense of these primitive sensations by weaving them into nuanced feelings, perceptions and cognitions.
>
> Restoring the balance and rhythm between instinct and reason also plays a central part in healing the mind/body split.[97]

The primary channels can also be needled as they deal with ying and wei (and yuan, to some degree) and can be added as support for luo issues, some of which mediate ying and wei (e.g., longitudinal), and others which resonate towards the yuan (transverse luo treatments with the addition of primary channel source points).

Luo vessels: Just tapping the surface

Thus far I have presented a brief introduction to the luo vessels, their functions and physiology, differentiations in terms of longitudinal and transverse luo as well as their associated symptoms, and a basic paradigm for treatment. This, however, is just tapping the surface of this channel system, and there is much more to be said about them. However, my goal is not to provide a full teaching on the luo but rather to provide enough of an orientation so that one can utilize these concepts in the treatment of Heart Shock and trauma and its sequelae. As such, there is much that must be left out in the service of staying on topic. Some of the additional uses of the luo include the energy transfer theory of the luo vessels, the use of the luo vessels for the treatment of the digestive system and its internal disorders, as well as an alternate progression theory from the sinew meridians as the wei level internalizes to the ying. I am hopeful that these will be addressed in further writings in the near future.

The use of luo vessels in treating Heart Shock

Applying all the foregoing from this chapter, I'd like to suggest a few options for the use of the luo vessels in the treatment of trauma and its varied expressions. One of the major implications of the luo and Heart Shock is that we have stagnant blood. With the help of the luo channels, we start to release that stagnant blood, which has the impact of freeing the shen, as well as the memories and deeper suppressed emotional components of the traumatic event. At times, these emotions can become overwhelming, and patients may even begin to relive some of the memories and traumas of their past. The luo vessels can help with the processing of, and moving past, these difficult emotions.

Mood, emotion, and temperament

First, we need to distinguish between mood, emotion, and temperament. One's mood is more a reflection of wei energetics and doesn't have consciousness. One may feel angry, irritated, sad, etc. and not know why. It comes over one independent of reasoning. With an emotion, one has knowledge and understanding of what is making one feel the particular emotion. As such, it has more blood (conscious awareness) attached to it and is reflective of the ying level. As the emotion is fueled by the thought process to some degree, at this stage there is also some degree of control over the emotion or, in the very least, some power of decision making allowing the emotion to be experienced. This comes from the Spleen and the contextualizing of what is making one angry, sad, etc. Temperament is generally a reflection of one's stance in the world and stems from yuan qi energetics. It is formed very early on and often stems from old repressed emotions impacting how one views the world. To some degree, there are also constitutional elements at play (e.g., wood personality whose stance in the world may be aggressive as the person feels compelled to achieve).

Utilizing this model in treatment relies on whether the patient is experiencing difficulty based on a mood, emotion, or temperament and whether she is expressing the feelings, suppressing them, or repressing them. Emotional expression utilizes the wei qi to release it, suppression relies on the ying qi and blood to contain it, and repression buries the emotions in the jing level. The wei level is associated with the Lungs and Liver, the ying level with the Spleen and Heart/Pericardium, and the yuan-jing level with the Kidneys and Triple Burner.

The emotions themselves also have associations with the elements/phases and organ systems, e.g., wood: anger; fire: anxiety, excitement, mania; earth: sympathy, pensiveness, obsessiveness; metal: grief, sorrow, sadness; and water: fear, paranoia, phobias, etc. Within this simple but effective model, one uses (needle or bleed) the luo points of the yin meridians that deal with the status of the emotions (where it is being held: expression, suppression, repression), and bleeds the yang luo point of the elemental emotion being experienced. Bleeding can be done with the lance needle and 7 star hammer, or, if the patient is too sensitive, gua sha can be used. For example, if a patient comes in expressing a lot of anger that needs to be released, the treatment based on this model would be to needle or bleed LU 7 and LR 5 (because they are expressing the emotion and aware of the mood), and bleed GB 37, the yang luo point associated with the elemental expression of anger.

Another example is a shy timid person presenting with a dark tongue, dark distended veins, Tight, Choppy pulses reflecting qi and blood stagnation, and demonstrating repressed fear with a history of abuse and trauma. A treatment option would be to needle or bleed KI 4 and SJ 5 (level of repression) and bleed BL 58 to release that fear. And as always, we are using this as an opportunity to communicate with our patients, deepen the therapeutic relationship, establish trust, and address the emotional roots of the pathology.

Diagnosing and treating the luo from the psycho-social profiles

All of the psycho-social profiles listed and detailed earlier have relevance to patients suffering from Heart Shock. From the Lungs through the Liver and into the great luos and the Ren and the Du, one will confront all of these profiles to some degree and often multiple profiles will be present in any given patient. I do, however, want to highlight some of the most common aspects.

The Lung luo has two components. With fullness, we see a lot of hyperactivity, fidgetiness of the hands, etc. from heat that has built up in the chest. This manifests with excessive touching and physical as well as emotional neediness to bond with others. The Lungs deal with wei qi and provide a boundary to the external world (skin). With fullness of the Lung luo we may see a lot of inappropriate behaviors, engaging in frequent, often unsatisfying, sexual encounters, and otherwise engaging in relationships that do not always have one's best interests at heart. As the wei qi which homes to the chest becomes stagnant and creates heat, it harasses the spirit and prevents proper internalization of the ying qi to nourish oneself. Instead, patients seek external relationships in an attempt to satisfy this need. Treating a fullness of the Lung luo by bleeding LU 7, LU 10, and PC 8 can release the stagnant qi and blood and resultant heat, allowing wei qi and ying qi to home back to the chest. As the stagnation in the chest (which is the home of wei qi) can also create muscular tension and armoring, the sinew channels can also be added to this treatment when such symptoms are present.

Emptiness of the Lung luo is often the result of traumatic experiences which were so painful as to dull and dim the spirit. We may see a loss of animation and an inability to get in touch with our senses and feel things deeply. The pain of many traumatic experiences, especially the loss of a loved one resulting in grief and sadness, can cause one to shut down emotionally. Nothing seems important, and caring can even seem dangerous as one has realized that to love and lose is too painful to risk opening one's Heart again. Using the Lung luo can assist in releasing the pain while providing the yang necessary to rekindle the animation and recharge the spirit by bringing yang back into the chest. With this treatment, I often recommend using moxibustion on LU 7 as well as PC 8 (palace of weariness), and even Ren 17, to spark the pilot light back to its original flame.

The Large Intestine, Stomach, and Spleen luo profiles are also commonly present in the clinic. Trauma often has the impact of affecting one's ability to handle stimuli. As the nervous system is often destabilized post trauma, patients often find it hard to process and assimilate lots of information. The cacophony of sounds and all the varied sights one is confronted with (think of the amount of images, colors, and sounds that one is exposed to in the course of a day; even a television show or while surfing the internet) is like an assault on one's being. The Large Intestine luo becomes easily overwhelmed, requiring repetitive attempts to process, and the eventual retreat from stimulation and inability to animate one's feelings. Typically, in these scenarios one finds lots of spider veins and broken vessels and visibility around the cheeks, especially common in children that have been traumatized. The cheeks reflect the center point between the sensory orifices with the eyes above, the ears laterally, and the nose and mouth medially. As such it has a strong impact on one's senses and the ability to clearly perceive our external world. Bleeding these luo, or with children using gentle gua sha or cupping, or creating a liniment with essential oils, can be effective in reducing this sensitivity.

This blockage in the Large Intestine luo sets the stage for pathology in the Stomach luo. Our external senses have now been impacted and our threshold for stimulation maxed out. Heat in the yangming results from this stagnation and the patient now becomes highly reactive and emotional. We may see explosive reactions and with children the whole gamut of temper tantrums and lack of control, insomnia, impulsivity, etc. In the extreme one sees the dian kuang syndrome with mania, anxiety, and bipolar syndrome as the Stomach channel reaches to the brain and crosses over to create polarity. There are also relationships to the eyes, BL 1 (confluent point for the Stomach divergent channel, and Qiao mai point), the Liver and hyperactivity of wei qi (overstimulation, anger, irritability, etc.), and the Stomach's influence over the upper portals. Ling Shu Chapter 22 on dian kuang discusses the relationship of this disorder and the portals as dian kuang is manifested through the eyes:

In the beginning of the dian disease (disorder of the head), the patient appears to be unhappy, his head is heavy, his two eyes are red and stare straight forward. When the disease is severe, the patient will have the feeling of oppression over the chest and restless. When one examines the expression between the two eyes and the eyebrows of the patient, he can predict the attack of the disease.[98]

A branch of the Stomach luo also follows the Kidney luo from the abdomen up to the chest. This branch creates symptoms akin to running piglet qi and the ability to lose control and react with extreme results from an episode of fear causing a temporary insanity and irrationality. In this scenario, treating both the Stomach and Kidney luos would be warranted.

The Spleen luo furthers this pathology by creating distorted thought processes and becoming obsessive. One's narrative has been corrupted and they cannot let go of the turbidity in their lives. On a physical level we see blockage of the intestines and drumlike swellings, as well as the overall ability to take anything of value into one's life and make it one's own. Here, bleeding SP 4 and the rest of the luo channel can be accompanied by bleeding the preceding luo channels as they set much of the backdrop for obfuscating the senses. In addition, the first trinity of ghost points can also be treated, especially with moxibustion (see Chapter 9 for a complete discussion of the 13 Ghost points).

The Heart luo becomes activated when one experiences profound disappointments, betrayals, and other causes of Heart pain. In such instances people shut down their Heart to compartmentalize their pain and wounds, and separate it from their consciousness. But of course, when we close our Heart, not only can we not let out our pain, we also can't receive love and experience happiness. The chest feels heavy, and as the lymph all drain to the thoracic duct, we also experience a phlegmatic stickiness that weights down our shen and blunts our emotions. Stickiness in the chest means one is also stuck in their painful emotions, with an inability to fully express oneself and one's shen.

Emptiness of the Heart luo is the loss of one's (inner) voice and sense of self which often comes post trauma when the individual tends to act and think/perceive differently than they used to. Often the traumas are so painful or the patient is laden with guilt that he cannot bring himself to speak about it. Bleeding HT 5 starts to free up the chest, reinvigorate blood to open the Heart, and begin circulating its blood to the outside world (remember the Heart deals with peripheral circulation). The Heart luo also goes to LU 2 after HT 1, enabling it to come back in touch with the present moment (breath and the po) and re-engage with life. From there it moves to BL 1 and ST 1 and has the capacity to change the way one views and perceives the world as it rids the sticky phlegm and occluded blood from the luo. Other organs have the ability to process damp and phlegm. The Lungs expel it, the Spleen transforms it, and the Kidneys dissolve it. But the Heart is the only one with the capacity to vaporize phlegm and allow for instantaneous healing. The channel also passes through the throat, re-establishing the connection to the voice and one's self-expression.

The Heart luo can also manifest with rate and rhythm issues. Earlier in this text I detailed the impact and importance of rate and rhythm, especially in the context of Heart Shock. Treating the Heart luo is one such method for re-establishing proper rate and rhythm by clearing the obstructions of phlegm, heat, and blood stasis.

The Bladder and Kidney luo have great usefulness in treating Heart Shock as they are implicated directly with the treatment of PTSD and fear/fright. With the Bladder we see a constant setting off of the alarm which triggers a patient back into the state of the original traumatic event as if they were reliving it. As a baseline, these patients tend to be hypervigilant and we can see a relationship here between the Bladder luo and the Bladder sinew meridian where the muscles in the sinew channels are tense and prepared for fight/flight/freeze (or weak and flaccid if Kidney yang has been sufficiently drained over time). Those with active Bladder luo issues are constantly prepared as they are always re-experiencing their traumas. Like the Gall Bladder and Lung luo, the Bladder is a descending pathway. But, unlike the Gall Bladder and Lung which seeks to release the pathogen, the Bladder looks to deposit its pathology into the Kidney, looking for comfort from its yin counterpart. As discussed above, BL 58 is bled to release fear in the expression/suppression/repression model above. Those with emptiness of the Bladder luo tend to not know their limits and often engage in behaviors that are risky or inappropriate. The ability to say no and establish proper boundaries (taiyang function or protection) is compromised and these patients can find themselves in situations that allow for further traumas, abuses, betrayals, etc. as they have a hard time defending themselves and are vulnerable targets due to their need for love and connection. The patient–practitioner relationship is of crucial importance in modeling a healthy relationship with appropriate boundaries, and the practitioner should make sure to instill a sense of power and control in the patient. Bleeding the Bladder luo helps to release the perceived threat and modulate one's response, akin to what Peter Levine terms "pendulation," wherein, as he describes, "Where before, there was overwhelming immobility and collapse, the nervous system now finds its way back toward equilibrium. We cease to perceive everything as dangerous, and gradually, step by step, the doors of perception open to new possibilities."[99]

With the Kidney luo, patients are often paranoid and extremely fearful, deeply depressed, and often go to dark places, even inflicting self-harm. They are risk takers and tend to be obsessive. Bleeding KI 4 and all the spider veins and occluded blood around the ankle is important in dredging these toxic emotions. The Kidney luo channel follows the primary channel from KI 4 up the leg and into the lower dantian and the reproductive organs. It travels upwards to Ren 14 and KI 21 where it brings that fear up to the Heart and manifests with panic attacks and running piglet qi. From here it circles back inside and dives down to the lumbar region and the constitution, embedding these toxic emotions in the source qi and impacting the Triple Burner mechanism. Earlier I discussed the role of the Triple Burner and its dissemination of yang qi up the spine into the source points of the Bladder, directing the amount of yang qi into the organ systems. At the Kidney luo, fear has now corrupted and contaminated the source, altering the Triple Burner's dissemination. And the next channels to be impacted show reclusiveness (Pericardium luo), hollowness (Triple Burner luo), despair (Gall Bladder luo), and altered personalities (Liver luo). Treating the Kidney luo via KI 4 and the channel pathway and releasing the pathogenic fear (and associated traumatic experiences) can re-establish the proper yang qi rooting and dissemination, allowing for one's personality/constitution to re-emerge.

One example of using the Kidney longitudinal luo is from a patient I treated years ago. She was in her late twenties and experienced a tremendous amount of Heart Shock throughout the course of her life (multiple instances of abuse, physical and sexual, with frequent rapes and other violent experiences). She experienced tremendous emotional pain, often had dark thoughts, was very depressed, and frequently cut herself. I explained to her the concepts of blood stagnation and toxicity as well as the blood housing the shen and emotions, and how releasing blood can also release the pent-up emotions of fear, depression, and frustration. I utilized a Kidney luo vessel treatment and taught her how to bleed the luo vessels instead of her cutting herself.[100] I created a ritual for her where she was to set a certain intention before bleeding, including where to do it, the lighting of candles, and an invoking of the purpose of what she was doing by verbalizing it to herself. One of the biggest issues I find with women and men who cut is it becomes very shameful and secretive. They tend to do it in places where you can't see (e.g., under bra straps, and places that are never exposed). By making the bleeding ritualistic and something more positive and directed towards a state of wellness and treatment, it became a healing experience rather than something shameful. The patient did this treatment a handful of times for a few months after I taught her, and only when she felt the need to cut. Very quickly it had an impact, and after bleeding her luo a few times, she ceased needing to cut herself.

The great luo of the Spleen has tremendous and varied usefulness in the treatment of Heart Shock. The dynamics of the great luo of the Spleen include the wrapping known as Da Bao which surrounds the body from front to back, much like Dai mai in the belt area. It covers the area around one's rib cage as well as much of the energetics of the diaphragm. As such it has a strong impact on blood circulation, and bleeding or needling this channel can release stagnant blood and provide a much-needed release to one suffering from trauma. As the origination point is on the earth channel (SP 21), it can serve much like a motherly embrace to a child in need of comfort.

The great luo of the Spleen has further connections as it communicates with the Bao mai, the internal channel system which connects the Heart and Kidney

(Heart to the uterus), as well as the Dai mai. In Chapter 3, I discussed one of the Classical treatment strategies for shen disturbances as addressing the relationship of the uterus to the Heart and brain with emotional disturbances. The great luo of the Spleen, with its connection to Bao mai, provides us with one opportunity to address this linkage. As the Bao mai also connects with and links up to the Dai mai, one has a powerful energetic circuit in which to tap into and treat all the emotional and physical implications that trauma has on the Heart, diaphragm, ribs, pelvis, and communication between the Heart and Kidneys. Very often one will find spider veins and broken blood vessels throughout this area. I have found over the years that tapping into this trinity of channels can have a very powerful impact on releasing blood stagnation from all three burners while simultaneously calming the shen, relieving tension, and providing a much-needed grounding.

It should be noted that originally the great luo of the Spleen's luo point was GB 22. In Chapter 4, I discussed a bit about the dynamics of this point as a meeting point of the yin arm sinew channels and its importance in treating pain, internalized pathogens, Heart pathology, etc. In the divergent chapter, one will also learn about the importance of this point as a confluent point on the Small Intestine/ Heart divergent channel, its relationship to blood, fluid (and hormonal), and lymph dynamics as well. Commonly, when I treat the great luo of the Spleen, I will either include both GB 22 and SP 21 or treat whichever is more reactive (sensitivity or visibility) or which point dynamics/functions are most appropriate to the strategies I am employing in any given treatment.

Whether we're looking at the luo point being GB 22 or SP 21, the general dynamic of this channel is that it wraps all the way around the chest and back, and from Ren 15 goes down into the uterus (connecting with Bao mai) and then wraps around the waist (with its connection to Dai mai). As mentioned, it creates a communication between the Heart and Kidneys, deals with mental-emotional issues, and can clear heat that has been harassing the Heart. Opening up the Dai mai portion of this relationship allows qi to ground and root in the abdomen by releasing the stagnation preventing this. This can prevent qi rising up and running piglet syndrome. One should also remember, and more will be discussed in Chapter 8, that the original Dai mai consisted of wrapping around the waist with SP 15 and ST 25 (LR 13 and GB 27–28 were added later in history). Thus, utilizing the Dai mai with the great luo of the Spleen can release more stagnant fluids and blood (Gall Bladder 27–28) or secure more qi and consolidate with SP 15 and ST 25. Either treatment should start with needling or bleeding SP 21 and/or GB 22, Ren 15, and KI 16, as well as Ren 2 (or Ren 3). From there we can utilize the Dai mai component and open up with GB 41 (left for men, right for women), followed by points on the Dai mai (or other Gall Bladder points such as GB 34 which has a strong dynamic on treating/releasing the chest). Here is where, if one uses SP 21 as the luo point, one can also choose to add in GB 22. And if there are signs of visibility on the chest and/or diaphragm, I often will add in LR 14 or GB 24 to the treatment.

The great luo of the Stomach also has a relationship to the diaphragm and as such helps to mediate blood circulation from the abdomen to the chest. The diaphragm is also a location that can shut itself down (under the direction of the Liver) to prevent passage into the internal organs. The Stomach's great luo is located right near LR 14 on the left side by the apex of the Heart and can also be implicated when heat in the Liver (from stress, suppressed emotions, hypervigilance, etc.) harasses the Heart. As the area of LR 14 also communicates to the Lung channel (exit-entry), this channel will also have a direct relationship on the energetics of the Lung system, including regulation of the heartbeat (both the Liver and Lung's relationship to wei qi). Symptoms that are typically present are tachycardia and arrhythmias, irregular breathing, rapid breathing, chest congestion, and congestive heart failure. The great luo of the Stomach can be bled to release the suppressed stagnation and toxic heat that has accumulated, help to calm the Heart and shen, and invigorate blood throughout the diaphragm and chest.

The other luo channels play a vital role as well (e.g., the Small Intestine luo and trusting oneself, the Triple Burner luo with fixed attitudes, indifference, and depression, the Gall Bladder luo and despair, and the Liver luo and destructive behavior), but the foregoing are the ones I most often use clinically. Treating those channels mentioned in the parentheses is done in the same manner as the others: bleeding the luo points and following the methods outlined above for fullness or emptiness. All of the aforementioned psycho-social profiles within this chapter can be sufficient diagnostic evidence to warrant treating the luo vessels they represent. The more corroborating signs one perceives, however, e.g., luo vessel pulses, visibility, and physical symptoms of the longitudinal luo (including rebellious qi symptoms) and transverse luo, the more pressing the body and mind are directing one to treat with this channel system. One has multiple diagnostic parameters within the luo channels with which to interpret a luo pathology and whether or not one would prioritize the luo (over another channel system) in treatment.

Using the luo vessels in the treatment of physical trauma

The luo vessels, like the sinew channels, have a place in the treatment of pain and physical traumas. It is important to remember, however, that they do not enter the joints themselves. Nonetheless, their use in treating pain from injuries can significantly aid the healing mechanisms. At the onset of a traumatic injury, wei qi and yang qi respond by traveling to the site of injury which causes a certain degree of inflammation. Ying qi also responds bringing blood and fluids to the area, and this results in swelling. When one is prepared for a trauma (i.e., has time to brace for an impact, or is aware of an impending surgery), wei qi will already be at the surface. When a trauma happens accidentally, and one is unprepared, wei qi will need to be mobilized to the area and the body responds more slowly. In this case it may take a bit longer for a bruise to become manifest. In the initial stages of a traumatic injury, the goal is to speed up the healing process by mobilizing blood and fluids to the area to protect and stabilize the injured area. The next stage of healing is to eliminate the buildup of fluids and blood by invigorating it away, reducing pain and inflammation, and restoring normal physiology.

As discussed in Chapter 4, often injuries can combine with a climatic component (usually some combination of wind, cold, or damp) when wei qi is weak. There is usually a predominance of one over the other, and the needling technique is different. With a predominance of wind you tend to needle the point, reduce it, get de qi, and remove the needle; with damp, you needle followed by moxa on top to dry the damp; and with cold you tend to use direct or indirect moxa over the point. Then one tonifies wei qi. And we never use ice as it has the nature of contracting and constricting and our goal is to facilitate circulation to allow for healing to take place. We can, however, use some type of alcohol-based liniment to invigorate the blood, warm the channels, disperse the wind, etc. by massaging with circular movement, increasing the circumference to assist with dissipating it. When pain is just due to climatic factors, a sinew treatment is sufficient. When it is chronic (implicates blood), then the luo becomes instrumental in the treatment.

When approaching physical trauma it is best to treat both the sinews and the luo as we want to bring blood to the area. To accomplish this, one should needle the luo point that relates to the affected sinew meridian toward the site of the injury with a tonification technique to bring blood there. Next, one needles the point proximal to the he-sea, to regulate the blood within that channel. This is followed by the sinew channel treatment and described in the following example:

A patient presents with shoulder pain near LI 15 area and is worse with damp, and aggravated when the arm is extended and rotated. From the previous chapter we would associate this with a shaoyang pathology of the Triple Burner sinew channel. As the injury is on the LI channel one should needle the LI luo point, LI 6 (with tonification), towards LI 15, to bring blood to the injured site, followed by needling LI 12 (one point proximal to the he-sea) to regulate blood (with an even technique). At this point, the sinew treatment would be added and would consist of local ashi point needling, needling obstructions along the channel and areas of knotting, along with releasing the Triple Burner jing-well point, SJ 1. And because damp is involved, we can utilize moxa.

The second stage, as the injury begins to heal, requires that we move blood away from the area. One can plum blossom or needle with a strong dispersal technique on the luo point of the affected sinew channel, LI 6 in the example above, in addition to needling or plum blossoming away from the site of the injury. Next, one needles one point proximal to the he-sea point to regulate the blood and follows with the rest of the sinew treatment. The sinew part of the treatment remains the same, while adding in the luo vessel aspect of either bringing blood to the area or trying to disperse blood away from the area as needed.

Luo vessels for pain from traumatic injury protocol

1. Determine the sinew channel involved.
2. Determine the type of movement that exacerbates pain (see Chapter 4).
3. Needle the luo point on the affected sinew channel:
   a. Towards the area of pain for the initial stage
   b. Away from the area of pain for the secondary stage.
4. Needle one point proximal to the he-sea point of the affected channel.
5. Needle ashi points.
6. Needle the jing-well point that relates to the movement which causes pain.

Using the luo vessels for pain from emotional trauma

Pain is not always from physical trauma; often it has an emotional origin. Treatment is very similar to that for pain from physical trauma, without the need to evaluate for any type of climatic factor. Instead, we are to utilize the bloodletting of the yang luo point related to the suspected emotional issue. For example, if we suspect that fear is the root cause of the pain, we would bloodlet BL 58; if it was anger that was relating to the pain then we can do GB 37. We're treating the emotions from the yang luo channels just as in the model discussed above with the expression, suppression, and repression aspects of releasing the mood/emotion/temperament. Using the same example above, with pain at LI 15, here we are determining the root as being from an emotional origin of grief and sadness. Like above, needling or plum blossoming LI 6, plus needling LI 12 to harmonize the blood, followed by needling ashi points, and ending with bleeding LI 6 (yang channel related to emotion of sadness and grief) (already being bled due to channel trajectory).

Luo vessels for pain from emotional injury protocol

1. Determine the sinew channel involved.
2. Needle the luo point on the sinew channel affected.
3. Needle one point proximal to the he-sea point.
4. Needle ashi points.
5. Bleed the yang luo point associated with the emotional root cause of the pain.

Using the luo vessels to treat personality disorders

Personality disorders are characterized by internal shifts causing changes in one's personality or behavior. This can be due to genetics, extreme mental and emotional stress, or traumas that block the typical dissemination of jing and irrigation to the Bladder shu points. From a Chinese medicine perspective we see a breakdown in the communication between the Heart and Kidneys. Our Heart governs the curriculum of our lives, and when our desires and actions are not being used to express our internal nature we see the backdrop of pathology develop. Alternatively, one may have diminished resources/water to create new possibilities, resulting in frustrations and irritability. Early signs of the Heart and Kidneys not communicating include insomnia (reflecting the inability to quiet our desires) and lower back pain (demonstrating a lack of structure and integrity in how we stand up to ourselves and the world).

A model that can be used for accessing the level of the blood to treat shifts in one's personality incorporates the Bladder back shu points. The Bladder shu points that deal with blood, carrying the shen and one's experiences of life, are related to the Spleen, Liver, and Heart. They also help to treat the visceral agitation (zang zao) that often leads to psychological and emotional imbalances. The Bladder shu points represent the unfolding of water (yang of water) which assists in irrigating the dryness associated with zang zao. The treatment includes the use of BL 20, BL 18, and BL 15, which are Classical points to treat visceral dryness (which shares a similarity to personality disorders).

In addition to these three points, points to impact the level of blood and one's consciousness can be used. Pericardium channel points can be used to address the specific profiles presented. The Heart and Pericardium have nine points and they associate to the "nine Heart pains." In a very simplistic way Heart pain can refer to some type of trauma to the Heart which has shifted one's behavior. The use of Pericardium points helps one to work out and manage the stress/trauma. Additionally, we open treatment with either bleeding HT 5 (used when there has not been any external trauma) or ST 40 (for when there has been some external trauma).

The treatment begins with bleeding either HT 5 or ST 40, followed by needling of BL 15, BL 18, and BL 20 to reorient the blood and assist the patient with shifting his perspective. BL 15 is known to calm the shen, treat bipolar disorder and manic-depressiveness, palpitations, insomnia, etc. BL 18 can treat visceral agitation, epilepsy, mania, dementia and loss of memory, confusion, as well as calming the shen, and nourishing and invigorating blood. BL 20 is for a person who is lethargic, distrustful of others, uncaring, disengaged, etc. BL 23 can also be added to these points for its association with the Kidneys and water and the source of the Triple Burner's dissemination. Direct moxa from the top to bottom of these shu points can be done as well to use heat to clear heat from the organs. Three to seven cones are used, and if that doesn't provide sufficient results, one can moxa until the area becomes red and irritated (use burn cream to prevent burning the skin) to keep the area stimulated. The appropriate Pericardium point can be added based on the profiles as noted below.

Pericardium points based on psychological profile[101]

Pericardium 8: Kidney and paranoia/distrust of others

Pericardium 5: Heart and the egoistic personality (narcissist)

Pericardium 4: Spleen and the schizoid personality (detachment)

Pericardium 7: Lung and the avoidance personality (vulnerability)

Pericardium 6: Liver and the borderline personality (impulsive/self-destructive)

The luo vessels and Wang Qing-ren's cardiovascular model

In Part I, I referenced Wang Qing-ren and his theories on the physiology of blood circulation. These concepts are applicable to luo vessel treatments for Heart Shock, as one of our main strategies is to address blood stagnation. Wang Qing-ren lived in the 18th century and was one of the first practitioners to integrate Chinese and Western medicine. Wang Qing-ren saw luo circulation as describing basic aspects of the cardiovascular system, with the Heart being responsible for arterial circulation, and the Pericardium for venous circulation. He also noticed a very intimate relationship between the curious organs and cardiovascular issues, in particular the connection of the brain with Heart pathology, which of course is mediated through the blood vessels as another curious organ. We also have a connection between the blood and the Spleen, which makes the gu qi and ascends it to the chest and Heart for final production into blood, and then circulates it to the Liver for storage via the Pericardium, its jueyin pair.

A treatment option applying this is to needle SP 21, HT 1, and then LR 13 to assist in the Spleen's production and ascension to the Heart as well as its storage in the Liver. Thus we can promote blood production, management, and storage to accompany a whole host of other presentations. One can also combine this basic building block protocol with other points, depending on other diagnoses. For example, if a patient presents with peripheral circulation symptoms (e.g., Raynaud's syndrome or poor circulation secondary to physical traumas) such as pain, cold hands and feet, numbness of the extremities, etc., HT 5 can be bled and its luo channel treated (spider veins identified, bleeding or plum blossoming to stimulate wei qi and release wind, etc.). PC 6 is used for more systemic circulatory issues within the chest itself, e.g., angina or plaque. One can tonify Ren 15 if there's a yin deficiency underlying or do moxa on Du 1 to strengthen yang qi. If one is treating issues of peripheral circulation (with HT 5), the treatment is ended with LU 7 as it deals with wei qi which helps set the rhythm for the heart rate (see Part I). If treating a more systemic or internal circulation, one uses PC 6 and ends with GB 37, which travels to ST 42 creating a relationship with the Chong mai to strengthen and solidify treatment. Tying in the brain with shen disturbances, ST 40 goes to the brain via Du 20 in terms of its luo vessel trajectory and also addresses the shen. So, one can always add the Stomach luo to treatments if there are psycho-emotional symptoms present.

As a case example, a patient presents with palpitations, insomnia, anxiety, Changing Amplitude and Intensity over the entire pulse, Feeble left distal position, and heart rate of 50 bpm 30 years after the trauma of her mom suddenly dying. As the Heart qi is deficient, one can needle/moxa Du 1 to tonify the qi, bleed/7-star/gua sha HT 5 and treat the rest of the Heart's luo channel (potentially adding moxa), needle SP 21, HT 1, and LR 13, and bleed LU 7.

Cardiovascular treatment model

1 Bleed HT 5 (peripheral circulation) or PC 6 (systemic)
2 Bleed, needle, or moxa either Du 1 (yang deficiency) or Ren 15 (yin deficiency)
3 Needle and retain SP 21, HT 1, and LR 13
4 Bleed either LU 7 (if HT 5 is used) or GB 37 (if PC 6 is used)

Luo vessel herbal formulas: Invigorating the spirit, changing perceptions

Luo vessel theory lends itself readily to herbal medicine, and much of its focus is on addressing blood stagnation and its sequelae.

Wang Qing-ren

As discussed just above, Wang Qing-ren was instrumental in breathing life back into the luo vessel theories and applications. This was particularly evident in his contributions to herbal medicine. A number of his formulas are applicable to the treatment of trauma and have a strong focus on invigorating blood. Below are a few of these influential formulas.

Xue Fu Zhu Yu Tang (Drive Out Stasis in the Mansion of Blood Decoction)

Tao Ren
Hong Hua
Chuan Xiong

Dang Gui
Sheng Di Huang
Chi Shao
Chai Hu
Zhi Ke
Gan Cao
Chuan Niu Xi
Jie Geng

Xue Fu Zhu Yu Tang is the archetypical formula for blood stasis in the chest with impaired circulation above the diaphragm. This pattern is complicated with Liver qi stagnation and prevention of the clear yang of the Stomach from rising as well as descension of the Stomach's turbidity. The stasis in the chest and the obstruction in the diaphragm prevent the proper communication of the Liver to the Heart (the Liver's blood being essential to the production of the Heart's qi) and can manifest in mental-emotional symptoms. Often there will be symptoms of chest and rib pain, headaches, insomnia, palpitations, depression and irritability, etc. From our Heart Shock perspective, we can see many of the treatment strategies at play, including: nourishment of Heart yin (Sheng Di Huang), invigorating the blood (Tao Ren, Hong Hua, Chuan Xiong, Chi Shao, Chuan Niu Xi), regulating qi in the chest (Chuan Xiong, Chai Hu, Zhi Ke, Jie Geng), strengthening Heart qi (Gan Cao, Dang Gui, and Sheng Di Huang via Liver blood ascending to nourish Heart qi), clearing heat and calming the shen (Sheng Di Huang, Chi Shao), and regulating the Spleen and Stomach (Zhi Ke, Chai Hu, Gan Cao). This formula is easily modified to accommodate other signs and symptoms as well as adjusting dosages to highlight or prioritize other treatment strategies.

Xue Fu Zhu Yu Tang can also be considered an archetypal luo vessel formula with a strong influence on invigorating blood in the Liver and Pericardium (jueyin), chest, and diaphragm. As these areas are primary influencers of blood circulation systemically, Xue Fu Zhu Yu Tang can be used to treat a wide range of disorders. As a luo vessel formula, its actions have similarity to the great luo of the Spleen. Earlier, I discussed the use of the luo vessels in treating specific emotional states, e.g., anger, sadness, etc. This formula can also be used in a similar manner. The formula's actions can be modified and enhanced to treat any of the five emotions by simply adding in directionality via herbal substitutions and additions or changes in dosage. For example, if the prevailing emotion is sadness, which depresses and weakens the qi, herbs to strengthen and/or lift the qi like Zhi Ke, Huang Qi, Jie Geng, etc. can be added and/or increased in dosage. Or if anger is dominating, using herbs to descend like Niu Xi (increase dosage), Xiang Fu, Mu Dan Pi, etc. can be incorporated. Thus, one is able to treat the root blood stasis condition as well as the specific emotional manifestation in order to ease the patient's suffering.

Tong Qiao Huo Xue Tang (Unblock the Orifices and Invigorate the Blood Decoction)

Tao Ren
Hong Hua
Chi Shao
Chuan Xiong
Cong Bai
Da Zao
Sheng Jiang
She Xiang

Tong Qiao Huo Xue Tang treats the accumulation of blood stasis in the head, face, and upper body. One may experience headaches, vertigo, hair loss, purplish discolorations, chronic disorders with underlying blood stasis and exhaustion of blood, dark eyes and complexion, etc. Analyzing the formula, one can see that a number of our Heart Shock strategies are missing, so modifying this would be warranted, but it can make up the base of a formula and be very suitable with some alterations, namely adding herbs to nourish Heart yin as well as to calm the shen. What this formula does have that the previous formula does not, however, is a herb to open the orifices (She Xiang), as Wang Qing-ren is attempting to affect the circulation of the head and release obstructions.

Ge Xia Zhu Yu Tang (Drive Out Blood Stasis below Diaphragm Decoction)

Chao Wu Ling Zhi
Dang Gui
Chuan Xiong
Tao Ren
Mu Dan Pi
Chi Shao
Wu Yao
Yan Hu Suo
Gan Cao
Xiang Fu
Hong Hua
Zhi Ke

Ge Xia Zhu Yu Tang treats blood stasis and Liver qi stagnation below the diaphragm with painful abdomen, including palpable masses that may be visible when lying down. As with the prior formula, we are lacking many of the necessary treatment strategies to classify this as a Heart Shock formula, but it is easily modified to accommodate that diagnosis by adding herbs to nourish Heart yin and strengthen Kidney yang. In this formula Gui Zhi and/or Rou Gui would be a good addition for the Kidney and Heart qi, Gan Cao can be substituted with Zhi Gan Cao to further strengthen the Heart and Kidneys, and one can add an additional herb for Heart yin such as Bai He which will also calm the shen and release emotions such as sadness and grief which trap qi and blood in the diaphragmatic area.

Shao Fu Zhu Yu Tang (Drive Out Blood Stasis in Lower Abdomen Decoction)

Chao Xiao Hui Xiang
Chao Gan Jiang
Yan Hu Suo
Dang Gui
Chuan Xiong
Mo Yao
Guan Gui
Chi Shao
Pu Huang
Chao Wu Ling Zhi

Shao Fu Zhu Yu Tang treats blood stasis accumulating in the lower abdomen with palpable abdominal masses, painful menstruation with dark blood and clots, low back pain, etc. It is an excellent formula that warms and moves the blood, but one that only addresses some of our Heart Shock strategies. Using this formula is part of the symptomatic presentation only when blood stasis in the pelvis is secondary to trauma. Otherwise, one must modify it accordingly, or, alternatively, use some other modality to address the other strategies, e.g., essential oils, dietary therapy, acupuncture, etc.

Shen Tong Zhu Yu Tang (Drive Out Blood Stasis from a Painful Body Decoction)

Qing Jiao
Chuan Xiong
Tao Ren
Hong Hua
Gan Cao
Qiang Huo
Mo Yao
Dang Gui

Ling Zhi
Xiang Fu
Chuan Niu Xi
Di Long

Shen Tong Zhu Yu Tang treats blood stasis throughout the body manifesting with bi-syndrome in the joints with symptoms such as low back pain, chest pain, joint and limb pain, etc. Like the previous formula, however, many of our Heart Shock strategies are lacking and one needs to modify this to make it appropriate for trauma as the etiology of the blood stasis and bi-syndrome.

Luo vessel formula base

The general marking of a luo vessel herbal formula is one that should have an impact on the level of blood and the jin-ye. To a large degree, these formulas prioritize the treatment of blood stasis, but they can also regulate the fluid dynamic as well. And as part of the sheng-hua theory (an important theory within gynecology), whenever one moves the blood, one should nourish it, and whenever one nourishes the blood, one should move it. So, ideally, herbs that invigorate should be combined with herbs that nourish the blood. This is important, as blood stagnation results in deficiency as well as damage to the tissues which rely on the blood and jin-ye for its continued nourishment. Likewise, blood deficiency leads to stagnation and the accumulation of toxins and gases as discussed in Part I. Looking at one of the most famous of blood formulas, Si Wu Tang (Four Substance Decoction), we see a blend of these two treatment strategies inherent within.

Si Wu Tang (Four Substance Decoction)

Shu Di Huang
Dang Gui
Bai Shao
Chuan Xiong

Thus, Si Wu Tang can serve as the basis for the creation of a luo vessel formula. This formula serves doubly the purposes of Heart Shock as it also contains additional treatment strategies, such as nourishing yin (Shu Di Huang and Bai Shao), calming the nervous system (Bai Shao and Chuan Xiong) and, to some degree, the shen (Bai Shao), regulating qi in the chest (Chuan Xiong), and nourishing Heart qi (here, indirectly with Dang Gui, Bai Shao, and Shu Di Huang nourishing Liver blood and moving it to the chest with Chuan Xiong). Additional treatment strategies that still require attention include opening the orifices, strengthening the Spleen and Stomach, and nourishing/anchoring Kidney yang. Adding Si Jun Zi Tang (Four Gentlemen Decoction) and creating Ba Zhen Tang (Eight Treasure Decoction) can provide some of these strategies, e.g., strengthening Heart and Kidney yang (Ren Shen and Zhi Gan Cao) and strengthening the Spleen and Stomach (Bai Zhu, Fu Ling, Zhi Gan Cao).

Si Jun Zi Tang (Four Gentlemen Decoction)

| Ren Shen |
| Bai Zhu |
| Fu Ling |
| Zhi Gan Cao |

Ba Zhen Tang (Eight Treasure Decoction)

| Shu Di Huang |
| Dang Gui |
| Bai Shao |
| Chuan Xiong |
| Ren Shen |
| Bai Zhu |
| Fu Ling |
| Zhi Gan Cao |
| (Sheng Jiang) |
| (Da Zao) |

With the additions of Sheng Jiang and Da Zao, we can also strengthen the relationship of the formula to the regulation of the ying and wei levels (Sheng Jiang) and also help nourish more blood, while calming the spirit (Da Zao). Both of these additions assist the Spleen and Stomach to digest and assimilate the formula more easily, especially as Shu Di Huang can be cloying for those with weak digestive systems.

Ba Zhen Tang can be modified in numerous ways to highlight any of the various treatment strategies within a Heart Shock diagnosis. Simply by tweaking dosages, one can prioritize blood movement or nourishment or strengthening of Heart or Kidney qi-yang, or regulating the Spleen and Stomach. Additionally, any of these herbs can be replaced with other herbs that have similar functions and also satisfy additional strategies. For example, Yu Jin can be used in place of any of the blood movers, and this will also add in a treatment strategy of opening the orifices of the Heart. It can also simply be added to the formula. Similarly, Fu Ling can be replaced with Yuan Zhi and Shi Chang Pu which also harmonize the middle jiao and transform turbidity while also opening the orifices, calming the shen, and quieting the spirit, while additionally providing communication between the Heart and Kidneys. To create an even stronger impact on calming the spirit, while also maintaining focus on invigorating the blood and qi within the channels and connecting vessels, we can substitute Dang Gui with Dang Gui Wei and also replace Shu Di Huang with Ji Xue Teng and/or Ye Jiao Teng. The amount of modifications is almost limitless and only restricted by one's creativity and the herbs one stocks in the clinic pharmacy.

Looking at some of the representative formulas like Si Wu Tang and Ba Zhen Tang as models that can be modified and altered to suit the specific needs of our diagnoses is very helpful. We must simply understand the strategies at play within any of these formulas and utilize herbs that serve the manifold functions we seek within those strategies.

There is another trio of herbs that is also commonly used to provide access to the luo vessels. These herbs include: Tan Xiang, Dan Shen, and Sha Ren; they make up the Classical formula Dan Shen Yin (Salvia Decoction). Collectively, these three open the chest to release the qi dynamic (Tan Xiang), clear heat and invigorate blood in the chest and soothe irritability (Dan Shen: Liver, Heart, and Pericardium), as well as strengthening the Spleen and Stomach, manage the fluids, and address its transformation and turbidity (Sha Ren). This trio can be used as a base formula to drive the overall energetics toward the luo vessels, and modified according to the other strategies of Heart Shock. It can also be added directly to the Ba Zhen Tang formula above or modified within it.

Dan Shen Yin (Salvia Decoction)

Dan Shen	30g
Tan Xiang	4.5g
Sha Ren	4.5g

Formulas for traumatic injuries

As described in Part I, traumatic injuries that are chronic and repetitive can have significant sequelae, over time consuming the Heart qi, impacting the Lung and wei qi circulation, and damaging the blood circulation. Symptoms of Heart qi deficiency are common, as are a number of other signs of taxation over time. The following formula is used for such a situation wherein blood dryness and stagnation have accumulated causing chronic diseases with underlying weakness to the organ systems, as well as yuan qi.

Da Huang Zhe Chong Wan (Rhubarb and Eupolyphaga Pill)

Da Huang	300g
Tu Bie Chong	30g
Tao Ren	60g
Gan Qi	30g
Qi Cao	60g
Shui Zhi	60g
Meng Chong	60g
Huang Qin	60g
Xing Ren	60g
Sheng Di Huang	300g
Bai Shao	120g
Gan Cao	90g

Da Huang Zhe Chong Wan strongly prioritizes breaking up blood stasis while also generating new blood. My colleague Brandt Stickley describes the formula as treating "excesses" that have led to a state of extreme deficient taxation, the bugs acting on behalf of the earth to digest all of the stagnation which eventually gets liberated by Da Huang.[102] Freeing up the blood stagnation, engendering new blood, and eliminating the taxation on the Heart and organ systems, Da Huang Zhe Chong Wan can be used in severe cases of Heart Shock from traumatic injury with damage to the blood circulation, causing emaciation, extreme fatigue, weakness, skin disorders, and of course pain. Its robust dosage of Sheng Di Huang and Bai Shao make sure to protect the yin and blood while invigorating, but care should be used with this formula due to the strong nature of its ingredients.

Fu Yuan Huo Xue Tang (Revive Health by Invigorating the Blood Decoction)

Dang Gui	9g
Tao Ren	9g
Hong Hua	6g
Chuan Shan Jia (substitute with Wang Bu Liu Xing or Lu Lu Tong)	6g
Ji Zhi Da Huang	30g

Tia Hua Fen	9g
Chai Hu	15g
Gan Cao	6g

Another formula to treat traumatic injuries, Fu Yuan Huo Xue Tang strongly invigorates the blood to overcome blood stasis, especially when trauma occurs to the chest, hypochondria, and flank. Additional herbs will be needed to round out this formula to accommodate a full Heart Shock protocol. Yin is moistened by Tian Hua Fen (the Lung and Stomach, so additional herbs can be used to bring yin to the Heart), and with the amount of blood invigoration, herbs to strengthen Heart and Kidney qi should be incorporated, as should herbs to impact the portals.

Dang Gui Si Ni Tang (Tangkuei Decoction for Frigid Extremities)

Dang Gui	9g
Gui Zhi	9g
Bai Shao	9g
Xi Xin	3g
Zhi Gan Cao	6g
Da Zao	25pcs
Mu Tong/ Tong Cao	6g

Dang Gui Si Ni Tang is used for blood deficiency and cold in the channels with cold hands and feet from poor circulation, as well as joint pain, menstrual irregularities, etc. It can be used in the context of Heart Shock where long-term stagnation from traumatic injuries damages the circulation. Additional nourishment to Heart yin can be warranted, as can further Kidney yang tonification as needed (Xi Xin warms the yang). The chest is opened with Gui Zhi and Mu Tong, blood nourished by Dang Gui, Bai Shao, and Da Zao, and invigorated by Dang Gui, Gui Zhi, and Mu Tong, the Spleen and Stomach addressed with Zhi Gan Cao and Da Zao, the portals opened by Xi Xin, and the nervous system calmed by Bai Shao.

Luo vessels and essential oils

The use of essential oils can be very powerful in the treatment of Heart Shock and there are many ways one can specifically address luo vessel energetics with this modality. As essential oils are the life-blood of the plants, they have a strong resonance to the blood and ying level. With an understanding of the acupuncture energetics as well as the functions and uses of essential oils, the combinations and possibilities for using oils on the luo points and channels are diverse. Below are some suggestions, many of which have come from Jeffrey Yuen's teachings and been utilized by me (and others) over the years.

With essential oils we want to create signatures that resonate with the level of blood. Generally, for a fullness condition of the longitudinal luo, a base formula would include myrrh; if there's an emptiness, parsley. Other oils to choose from include ones that affect the blood such as frankincense, styrax, cumin, litsea, camphor, etc.

To use the oils, one most often creates a blend, typically a 6–8 percent dilution for luo vessel energetics. The carrier oil I typically use is safflower oil as it will invigorate the blood. Occasionally, especially with an injury that involves redness and swelling which implicates involvement of the luo, I will mix the safflower oil with rice wine or grain alcohol to potentiate its impact on invigorating the blood. And as luo formulas promote internal movement of blood, adding oils to promote elimination, usually via the bowels or urinary tract, can be helpful. If the patient experiences constipation, the blend can be used as a compress to help descend qi and induce peristaltic activity, and the oils can be massaged in with strong acupressure to encourage movement. The luo blend can be applied to the luo points and the implicated channels, especially over areas of visibility. If there are nodules (emptiness of the luo), oils to treat phlegm stasis should be used such as grapefruit, bay laurel, eucalyptus smithii, eucalyptus polybractea, etc. Caulophyllum (tamanu) can also be used as a carrier oil to break up stagnation and scar tissue if any is present.

There are a number of factors that should be considered when choosing oils and strategies for the blend. The first is whether or not there are deep-seated wounds involved, typically from an internal pathogen or trauma; if so, resins are included within the blend. Second, one must assess the quality and quantity of blood as a resource and choose oils that nourish and move the blood accordingly. Common oils to nourish the blood include angelica seed, carrot seed, savory, thyme geraniol, geranium, etc. Third, if there is a fullness condition of the luo, we should determine if there is any blood heat and, if so, add oils to cool the blood. Oils that can accomplish this are rose and vetiver, helichrysum, ylang ylang, clary sage, melissa, mimosa, etc.

Once the blend is created, it is applied to the luo points and impacted channels.

Essential oil strategies for luo vessels

- Resonate to the level of the luo:
  - Fullness: myrrh
    - If blood heat present, add oils to cool blood: rose, vetiver, helichrysum/everlast, ylang ylang, clary sage, melissa, mimosa
  - Emptiness: parsley

- – If blood deficiency, nourish blood: angelica, carrot seed, savory, thyme geraniol, geranium
  - – If nodules, add grapefruit, bay laurel, eucalyptus smithii, etc.
  - ○ Other oils include: frankincense, styrax, cumin, litsea, camphor
- • Resins for deep-seated wounds and traumas: myrrh, elemi, benzoin, etc.
- • Other oils for trauma strategies:
  - ○ Communicating Heart (yin) and Kidney: rose, geranium, clary sage
  - ○ Strengthen Kidney yang: fennel, cinnamon bark
  - ○ Open portals: eucalyptus, rosalina, basil, peppermint, angelica archangel
  - ○ Calm the nervous system: chamomile, orange, rosemary, lavender.

Different essential oils can have resonance with specific luo points, allowing one to create a signature blend with certain characteristics or personalities. Thus, blends can be tailored to the psycho-social profiles of a Lung luo or Spleen luo, etc. These associations are listed below.

Essential oils for specific luo points/channels

LU 7:

Fullness: ravensara, myrtle

Emptiness: pine

LI 6:

Fullness: orange, tea tree

Emptiness: clove

ST 40:

Fullness: mimosa

Emptiness: cedarwood

SP 4:

Fullness: rosewood, ho leaf

Emptiness: violet

HT 5:

Fullness: lemon verbena

Emptiness: violet

SI 7:

Fullness: onion

Emptiness: cumin

BL 58:

Fullness: styrax

Emptiness: basil

KI 4:

Fullness: niaouli

Emptiness: anise seeds

PC 6:

Fullness: melissa

Emptiness: clary sage

SJ 5:

Fullness: petitgrain

Emptiness: thyme thujanol

GB 37:

Fullness: rosemary

Emptiness: vetiver

LR 5:

Fullness: German chamomile, turmeric

Emptiness: carrot seed

SP 21:

    Fullness: rose

    Emptiness: oakmoss, cumin

Ren 15:

    Fullness: sandalwood

    Emptiness: niaouli

Du 1:

    Fullness: fennel, larch

    Emptiness: spikenard

CHAPTER 6

Primary Channels and Five Element Model

The primary channel perspective within mainstream acupuncture is much more familiar than the secondary vessels, and as such requires perhaps less of an introduction and background. Each channel system, according to modern acupuncture, has its own functions and indications, though of course each channel has numerous interrelationships. For the purposes of this book, detailed exploration of the primary channels is unwarranted; however, to orient one towards their usage in the treatment of Heart Shock, I will briefly explore the main energetic functions of each of the primary channels, then present the most common points that I use in the treatment of trauma.

As the Five Phases theory for many is embedded within their understanding of the primary channel system, I will also touch on the Five Phases character traits and their psychology. The psychology of Chinese medicine is a profound topic and one that cannot be discussed without referencing a major contribution on this subject, Dr. Leon Hammer's *Dragon Rises, Red Bird Flies* (hereinafter "DRRBF"). In addition to being one of the foremost experts in Chinese medicine and Chinese pulse diagnosis, Dr. Hammer is also a psychiatrist. His experience as an expert in both the fields of Western psychiatry and Chinese medicine has allowed him to expand upon the more basic concepts elaborated in the traditional Five Phases.

Based upon my training with Dr. Hammer, I will elaborate on the Five Phases theories while explaining their emotional components.[103] It should be noted that there are many psychological models within Chinese medicine, and what I am describing is but a piece of the larger whole. As I have begun presenting (and will continue in the following two chapters on the divergent meridians and 8x channels), each channel system has its unique psychological profiles. I am placing the Five Phases and DRRBF models within the primary channel chapter to differentiate them from the secondary vessels, though one will see some overlap does exist. Also of note is that the DRRBF personality types tend to develop early in life (even in utero with Water phase insults) as adaptive responses to challenges faced. Thus, they mark, to a large degree, experiences and adaptations to normal development. These play an important role when looking at the organ system and Five Phases personalities via the lens of Heart Shock, in which often these personality types are more severe and entrenched.

A Classical Daoist approach (via the teachings of Jeffrey Yuen) on using the primary channels is one that sees the movement through the primary channels as a continuum and progression of illness from its most exterior aspect, the Lungs, to its deepest, the Liver, wherein pathology moves into the jing and impacts one's next incarnation. I will briefly present an overview of this approach, as well as the overall nature of the three trinities combined within, i.e., the first trinity (LU/LI/ST/SP), the second (HT/SI/BL/KI), and the third (PC/SJ/GB/LR).

Thus, the first part of this chapter will briefly discuss the energetics of the primary channels from modern acupuncture, followed by the continuum approach, the Five Phases, and DRRBF emotional character traits. Within this section, I will offer acupuncture point suggestions for the treatment of Heart Shock, the bolded ones reflecting my more commonly chosen points. Second, I will present specific treatment ideas from Sun Si-miao and Ge Hong that I have found useful over the years. Next, a slew of herbal formulas, both from the Shen-Hammer and Classical lineages, will be discussed and analyzed for their usefulness in treating Heart Shock. Lastly, I will present essential oils useful for a host of emotional and psychological conditions relevant to Heart Shock. I will begin the discussion with the Metal phase and Lung/Large Intestine channels and follow the primary channel sequence through the channels, rather than the creation cycle of the Five Phases. Channel pathways will not be discussed for the primary channels as sources abound covering this information in detail.

Metal phase
Lung channel functions

- Rules/dominates/circulates qi:
  - Circulates wei qi to skin to protect against EPFs, regulates body temperature, controls opening and closing of the pores, treats mood disorders
  - Regulates circulation of wei qi in the chest: wei qi in the chest helps to regulate heart rate and rhythm via its control of the smooth muscle contractions.
- Diffuses and descends qi: the Lungs diffuse wei qi to the exterior and descend to the lower body. Its ability to diffuse assists in the opening of the lower orifices, i.e., colon and bladder.
- Upper source of water: the Lungs regulate body fluids in the upper body and diffuse them to the skin, body hair, and sensory orifices above and descend to the Kidneys to recirculate.

- The Lung channel can treat pain and other pathologies in areas that its channel circulates.

- Opens to the nose: draws in zong qi from the environment; part of wei qi's first defense from exterior pathogens.

Lung channel continuum approach

The primary channels as a continuum represent the fact that life is about survival, interaction, and differentiation. We need to breathe, eat, digest, eliminate, and sleep, and these functions are assisted by the Lungs/Large Intestine and the Spleen/Stomach (and a bit from the Heart). Interaction is mediated by the second trinity of channels, the Heart, Small Intestine, Bladder, and Kidneys, wherein one communicates with the world and learns about one's true self, individuates and learns lessons, and follows the curriculum of an individual's life. Differentiation occurs when we habituate, form judgments, and separate ourselves from many aspects of the world to focus on the things we want to enjoy and cultivate and begin to relinquish control of that which we recognize cannot be changed. This is regulated by the Pericardium, Triple Burner, Gall Bladder, and Liver channels.

The Lungs within this continuum deal with many aspects one would consider instinctual, wei qi associations, like sweating when one is hot, shivering when cold, and adjusting to the varied changes one is exposed to. Psychologically, it reflects the process of letting go of that which is no longer needed. Physically, this layer manifests with symptoms from exposure to wind-cold. The Lungs' ability to diffuse and disperse to the exterior is their main function and concern. To do this, they must be able to unbind the chest and rid stagnation. Next, they must be able to descend qi to the Kidneys, Bladder, and Large Intestine.

Large Intestine channel functions

- Receives from the Small Intestine, re-absorbs water, eliminates waste, and assists with wei qi/smooth muscle/peristaltic movement.

- Circulates wei qi to the head, face, sense organs, and throat.

- Regulates the body fluids.

- Circulates qi throughout its channel pathway.

- As a yangming channel, can clear heat from the blood and channel.

- Tonifies qi and blood: tonifies and promotes circulation of qi and blood.[104]

Large Intestine channel continuum approach

The LI channel becomes activated as the pathogen begins to move internally, transforming from wind-cold to wind-heat. It makes contact with Du 14 (connecting to yang) and ST 12 (where pathogens internalize). Psychologically, the Large Intestine represents how a person positions himself in and interprets the world around him. A world seen as hostile will generate a need to be hypervigilant and combative or rebellious. The Large Intestine promotes sweat, clears heat, orders and descends the qi, impacts the face, and clears the orifices.

Five Phases

The Metal phase is most active seasonally in the autumn and represents the internalization/descension of energy, decay, rotting, and turning over of the life cycle. It represents things coming to an end, and as such it is associated with grief and sadness. The Metal phase is associated with the Lung and Large Intestine organs and energetically controls the ability to take in the pure (emphasis on beauty and idealism) and let go of the turbid and that which no longer serves. It deals with the rhythms and natural flow of our breathing cycles.

DRRBF[105]

The Metal phase builds on the bonding of the Earth phase and transforms and expands relationships through appropriate letting go and re-attachments. Metal allows for the investment of authority in oneself tested through life struggles and the eventual individuation to find one's life path/destiny. Ultimately, it brings awareness of the heavenly nature of all things. There are four major patterns, as follows.

Metal yin (Lungs) deficiency

The individual has difficulty forming and/or maintaining bonds due to a poor self-worth and failure to individuate. Unable to contribute, he relies on others, is uninspired, and tends to have a flat affect.

Metal yin excess

He tends to be overbearing and dominating, creating bonds which calcify and harden, and challenging others when they desire to leave the relationship. Due to his extreme possessiveness, partners and close relationships often become drained and monopolized.

Metal yang (Large Intestine) excess

The individual will be forever discarding her bonds in search of the newness and excitement of new relationships. The tendency is to get caught up in the moment, often having a scatter-brained/"grasshopper" mind. Relationships tend to be short-lived for fear of true intimacy and settling down. Depression can set in when she becomes aware that lack of meaningful relationships creates emptiness within.

Metal yang deficiency

This person lacks the strength to leave an unfulfilling relationship. She clings to the safe and familiar and cannot let go. This inability to leave the old and bring in the new creates the inability to grow (emotionally and intellectually), creating anxiety when life presents this need.

Metal acupuncture points for trauma

The Lungs provide the wei qi which assists the Heart in its pumping and moving of the blood. It provides organization and sequencing (e.g., rate and rhythm), and is often implicated when a patient does not feel his life is in order. As chaos is a marked feature of Heart Shock, Lung points which regulate/rectify qi are very useful. Many points on the metal channels assist in opening up the chest, transforming and expelling phlegm, and clearing heat that is harassing the spirit. Many also have an impact on the portals.

Lungs

LU 1: Front mu point of the Lungs, assists in freeing circulation of wei qi in the chest; diffuses wei/Lung qi; assists in regulating heart rate and rhythm; can clear heat from the chest. As the first Lung point, LU 1 can help the patient reconnect with heaven, one's destiny, and allow for a clearer vision and inspiration.

LU 2: LU 2 is often used in combination with ST 25 to anchor the wei qi to the lower burner, ST 25 being the front mu of the Large Intestine, but also having a strong energetic impact on the Kidneys and source qi. Where wei qi is hyperactive and chaotic, LU 2 to ST 25 can anchor and root back to yang. LU 2 is also an excellent point in the treatment of grief and depression where one walks around as if a dark cloud is over his head. Reducing this point disperses the cloud, allowing heavenly qi to enter.

LU 3: A WOS point which helps to clear the portals, especially effective in assisting with the processing of grief and loss and the promotion of forgiveness, it can also treat possession and mental confusion. As one of the points proximal to the he-sea point (LU 5), it is also helpful in moving the blood (with the help of wei qi) and can regulate rate and rhythm issues (as can LU 4).

LU 5: Clears heat and Lung fire in the upper burner, relaxes the sinews, downbears counterflow, and descends Lung qi. Excessive wei qi in the chest from prolonged grief or worry can create tension in the chest and pectoralis which over time creates heat and harasses the spirit. LU 5 relaxes the chest and provides the cooling impact to calm the shen, and, as a water point, allows descension to the Kidneys to root and anchor the qi.

LU 6: As the xi-cleft point, LU 6 stops bleeding, the psychological expression of which can be intense emotional pain (especially grief, sadness, and depression), especially when accompanied by chest pain. It is also used to stop palpitations, especially when caused by excessive sweating (a common occurrence in those who are nervous post trauma).

LU 7: With varied uses in Heart Shock patients, LU 7 can free and diffuse wei qi, release the chest from pent-up emotions, and release to the exterior. As a luo point, the Lung luo helps to clear heat in the chest and calm the shen. As a Ren mai opening point, it taps into the energetics of the Ren, governing bonding and security. As mentioned in the DRRBF section, from a primary channel and Five Phases perspective, bonding and boundaries are established in the Earth phase. From an 8x point of view, Ren mai maintains this role. The Lungs and the Metal phase are responsible for expanding these bonds and individuating. LU 7 is an important point for securing Ren mai, garnering the bonding energies, so that the patient can build thereon, find security, and individuate, becoming his own person.

LU 9: A yuan-source point that can tap into the yuan level and calm hyperactive wei qi. LU 9 also has the functions of diffusing Lung and wei qi and opening up the chest. As the influential point of blood, it strongly promotes circulation and, as the blood contains the shen, has an impact on one's psychological state. As it can also treat phlegm in the chest, it can have a profound impact on symptoms such as palpitations, shortness of breath, congestion, and feelings of resignation.

LU 10: The ying-spring fire point, LU 10 clears heat in the chest (e.g., anxiety, insomnia, irritability, etc.). A point on the Lung luo channel, it is often bled for this function.

LU 11: As a jing-well point, LU 11 can be used to open the portals and clear the senses. It has a classical function of restoring consciousness and is one of the 13 Ghost points and part of the first trinity (it will be discussed later in Chapter 9).

Large Intestine

LI 1: As the jing-well point, LI 1 can be useful for calming the nervous system, especially for the agitated yangming wind-heat-type personality. It also clears heat in the portals and can assist with proper perceptions, especially when combined with points such as LI 20, ST 8, and Du 24.

LI 4: As a source point and command point for the face, LI 4 can be useful for ascending the pure yang of the Stomach up to the sensory portals. LI 6 and ST 42 can be useful additions in this regard, especially if one is combining this point with the Stomach/Spleen divergent channels. LI 4 can also ascend the Lung qi and open the clavicle, an important area where pathology internalizes (ST 12 area). As it can access internalized pathogens as well as coursing and ridding exterior wind, LI 4 is useful for eliminating pathogens and letting go of that which is unwanted or no longer needed in one's life. And, of course, LI 4 is very useful in quickening the connecting vessels, relieving pain, and quieting the spirit.

LI 6: The luo point LI 6 is useful for treating pain and heat that has entered the channel. It also regulates the waterways and, with LI 4, ascends the pure yang of the Stomach for clarity in the sensory orifices.

LI 10: LI 10 is a good harmonizing point, especially with ST 36, to nourish patients who have been depleted by long-standing traumas, especially when nervous system tension impacts and overacts on a weakened digestive system. It has also been reported as having the empirical function of releasing negative energy.

LI 11: Can clear pathogenic heat internalizing via yangming, and can cool the blood. Often with long-term Heart Shock patients, heart rates have become elevated and heat becomes generated internally. Eventually, that heat begins to compromise the fluid and the blood begins to get hot. Over time, this creates thickened, more viscous blood, putting more work on an already taxed cardiovascular system, leading to atherosclerosis. LI 11 is a good point to assist with clearing heat from the blood and, as it also regulates the jin-ye, can be combined with other points to begin to nourish back the fluids.

LI 15: This is a major point for clearing yangming heat, often gua sha'd as part of the "ring around the neck" treatments (see divergent chapter). As a shoulder point, energetically it also helps to clear phlegm from the chest and can be useful for treating symptoms of the upper back (internal connection to Du 14), neck, throat, and chest.

LI 18: A WOS point which helps to open the portals and let go of old grief, sadness, and trauma. It is also the upper confluent point of the Large Intestine and Lung divergent channels (more information on its use in Chapter 7).

LI 20: This point opens the orifice of the nose and sense of smell, which impacts the most primitive areas of the brain and deep-seated emotions. It's a point perfectly suited for the use of many essential oils that have been discussed (and soon to be discussed) to impact the psyche (moods, emotions, and temperaments). As the final point on the metal channels, it can assist with letting go. And when needled up towards BL 1, it can make the eyes tear, releasing long-standing chronic emotional states and clearing the vision.

Earth phase
Spleen and Stomach channel functions

- Promote and regulate the digestion and absorption of food and drink.

- Regulate the transportation of body fluids and prevent the formation of dampness in the middle burner.

- Tonify qi and blood.

- Raise and stabilize the qi.

- Nourish the muscles and extremities.

- Manage the blood.

- House the Yi.

- Open to the mouth and manifest in the lips.

Spleen channel continuum approach

At the SP channel, we have the internalized pathogen that becomes accommodated and adapted to. Dampness begins to form in response to the heat, to quell and pacify it. Qi, blood, and fluid stagnation occurs, and the Spleen represents the beginning of chronicity of disease.

Stomach channel continuum approach

The ST channel represents the internalization of the pathogen and internalized heat. The main branch of the ST channel represents the sensory orifices and one's perceptions (deposited into the brain at Du 24). Heat/inflammation here impacts the portals, creating irritation. A branch moves down the throat into the chest allowing for internalization of the heat pathogen and a scorching of the internal domain. Irritability, anxiety, and panic are common as this occurs.

Five Phases

Earth as the "mother" favors neither yin nor yang and nourishes all equally. The Earth represents the transition between all seasons wherein everything returns for restoration. Where Wood is the birth, and Fire is full growth, Earth represents the harvest wherein one reaps what one has sown. The Earth, and its associated organs the Spleen-Pancreas (hereinafter "Spleen") and Stomach, is responsible for the transformation and transportation of acquired nourishment to the rest of the body. As the mother, Earth energies in balance enable one's caring and concern for others, and out of balance create worry, over-thinking, and pensiveness.

DRRBF[106]

From this perspective, the Earth element's natural functions are the formation and maturation of bonds, as well as capacity to understand boundaries. These have their roots at the earliest possible time during conception and the bond of the sperm and egg, bonding of the placenta to the uterine wall (a crucial aspect for the proper nutrition and health of the fetus), as well as the integrity of the placenta to provide a boundary between mother and fetus. These energies are imperative for the knowing of who one is, where one leaves off, and where others begin. Some imbalances that can result from a breakdown of this basic boundary include the Rh factor (which can result in brain damage to the fetus or death to the mother) as well as schizophrenia (unstable boundaries of self versus one's environment and others). Varied personality types can develop from weakness or excess in the Spleen and Stomach. It is important to note that the personality types and signs and symptoms that can often present with them can be the result of insults early in life and/or crucial stages of development, or can develop after a deleterious lifestyle, habits, and behaviors which have the effect of weakening these organ systems. So, it is possible for a deficient personality type to develop from the death of one's mother early in life or repetitive long-term use of antibiotics which damage the digestive energies. The earlier in life the insult, the more profound the imbalance will become.

Spleen deficiency

Schizophrenia: This is caused by early life trauma or genetic and intra-uterine deficits. The person generally has a blunted affectation, bizarre behavior and speech, delusions, hallucinations, etc.

Oral personality: Typically, there is either a parental abandonment or inadequate parenting, making the parent unavailable to the needs of the child. As a result, the child becomes dependent with poor self-esteem and feelings of inadequacy. The personality is always demanding from others the care and attention that they felt so deprived of. They are often described as obsessive and very clinging.

Avoidant personality: Typically caused by parental permissiveness, this person never learned the ability to test him/herself to gain the requisite skills. Poor role modeling creates a person unprepared to cope with pain, frustration, and the stresses of daily life. This person has a low self-esteem and seeks escape, often through drugs.

Spleen excess

Narcissistic personality: Very different from the preceding pattern, here the parents give the child a false sense of infallibility, making the child believe she is the center of the world. This spoiled, self-centered person is actually ill prepared to face the world as nothing has ever been expected of her and she falls prey to anxiety and confusion when she realizes her helplessness. She can be manipulative and very frustrated.

Stomach deficiency

Symbiotic personality: This person experienced an overly strong bond with a parent or caregiver and winds up living with one's parent their entire life. The main relationship is with the parent.

Stomach excess

Ruthless personality: The ruthless, competitive, power-hungry person was forced to fend for himself after being rejected by his parent(s) between the ages of 2½ and 5 years old. His Heart is armored and he often falls into gangs and criminal behavior.

Earth acupuncture points for trauma

Spleen

SP 1: The jing-well, wood point, SP 1 can clear heat in the Heart, stabilize the shen, and restore consciousness. It can be useful for heat in the blood as well with symptoms such as restlessness and acute insomnia. Also an excellent point to stop bleeding when the earth loses its boundaries and its management of the blood. Its communication to LR 1 via a branch of the Chong mai strengthens its influence over blood production, especially when combined with ST 42 and ST 30.

SP 2: The ying-spring, fire point, SP 2 can treat heat burning up the fluids (including the endocrine and the thyroid), potentially with hyperthyroid symptoms. A good point to assist the Heart and Small Intestine when damage to the ye exists.

SP 3: The shu-stream, earth, and source point, SP 3 treats all insufficiencies of the digestive system as well as regulating qi throughout the middle and regulating damp. It also has an impact on the spine (see collateral pathways from prior chapters), thus impacting lower back pain and Kidney energetics. SP 3 also treats obsessiveness, cloudy and confused thinking, as well as the clingy, oral, and symbiotic personality types.

SP 4: The luo point and confluent of the Chong mai, SP 4 is multi-faceted in its reach. It supports the Spleen and Stomach, rectifies the qi dynamic, regulates the Chong, and stops bleeding. It is often combined with PC 6 and the Yin Wei mai to invigorate blood and provide a greater influence over the pelvis as well as the chest. Its name grandfather-grandson reflects its use in treating one's blueprint and heredity. It can treat damp-phlegm and obsessive thinking, being stuck in old patterned and habituated thought processes, re-invigorating a sense of self and purpose. Its uses are further explored in Chapter 5.

SP 5: The jing-river, metal point, SP 5 manages dampness and phlegm and can treat obsessiveness, distrust, and jealousy, and is useful for the overly judgmental person.

SP 6: The 3 yin of leg intersection point, SP 6 has a relationship to a majority of the Heart Shock strategies, including influencing the Heart (via a subbranch from the Spleen to Stomach to diaphragm to Heart), where the production of blood becomes finalized, regulating the blood, nourishing blood and yin, strengthening the Kidneys, supplementing the Spleen and Stomach and regulating fluids, impacting the uterus, strengthening the Liver, cooling the blood, and calming the shen.

SP 7: Used mostly in relationship to leaky gut syndrome and the gu treatment protocol (discussed in Chapter 9).

SP 8: A main gu treatment point (see Chapter 9), SP 8 assists in digestion (of thoughts and food) and is important for leaking/prolapse of Spleen qi. SP 8 is also used to strengthen the Kidneys, and can bring Kidney yang into the earth via the KI 2 to SP 8 branch.

SP 9: The he-sea, water point, SP 9 is used mostly to consolidate the Spleen and Stomach, strengthen the earth, and manage damp, especially as it clouds the mind and thinking. In this regard, I often combine it with ST 8 and Du 24.

SP 10: As one point proximal to the he-sea, SP 10 can harmonize the blood, strengthening it, invigorating it, and/or clearing heat. As such it has a strong impact on calming the spirit/shen. It can treat a rapid heartbeat, insomnia, overthinking, and skin disorders amongst other things.

SP 12: A Chong mai (and for many a Yin Wei mai) point, SP 12 can treat the toxins that have internalized to the constitution, damaging one's essence. It can nourish yin-essence, especially nourishing Liver and Kidney yin, thus making it a good point to induce latency (see Chapter 7). SP 12 also helps to open the region of the breasts and promotes breast milk. It can also treat Liver-invading Spleen symptoms, or NST overacting on DSW. With its ability to treat the breasts as well as ameliorate Liver-invading Spleen symptoms, SP 12 can be useful in treating the process of breast cancer. (See the LI/LU divergent channel description in the following chapter for more detail.)

SP 15: As a Dai mai point, regulates the middle burner, a point on the Yin Wei mai; from a psychological perspective, treats overthinking and, when the mind goes blank, anxiety from overconcentration; affects the chest; and regulates peristalsis and transformation/transportation. As a Spleen point, will treat the further penetration of heat and the creation of dampness; treats leaky gut and the inability to assimilate.

SP 20: With an internal branch to the Lungs, SP 20 brings post-natal qi from the Spleen to the Lungs at LU 1. When needled towards LU 1, it can diffuse Lung qi and stimulate wei qi, making it effective for releasing the chest, letting go, and an overall immune system tonic.

SP 21: The great luo of the Spleen, SP 21 was discussed in detail in the preceding chapter. Briefly, it regulates qi and blood, impacts the sinews and bones, moves blood in the luo vessels, and has a strong influence over the chest, hypochondriac region, Da Bao, Dai mai, uterus, and four limbs. It is also often combined with BL 53 gaohuangshu (another wrapping). It can treat running piglet qi, pain all over the body (both physical and emotional), weakness in the limbs and body, etc. SP 21 and the great luo can be likened to the comfort and nourishment given by a mother as she embraces and soothes her child.

Stomach

ST 1: ST 1 can brighten the eyes and open the portals. Starting at LI 20, the internal branch of the ST channel moves to BL 1, then ST 1, with a strong impact on the eyes. Using the metal energetics, it helps to release sorrow and let go of disappointments related to how one thinks their life should be. It can unblock the flow of tears to wash away suppressed pain.

ST 3: Mostly used as an alternate point of the yang leg sinew meridians' meeting point, which covers the area between ST 3 and SI 18.

ST 5: A point on the GB/LR DM, ST 5 is where heat begins to internalize to the throat (branch descends to ST 9). Often treated to release wei qi stuck in the head, and not able to internalize, with symptoms such as TMJ and teeth grinding at night with insomnia.

ST 7: Opens the portals and sharpens hearing; descends Stomach and rebellious qi.

ST 8: The meeting point for the three yang sinew channels of the arm, ST 8 clears the head and brightens eyes, releasing old perceptions, obsessions, and distorted narratives. Can be combined with Du 24 in this regard. The Stomach channel has classical uses for shen disturbances and dian kuang syndrome as the entire first and major branch of the channel encircles the face and head, ending at the ST 8 to Du 24 branch. One's perceptions and reactions are governed by the Stomach, which controls the yi and manages the blood.

ST 9: A WOS point, ST 9 treats heat internalizing into the throat and chest creating irritability and anxiety. Helpful for those who swallow their emotions and suppress feelings of resentment to avoid conflict. ST 9 can also treat heat that rises up to the throat from internal pathogens, with symptoms of the hyperthyroid such as tachycardia, nervousness and fidgeting, hypertension, and outbursts of anger. An excellent point for those suffering from spiritual starvation, despair, and frustration, or those feeling as if they are being smothered by others.

ST 12: At the canopy of the Lungs, ST 12 is an important gateway to/from the exterior/interior. It is a major point for diffusing (and downbearing) the Lungs and wei qi and regulating the circulation of qi and blood, especially when used with LI 4 which opens the ST 12 area. This relationship to the Lungs and the exterior makes is valuable for distinguishing boundaries and the ability to empty and externalize pathogens. An inability to do so creates a collapse of the canopy, depression, and oppression of the chest. ST 12 is also a crossing point for many of the DM channels, providing the ability to put pathology into latency or clear it from the body.

ST 14–ST 18: These are the Stomach chest shu points; like the Bladder shu points which deal with yang-qi, and the Kidney shu points (to be discussed in the Water section) that deal with yin, the Stomach shu points of the chest manage the resource of blood. The same reflexology pertains, e.g., from top to bottom, metal, fire, wood, earth, water. Thus, ST 14 deals with blood and the Lungs (can treat blood-streaked sputum), ST 15 Heart blood (can treat insomnia and daydreaming; also regulates the diaphragm), ST 16 Liver blood, ST 17 blood of earth (here the nipple, and the understanding that breast milk is the excess of blood transformation nourished by the mother to the baby), and ST 18 blood-essence of the Kidneys.

ST 21: An important point for creating stability, ST 21 harmonizes the Spleen and Stomach and strengthens the earth.

ST 23: Clears heat from the Heart and quiets the spirit; ST 23 treats irritability, mania, indigestion, and chaotic thoughts, assisting with integrating experiences and helping one move on in life.[107]

ST 24: Like ST 23 above, ST 24 clears heat from the Heart and is useful in treating mania.

ST 25: The heavenly pivot, and front mu of the Large Intestine, ST 25 can help move stagnation via coursing and regulating the Large Intestine, strengthening the earth, clearing heat, and regulating qi in the digestive system and chest. A great point for providing stability, ST 25 also strengthens the Kidneys and anchors yang to the lower jiao. I often use ST 25 with LU 2 (or LU 1) to anchor wei qi and root it in yang via the lower abdomen.

ST 29: Not as commonly used as the following point, I use ST 29 with SP 15 to tap into the curious organs as together they open the uterus, making it very helpful in warming and moving qi-yang in the reproductive organs and pelvis.

ST 30: An intersecting point with the Chong mai and Stomach sinew meridian, ST 30 is a versatile point that can soothe the sinews, regulate qi and blood in the pelvis and reproductive organs, strengthen qi and blood, and tonify the earth. Via the Chong mai and its influence on the blueprint, ST 30 can harmonize qi and blood, assisting one to find consistency in who one is internally versus the external world, thus rectifying guilt and allowing one to accept her life as it is, rather than how she thought it should be. ST 36 and ST 9 can assist with this process.

ST 34: The xi-cleft point, ST 34 regulates the Stomach and rectifies the qi, and can treat inflammation in the intestines, including altered microflora and turbidity in the gut. Amongst other things it also treats heat in the blood, thus making it useful for treating mania, irritability, and shen disturbances due to heat.

ST 36: The he-sea, earth point, and command point of the abdomen, ST 36 is perhaps one of the strongest and most commonly used points on the Stomach channel (and perhaps of all the acupuncture points in modern Chinese medicine). It strongly tonifies the earth and the Kidney qi, nourishes the production of blood, regulates qi and circulation in the GI and intestines, disperses stagnation, and breaks blood stasis in the chest (and can be used for insomnia and mania). It can be used to treat underlying deficiencies with an external pathogen, rid cold, and strengthen and raise the yang qi. A very strong point for stabilizing and grounding a deficient and chaotic patient, ST 36 is an instrumental point with an Empty pulse in the right middle position, or any time a patient's experiences have compromised his foundation and/or integrity to function optimally.

ST 37: The lower he-sea of the Large Intestine, ST 37 is useful for opening the chest and Lungs, facilitating the process of letting go (both from above and below).

ST 40: The luo point, ST 40 has been discussed in detail in the preceding chapter. It is well known for treating the feeling of oppression in the chest, able to treat phlegm (both hot and cold) and heat disturbing the shen creating irritability, anxiety, fear, and panic (branch of the ST luo that follows the KI channel). As it treats the damp and phlegm, it helps with obsessive thoughts and transforming that which has become burdensome.

ST 41: The jing-river, fire, and tonification point, ST 41 is most useful for clearing Stomach heat and heat in the chest (it can relax the area of ST 12 and ease breathing, regulating wei qi), stabilizing the shen, clearing the mind, and brightening the eyes.

ST 42: The source point, ST 42 has a strong impact on the jin-ye fluids and opening the portals. It strengthens the Stomach and releases the neck and throat (WOS point areas, thus impacting the portals). The GB luo ends at ST 42, and the ST/SP DM opening point, BL 1, is said to correspond to and open ST 42, allowing the pure yang of the Stomach to ascend and nourish the sensory orifices.

ST 43: The shu-stream, wood point, ST 43 can release the upper portals, especially the eyes. It is also useful in the Gu treatment protocol discussed infra.

ST 44: The ying-spring, water point, ST 44 strongly clears heat and is useful for treating insomnia, agitation, and agitated thinking. It can regulate and downbear Stomach qi, treat pain, and eliminate wind from the face and sensory portals.

ST 45: The jing-well, metal point, ST 45 is a main point for relaxing the nervous system when heat from yangming is harassing. It clears heat from the Heart and has a calming effect on the shen. As a jing-well point it resuscitates yang and impacts the portals, especially the eyes, which it brightens. Its uses are more fully detailed in Chapter 4.

Fire phase

Heart channel functions

- Governs the blood and the blood vessels.

- Circulates qi and blood, nourishes the Heart, and regulates all emotions.

- Helps regulate heat in the body with the other fire channels.

- Opens to the tongue and controls speech, expression, and articulation.

- Fluid is sweat, created by the steaming of Heart blood.

- Manifests in the complexion and eyes where the shen can be observed.

Heart channel continuum approach

The second energetic layer is about creating meaningful relationships and better understanding of oneself and the divine within. The Heart strives to establish purpose in one's life and to satisfy its curriculum, maintaining enthusiasm and withholding judgment despite the challenges confronted by the nine palaces. From the continuation of pathology, the Heart channel represents heat that has entered the chest and blood level.

Small Intestine channel functions

- Circulates qi along the channel to the face and head, including the sensory portals of the ears and eyes, as well as the lower burner.

- As a taiyang channel, it moves and strengthens wei qi to the surface and assists in protecting the exterior, and releasing it. It assists with moving out into the world and bringing back to oneself information to be assimilated and that is nourishing to oneself.

- Separates the pure from the impure (including stimulation and information); absorbs fluids and micronutrients.

- Regulates the ye-thick fluids, manages the hormones, and protects the Heart (by clearing Heart fire).

Small Intestine channel continuum approach

The Small Intestine, from a primary channel point of view, represents the beginning of latency, using the blood and ye-thick fluids as its resource. As a pathogen internalizes past Stomach yangming and compromises the thin fluids, we begin to see dampness to accommodate the pathogen at the Spleen. By the time the Small Intestine is reached, the ye fluids have been utilized and now one sees fever with the absence of sweat, no longer being able to use the jin fluids to move the pathogen out. As a result of the deficiency of blood and fluids, "flare ups" become common. The Small Intestine also has a role in protecting the Heart. Any heat that is produced with the potential to overwhelm the Heart becomes displaced to the Bladder (organ for disinhibition, or shu points for latency) to protect the heat from damaging the jing (now that the jin and ye have been depleted).

Five Phases

Traditionally, the Fire phase follows the Wood phase of birth and growth and represents full growth, maturity, and ripeness. Seasonally, it is associated with the summertime and heat. The Fire phase contains our shen-spirit which is seen, amongst other places, in one's complexion and through the glitter in one's eyes. It houses our consciousness and desire to communicate with others and be social, spontaneous, and enjoy life. The emotion associated with the Fire phase is joy, but also represents the imbalance of one who needs to constantly seek and experience pleasure, one whose desires are out of control. The manic hyperactive personality is another description of this "excess joy."

As Chinese medicine has evolved through Daoist and Buddhist ideologies, the belief is that one's spirit can only be content when the Heart is free from desire. Desire is seen as strengthening one's ego, one's selfishness, and results in a never-ending cascade of dissatisfaction and pain. Desire, as one of the roots of suffering, is one way of understanding how "excess joy" can create illness. By affecting the spirit, it can create restlessness and agitation, insomnia, and a profound "lack of joy" (one type of depression) when one ultimately glimpses the profound emptiness resulting from a lifetime of want.

On a physical level, anything affecting the Heart will ultimately affect one's circulation with all its potential manifestations: chest pain, angina, arthritic conditions, premenstrual syndrome and irregular periods, dizziness, hypertension, arteriosclerosis, etc.

When the Fire phase is balanced, one experiences a unity in all things, with an ability to communicate and be social and act spontaneously from the Heart. When taxed, one experiences a lack of spirit or feeling a part of something.

DRRBF[108]

From this perspective the Fire phase (which is comprised of four organ systems in Chinese medicine: the Heart, Small Intestine, Pericardium, and Triple Burner) deals with the emotional, mental, and spiritual aspects of each individual. As such, if it is imbalanced, there will be disharmony throughout the organism. The Fire phase is also one's communication system, providing clues to the outside world of one's inner being. The yin aspect of the Heart provides one's ability for creative inspiration, while the yang allows for the expression and articulation of that vision.

Heart yang deficient

This individual, assuming their Heart yin is intact, will have the capacity for brilliant, innovative, and inspired ideas, but will lack the ability to express or communicate them. This, as one can imagine, will cause high levels of frustration and a deep sense of worthlessness. The Heart yang deficient person does not have the faculties to organize their mind and thus can never articulate their ideas into any purposeful or productive way. The frustration and worthlessness that develops over time can lead to significant anxiety when situations in life demand such articulation. A profound depression can result from these repeated failures, and suicide can be a strong possibility.

Heart yang excess

These are the people whose expression significantly outweighs the substance of which they express. In other words they are the compulsive communicators with little or no substance behind it. They are repetitive and constantly need an audience.

Heart yin deficient

Uninspired, boring, and bureaucratic, this person is simply occupied with the status quo and lacks any spontaneity or originality. This can be from a repressed excitement which will cause anxiety as one's armoring breaks down.

Heart yin excess

This person is hypersensitive and acutely aware. It is a life marked by chaos as one cannot control the impulses and flood of creativity which leads to over-stimulation and mental fatigue. These individuals are extraordinarily disorganized and fear losing their mind in the chaos.

Small Intestine deficiency

These people have difficulty separating their thoughts from their feelings; they are confused, with poor capacities to be analytical.

Small Intestine excess

This person is overly analytical, yet has little capacity to synthesize information. Things are perceived as either black or white.

Fire acupuncture points for trauma

Heart

HT 1: The first point on the Heart channel, HT 1 can revive qi and loosen the chest, freeing up the channel and allowing the Heart to experience and embrace the wonder and interconnectedness of life. It allows for nourishment to permeate one's chest, especially when combined with SP 21, the great luo. It can treat issues with intimacy, compulsive behaviors, insomnia, palpitations, etc. and provide trauma victims the memory and safety of life prior to damaging experiences.[109]

HT 2: As a point proximal to the he-sea, HT 2 can invigorate blood in the chest and is especially useful when patients are moving through transitions in their lives. It allows for forgiveness, and helps one to not get carried away with emotions, providing clarity and a state of calm.

HT 3: The he-sea, water point, HT 3 allows one to see a grander picture and gain perspective over where one finds himself in the larger cosmic plan. It can course the Heart qi, clear heat from the Pericardium and stabilize the spirit (e.g., palpitations, nervousness, insomnia, etc.), and remove obstructions from the channel, including phlegm (chest pain, angina, spasmodic pain and numbness of the hand and arm, etc.). It can treat Heart fire (e.g., insomnia, heat-causing wind symptoms such as epilepsy, tension around neck preventing wind from gaining access to the brain, etc.). HT 3 can help someone speak her mind and release tension around the throat.

HT 4: The jing-river, metal point, HT 4 can nourish the Heart qi and quiet the spirit, while also soothing the sinews (can treat joint pain, angina, etc.). It can show one his path and purpose in life, helping one to let go (metal) of pain and sadness, aligning oneself with a higher purpose.

HT 5: The luo point, HT 5 has been detailed in Chapter 5, but briefly, it can address qi and blood stasis, move qi and open the chest (relieving oppression and also allowing for greater intimacy with others), treat anxiety and insomnia, and allow for the Heart to express itself (e.g., stuttering, inability to articulate, etc.), quiet the spirit and strengthen Heart qi. Great for those who have diaphragmatic problems, and applicable to Dr. Shen's Heart closed and/or Heart small conditions, as well as peripheral circulation issues secondary to emotional or physical traumas.

HT 6: The xi-cleft point, HT 6 can strengthen Heart yin (as well as Heart yang collapse), astringe fluids, and treat chest pain, palpitations, rapid heartbeat, insomnia, etc. It also clears Heart fire and quiets the spirit. Great for those who sweat when they get nervous and whose hands and palms are always sweaty.

HT 7: The shu-stream, earth, sedation, and source point, HT 7 shen men can be tonified to strengthen the Heart, return wei qi and blood to the Heart, and provide comfort to the shen. It can nourish the Heart blood as well as opening the orifices. When sedated, can clear heat harassing the spirit (relieves anxiety, panic, insomnia, etc.), and assist with letting go of attachments (worldly as well as physical).

HT 8: The ying-spring and fire point, HT 8 can be dispersed to clear heat from the chest, Heart, and blood (e.g., anxiety, insomnia, itchy painful skin rashes or eruptions, etc.) as well as phlegm-heat harassing and obstructing the orifices. When tonified it can harness fire to promote optimism, interest (in oneself and relationships with others), and excitement in life, and treat depression and lack of will.

HT 9: The jing-well, wood point, HT 9 is a resuscitation point that can treat heat and/or wind-phlegm that is harassing the shen, palpitations, insomnia, tachycardia, arrhythmias, irritability, etc. Under root and termination, it homes to the throat (Ren 23 area), and also opens the chest (including the Chong mai Kidney shu points from KI 22 to KI 27) and the eyes.

Small Intestine

SI 1: The jing-well, metal point, SI 1 can clear Heart fire and move heat, as well as open the portals. Known to disinhibit breast milk, it can unblock stagnation in the channels of the chest. It can treat Heart Shock patients with impaired consciousness, insomnia, palpitations, tachycardia, red eyes, or clouded vision. Needled upwards, it can bring wei-yang qi to the chest.

SI 2: The ying-spring, water point, SI 2 can also clear wind and heat and treat the Heart (e.g., burning urination from Heart fire moving to the Bladder), but it is also used as a gu treatment point which has a strong influence on the esophagus and can separate the pure from impure (see Chapter 9).

SI 3: The shu-stream, wood, and confluent of the Du mai, SI 3 clears heat, calms the spirit, clears the mind, and rids interior heat, as well as being able to stabilize the exterior and eliminate wind from the Du mai. As it impacts and opens the Du mai and eliminates wind, it has a calming effect on the nervous system (Du mai and taiyang energetics), while also impacting the sinews. As it taps into the Du mai and yang qi, it can also be used to treat depression with a backdrop of Kidney yang deficiency and stimulate will power.

SI 4: The yuan-source point, SI 4 impacts the bone level, and can manage toxins (of which trauma is included) which have penetrated into the source. Helps to induce sweat, and bring things out of latency; can treat heat in sensory organs with yin deficiency moving to the organs themselves and/or to the five centers with irritability, agitation, and insomnia.

SI 5: The jing-river, fire point, SI 5 can quiet the spirit and clear/calm the mind (treating mental confusion) and nervous system, while calming wind. It also has usefulness in the gu qi protocol as it builds yang qi and strengthens the gut (described in Chapter 9).

SI 6: The xi-cleft point, SI 6 frees the channels, benefits the sinews and bones (and especially the lower back), and brightens the eyes. Often touted for the geriatric population, SI 6 can treat any age group when there is habituation preventing proper assimilation of new experiences, clearing stagnation, allowing forgiveness, and promoting clarity.

SI 7: The luo point, SI 7 has been detailed in Chapter 5, but briefly it can clear heat disturbing the shen, treats insomnia and anxiety from excessive thinking and obsessiveness, helps to resolve frustration and bitterness, and helps to calm the nervous system.

SI 8: The he-sea, earth, and sedation point, SI 8 is a strong point for clearing heat disturbing the shen and calming the mind and nervous system. It helps move the bowels and treats constipation (including that of one's thoughts). It can treat restlessness and promote enthusiasm that is focused (not distracted). With SI 11, it can also treat depression, especially if HT 8 is added.

SI 9: A main point near the scapula, SI 9 assists with reaching out into the world and helps one to handle external influences. It can also treat indifference and lack of enthusiasm.

SI 10: Another shoulder point, SI 10 can help one to handle difficult circumstances, treat anxiety and insomnia, and can also assist with the return of yang qi back to the chest and communicate with the Heart yin. SI 10 is a point on the SI/HT DM, and can release or anchor depending on its needling technique (see Chapter 7).

SI 11: The breast shu point, SI 11 diffuses qi stagnation and opens the chest and costal region. And as discussed in Chapter 4, this point (also SI 9) can treat symptoms and presentations of Heart fire. SI 11 and its impact on the breast, and milk in particular, represent a distillation and separation of the pure resources to provide nourishment.

SI 12: The 3-yang crossing point, SI 12 is a major point for wind and cold, thus making it an important invitation of change in one's life, and facilitates the process of letting go. Like the other scapula points, it allows one to extend out to the world and bring nourishment back to one's Heart.

SI 15: Not as commonly used in my practice, unless there are also neck/shoulder symptoms, SI 15 can diffuse the Lungs and help let go, transform phlegm, and brighten the eyes.

SI 16: A WOS point, SI 16 quiets the spirit and nourishes the Heart. SI 16 has the effect of directing Heart yin back to the chest, making it a prime point in the treatment of Heart Shock and one of my most commonly chosen points when employing a primary channel treatment. As it directs yin back to the chest it is very grounding and suitable for the daydreamer and those that stare off into space, perhaps even dissociating and losing contact with reality. It can provide clarity and assist with the SI functions of sorting. As a WOS point, it also impacts and opens the portals, and I find it to have a hormone-regulating effect.

SI 18: The three leg yang sinew channel meeting point, SI 18 lies directly in the center of all the upper portals, exerting a tremendous influence over the senses, how one perceives and responds towards stimuli, reevaluating what one senses, and releasing that which is stuck or pathological. SI 18 also treats heat that has consumed the fluids and degenerated the senses, as well as having a strong influence on cognition. It can also treat excessive wei qi accumulation in the face and hyper-reactivity towards the external world (especially when utilized within the context of a HT DM treatment).

SI 19: Directly in front of the ear, SI 19 opens the ear portal and strengthens visual and hearing acuity. It can treat those that hear but do not comprehend what is being spoken, often misinterpreting others, and often feeling as if others misinterpret them despite their lack of clarity. SI 19 can help patients hear things as they are without coloring communications based on past experiences/beliefs, as well as the ability to listen to their own hearts.

Water phase
Kidney channel functions

- The Kidneys are the root of yin and yang and store the jing/pre-natal energies.
- Stores the qi.
- Dominates the fire at the gate of vitality and is the root of metabolic energy and adrenal activity.
- Houses the lumbar and regulates the energetics of the lower back.
- Dominates water metabolism.
- Rules reception of qi/grasps the Lung qi assisting with inhalation and expanding the Lungs and diaphragm.
- Rules growth, reproduction, and development.

- Produces marrow and rules/governs bone and the spine.

- Opens to the ears and governs the capacity for hearing.

- Manifests in the head hair and maintains its health.

- Controls the "2 lower yin" (anus and urethra, and external genitalia) and the reproductive organs.

Kidney channel continuum approach

By the time the Kidney channel is reached, latent heat has been consuming the body's jing, creating yang deficiency and latent cold, and there is an attempt to hold onto and gather fluids to slow down progression, creating turbid damp, affecting the Triple Burner mechanism and the Lungs, Spleen, and Kidneys which deal with fluid metabolism.

Bladder channel functions

- Regulates the taiyang and controls the exterior.

- As the largest primary channel, it regulates the muscles, tendons, ligaments, and sinews.

- Via its pathway, it impacts the brain and can address mental-emotional symptoms and distributes qi to the head and sensory orifices.

- Governs the Bladder and Kidney organ functions.

- Via the dissemination of the Triple Burner, the Bladder channel connects with all the organs via the back shu points.[110]

Bladder channel continuum approach

At this point in the continuum, pathology has moved into the jing level and the Bladder channel attempts to move this internalized latent heat back out to the exterior. Symptoms include strong headaches, nasal congestion, painful dry eyes, etc., reflecting the heat and yin deficiency as the Bladder tries to externalize the pathogen with an underlying deficiency.

Five Phases

After the harvest has been reaped, nature prepares for dormancy, the process of storage and conservation of its energy and resources in preparation for the beginning of a new cycle of birth in spring. Water is associated with the winter and cold. It represents an inner strength and a focused willpower to achieve one's goals and fulfill one's destiny. Water always flows downward to its source and has an energetic for the lower organs, the Kidneys and Bladder. In harmony, it reflects faith in oneself and in a higher power; out of balance, one experiences fear.

DRRBF[111]

The two major considerations of the Water phase from this perspective are the sense of self, and fear of the unknown, especially the existential questions of who one truly is, and one's purpose. In balance, a healthy Kidney system provides antidotes to fear via faith (in a higher power, in others, and in oneself). The Kidneys provide a sense of reality in terms of our own importance and power, as well as that of others, and of the divine. This prevents the expansion of the ego and delusions of grandeur and helps to adapt and project our fears in service of controlling them.

As Dr. Hammer explains in DRRBF, the Kidney yin and yang are the life and force respectively in the life-force.[112] The yin represents one's genetic essence, as well as the central nervous system, our innate intelligence, and the substrate for all biochemical reactions. Yang is the genetic fire, force, will, and drive—the metabolic heat that drives the entire organism. Qi reflects our present and governs growth, reproduction, and development; it is a blending of the yin and yang and, as such, represents our intelligent will and our balanced healthy ego with an appropriate awe, acceptance, reverence, and humility, as well as faith.

Kidney yang deficient personality type

Here we see an unmotivated, cheerless individual with no goals or purpose in life. This person suffers from endogenous depression (unrelated to specific events), is petty, criticizes others, and is jealous due to their own inabilities. Anxiety presents itself when this person is in a situation that requires sustained effort or vigor that is not possessed. Fear accompanies all presentations of the Water phase.

Kidney yang excess

A human dynamo, but often presenting as tyrannical, egotistical, and controlling. Anxiety is produced when anything interferes with his will; and he becomes depressed when unable to assert his will and drive (even to the point of considering suicide).

Kidney yin deficiency

A ruthless competitor who lacks a social conscience as he is missing the capacity for divine love and faith. He identifies by seeking to dominate others and accumulate for himself. Endogenous depression is common, and anxiety will be experienced with any feelings or requirement of tenderness.

Kidney yin excess

This pattern has two subparts, a left brain dominant personality, and a right brain personality:

- Left brain: this person elevates man and material things, is logical, and distrusts instinct. Anxiety will be produced when she experiences situations that are considered illogical. Depression results from a realization that her life is empty, with logic not fulfilling her inner needs and desires.

- Right brain: this person elevates nature and spiritual considerations above all else, and reveres revelation and intuition as the main sources of acquiring knowledge. They experience anxiety when required to be logical and routined.

Kidney qi deficiency

This person lacks faith, awe, humility, and the ability to trust. She is arrogant, has a flat affect, and is extremely fearful, especially of confrontation. Anxiety is produced from challenges to their ego; depression from the thought or reality of their death.

Kidney qi excess

He is the fanatic (follower if more of a yin-type; and a leader if more of a yang-type), rigid and dogmatic. Anxiety is produced when beliefs are challenged, depression ensues if the belief system is rejected or collapses.

Water acupuncture points for trauma

As the Kidneys and Water phase is a direct area of impact in Heart Shock, these channels supply some of the most commonly used acupuncture points for its treatment. These points will have a major focus on anchoring Kidney yang, calming and strengthening the adrenals, allaying fear, relaxing the fight/flight/freeze response, disseminating yuan qi and correcting the Triple Burner mechanism, impacting the chest and Heart, etc.

Kidneys

KI 1: As the only point that is in contact with the ground, this point is wonderful for stabilizing the Kidneys and anchoring hyperactive wei and yang qi. It also tonifies yin and clears heat and is an overall calming point for the nervous system. Often combined with Du 20 and Ren 17 (and if the patient is amenable either HT 8 or PC 8), one can ground and calm a nervous hyperactive patient, relieve mania, anxiety/panic and/or depression, and open the portals (as a jing-well point it restores consciousness). KI 1 can communicate Heart/Pericardium and Kidney and treat fear, anxiety, and fright.

KI 2: The fire point on the water channel, KI 2 helps to anchor yang back to the Kidneys for patients with hyperactivity, floating yang (including Empty pulses in the proximals), insomnia, irritability, and anxiety (as it can cool the blood). As a point on the Yin Qiao mai, it can also impact the brain and shen disorders. Often combined with HT 3, one can create a communication between fire and water, Heart and Kidneys. KI 2 can be likened to the fire spirit herbal approach of using Fu Zi/aconite to anchor yang. I often needle this point first superficially and, when qi arrives, drive it down to the yuan level. With an internal pathway to SP 8, KI 2 brings yang to the post-natal environment to assist with assimilation of experiences and that which nurtures us.

KI 3: As the source point on the water channel, it can ground and internalize yang and yin back to its source. As an earth point, it can provide boundaries necessary to anchor and astringe qi back to the Kidneys. One can also tap into Kidney qi to arouse yang to mobilize activity for fear and paralysis of action. As it benefits essence, the foundation of the central nervous system, it can treat shen disorders and insomnia, as well as regulate qi throughout the portals, especially the ears. KI 3 can help with Heart and Kidney communication, treating such disorders as running piglet qi and hysteria; it can grasp the Lung qi and activate/regulate qi through the diaphragm.

KI 4: The luo point on the channel, KI 4 can assist with fear and paranoia, hysteria, and running piglet, especially when bled. It also has a connection to the lower back and ming men, and it is believed to impact the Dai mai (assisting with ridding one's baggage and clutter from life). Used often with BL 60 for assisting one in the dying process, KI 4 can help one to let go, forgive, and cleanse (hence its treatment of blockage in the two lower yin).

KI 6: A Yin Qiao mai opening point, KI 6 can impact the brain and orifices (especially the eyes) and help with self-esteem (how one sees himself). It nourishes yin and can calm hyperactivity in the nervous system and mind, cool the blood, as well as open the chest. As it penetrates the throat, it can also help the person to speak their truth and express their inner Heart.

KI 7: The tonification point of the Kidneys, KI 7 can strengthen yin or yang. As the jing-river it is also an important point for promoting circulation along the channel, thus being used to return proper flow and dissemination of yang. Its alternate name, waiming/beyond destiny, suggests that not returning back to one's curriculum in time may have created irreversible illness, wherein this point assists with the final transformation.[113]

KI 8: The xi-cleft of Yin Qiao mai, KI 8 is said to rid heat and stagnation from that channel, impacting the pelvis, including the Ren and Chong mai. In the context of Heart Shock, KI 8 provides the capacity of a patient to reaffirm faith, trust, and self-confidence, and reconnect one to the divine/Big shen.

KI 9: KI 9 is most often used in the context of Yin Wei mai's xi-cleft. It can calm fright and quiet the spirit. It is often needled with tonification, causing the point to pucker so that it can astringe qi and yin to provide comfort and anchor. Within the context of Yin Wei mai, KI 9 is often needled at the end of each pregnancy trimester to rid the negative karma of the parents. Within this idea, Yin Wei mai links together the most influential aspects/memories of one's life, traumas often being at the top of the list. Working with KI 9 and Yin Wei mai can help process these traumatic events, shaping one's personality and destiny. As Jarrett points out, the impact to the fetus can be metaphorical, serving as a time the spiritual embryo incubates, only to awaken towards a path of cultivation.[114]

KI 10: The water point on the water channel, KI 10 nourishes Kidney yin and helps to anchor floating yang. It is the he-sea point and can internalize yin and yang, bringing symptoms into remission (especially as it is the lower confluent for the Kidney divergent meridian and when needled with BL 10 and DSD needling (described in the following chapter)). It is commonly used to assist with Heart and Kidney communication.

KI 16: Directly adjacent to the lower border of the umbilicus, KI 16 strongly influences yuan-source qi and can anchor yang to the lower burner. It is a fantastic point for communicating Heart and Kidneys, especially as the Heart sinew channel binds here (the only actual channel communication that the Heart and Kidneys share). The name itself, huang, refers to the area between the Heart and diaphragm, also perhaps referencing the outer shu of the Pericardium, gaohuangshu. As a point on the Chong mai, it further strengthens this connection to the chest and Heart, giving it the function of impacting the shen. Communicating Heart, Kidney, and original qi via the umbilicus and nourishment to the fetus, KI 16 brings deep nourishment and connection back to one's original self.

KI 19: At the same level as Ren 12, I find KI 19 most useful in the context of Heart Shock to consolidate qi to the middle burner, especially in the context of a Triple Burner divergent meridian treatment. Connections to the Ren and Chong mai strengthen its impact on gathering qi and blood, and regulating the emotions.

KI 20: Often used to influence the middle burner, KI 20 is combined with points that treat gu syndrome (discussed in Chapter 9) as an etiology for trauma.

KI 21–27
The Upper Kidney Shu Points: these are related to the Heart and the mental-emotional and spiritual functions of arousing awareness, anchoring the spirit and allowing for full expression of one's shen. Each of the shu points resonates to a specific organ/Five Phases phase and mirrors that of the Bladder shu points. From top to bottom, KI 27 is the master shu point, KI 26 LU/metal, KI 25 HT/fire, KI 24 LR/wood, KI 23 SP/earth, and KI 22 KI/water. As the back shu represents yuan qi into the organs, the Kidney shu represents the yin component and anchoring/grounding, especially good for anxiety, panic, dissociation, etc. so common with Heart Shock patients.

KI 21 (Dark Gate): At the lower border of the ribs, just prior to entering the chest and the Kidney shu points, lies KI 21. It helps one become aware of and face the darkness of one's fears, terrors, and traumas. It is at this point that the Kidney luo channel internalizes and returns to the lower body communicating with ming men/Du 4, thus providing an additional incentive for this point's mental-emotional indications.

KI 22 (Walking Corridor): The water point, KI 22 is used for despondency and isolation. Needling this point towards the midline assists with astringing yin to the Kidneys and chest/Heart. Needling outwards disperses yin stasis and can resurrect the spirit overburdened by dampness.

KI 23 (Spirit Seal, Mind Seal): This point is used where the patient has lost the will to live, acting as a storehouse for the spirit. It is also effective at helping the patient who suffers trauma/terror to connect back to the divine.

KI 24 (Spirit Burial Ground): The wood point, KI 24 helps resurrect the spirit, especially for one who cannot let go grieving (either for a person who has deceased, or for one's own nature post trauma).

KI 25 (Spirit Storehouse, Mind Seal): The fire point, KI 25 represents the replenishment of spirit flowing back to provide purpose in the service of fulfilling one's destiny. This point seals the treatment to crystallize and allow for fruition. As a point that is related to the Heart, and as the Kidney shu points manage yin, KI 25 is one of my most commonly used primary channel points for Heart Shock. Needling it towards the midline can anchor and astringe yin back to the Heart.

KI 26 (Amidst Elegance): The metal point, KI 26 gently guides one towards individuation, and brings one back in touch with the present. Those whose ideals and illusions have been shattered by traumatic experiences can return to grace, finding internal balance, and being free from anxiety and anger.

KI 27 (Transporting Point Mansion, Store House): The master point, KI 27 provides the impetus towards change for those stuck in their past. It is the storehouse of physical, mental, and spiritual energy and gives motivation to all pursuits and can help with boosting the adrenal function. Consistent with the DRRBF conception of the Water phase energetics, it is said to enhance compassion and connection to others and the universe. According to Dr. Hammer, this point can allow for dissociation and for the spirit to leave the body under extreme circumstances and traumas in the interest of protection and survival.

Bladder

BL 1: As an intersection point for the Small Intestine and Stomach channels and with its location at the eyes, BL 1 is a profound point for opening the portals of perception. As discussed in Chapter 4, BL 1, upon exposure to light, activates wei qi and hence has a strong impact on the nervous system, as well as mood disorders (e.g., Seasonal Affective Disorder and the use of light in treatment). Its connection to wei qi activation brings strong influence to the Kidney yang and ming men (its alternate name), activating the dissemination of yang from storage. As the first point activated by the sun, BL 1 mediates and creates resonance and harmony as the internal landscape adjusts to the heavenly influence, providing clarity and aligning us to our true nature. As will be discussed at length in the following chapter, BL 1 is also the upper confluent point of the ST/SP and SI/HT divergent channels and impacts not only the jin-thin fluids, but also the ye-thick fluids and hormonal system. Via the SI/HT divergent channels, the impact on the chest and Heart is further strengthened, especially when combined with GB 22 (lower confluent of the SI/HT divergent channels). BL 1, brightness of the eyes, provides illumination and clarity in seeing and understanding, allowing one to look at life clearly. The Stomach and Small Intestine channels meet here, bringing their capacity to separate the pure from the impure. BL 1 also strengthens willpower (connection to the Kidneys) and brings a sense of belonging (connection to the outside world).

BL 2: While not as strong as BL 1, BL 2 can be used as an alternate point in those squeamish about having the inner canthus needled (or those practitioners not comfortable with needling it). From BL 1 and BL 2, experiences and perception can move to Du 24 and into the brain.

BL 3 through BL 6: While not as commonly needled in Heart Shock, these points can be effective in regulating circulation of qi throughout the head to open the orifices and impact thinking, hearing (internal narratives), and overall perception.

BL 7: This point can bring one's shen to the eyes and fluids to all the portals of the head, open the orifices, and resuscitate. It affects visual and sensory capacity, and in some traditions is used as a point of meditation to help bring the shen to a higher state of consciousness.[115]

BL 8: Considered the luo point of the brain, it deals with stagnation of fluids and blood with an impact on the shen and marrow.

BL 9: This point helps with insomnia, especially when caused by yin deficiency (Heart yin deficiency being the primary Heart Shock impact).

BL 10: As a WOS point, BL 10 helps to open the portals of perception. It also doubles as the upper confluent point for the BL/KI divergent channels, commonly used for traumas, especially ones that were life threatening and impacted the jing-essence. BL 10 is where the BL channel splits before descending the back and has tremendous usefulness for psychiatric conditions, especially when combined with the back shu points and/or outer shu points. It relaxes the sinews, thus calming an overactive nervous system, and can also descend hyperactive rising yang qi. As a point on the base of the occiput, it can provide support to stand tall and keep one's chin up in the midst of difficulties.

BL 11: This point is mostly used in conjunction with Heart Shock in connection with the BL/KI divergent channel treatments where there has been damage to the jing and bone level, with symptoms such as arthritis, especially with a loss of latency. It can also nourish the blood and be used in conjunction with BL 20, BL 18, and BL 15 in a primary channel treatment to bring blood to the chest and Heart. As a local BL channel point it has usefulness in relaxing the sinews in patients with a NST disorder.

BL 12: Where wind-cold penetrates, obstructing circulation within the channel, BL 12 can be used as a local point for relaxing the sinews and/or treating any attending pain. As wind-cold inhibits the circulation of wei qi, BL 12 can be used to free wei qi in the upper back as well as the chest, allowing the Lungs to diffuse. For this purpose, BL 12 can be needled or one can use cupping and/or gua sha.

BL 13/BL 42 THROUGH BL 25/BL 52

These points are used to access and utilize the dynamics associated with their respective organs, either nourishing, invigorating, or sedating as necessary within the Heart Shock framework. The outer shu points are often used for more mental-emotional symptoms that accompany the presentation. As these points have been discussed in multiple sources in the modern literature, I will present only a brief mention of their most common usages.

BL 13: As the back shu point of the Lungs, BL 13 can strengthen wei qi, diffuse Lung qi and open the chest, clear heat from the Lungs and chest, descend Lung qi to the Kidneys, etc. BL 13 allows one to forgive, let go, and live in the moment, providing a direct connection to one's breath.

> BL 42: The outer shu to the Lungs, BL 42 can open the chest and promote circulation. Related to the corporeal soul, it relieves grief, sadness, depression, and worry, and bring one into the present moment.

BL 14: As the back shu point of the Pericardium, BL 14 has a strong influence on the chest and Heart. It can also relax its jueyin pair, the Liver, and the sinews. BL 14 provides one with a stronger capacity for healthy socialization and problem solving, an intelligence of one's actions, and higher-level defensive/restorative mechanisms.

> BL 43: Gaohuangshu has long been considered a vital point in the treatment of intractable and deep-rooted diseases. As the outer shu point

of the Pericardium, the wrapping of the Heart, and the connection to the gao and huang, it helps with permeating qi through the chest and via the connection to jueyin, the diaphragm. BL 43 stabilizes the Heart, banks the Kidneys, and supports original qi and jing-essence. As an overall immune booster, it also supplements the Lungs and Spleen, and can invigorate the mind. Proper needling of this point requires the arms to be extended to open the scapula and reveal the point.

BL 15: The back shu of the Heart, BL 15 nourishes the Heart and shen and quiets the spirit, clears heat from the chest and stabilizes one's emotions, loosens the chest and regulates the circulation of qi in the chest, stimulates the brain and calms the nervous system, and invigorates blood. It allows a person to understand and come to terms with his desires, and sort out the distractions preventing the fulfillment of his curriculum.

BL 44: As the outer shu, BL 44 treats all the emotional counterparts to imbalances within the Heart, e.g., Heart qi deficiency and lack of joy-type depression, Heart fire and mania, cyclothymic depression, Heart blood stagnation and bitterness/vengeance, etc. The needling technique should be appropriate to the condition being treated, e.g., sedating for Heart fire, strengthening (perhaps even with moxa) for Heart qi-yang deficiency, etc.

BL 16: As the back shu for the Du mai, BL 16 is useful for calming hyperactive yang qi, especially in conjunction with a NST condition. It can be used to open up the chest and release wind (angina) as well as to treat running piglet qi.

BL 45: As the outer shu point to the Du mai, and being placed between the Heart and the diaphragm, BL 45 exerts an influence on the shen and blood. Jarrett notes the use of this point when one experiences shock in the form of receiving bad news, divorce, etc. and that it assists the individual drowning in sorrow and loss, preventing the pathology from entering and stagnating in the diaphragm.[116] Drawing on the yang from Du mai, this point can also stimulate Heart yang to vaporize phlegm obstructing the orifices. BL 45 also treats uncontrolled laughter or crying and talking to oneself (phlegm harassing the Heart and dian kuang), hallucinations and hearing voices, etc.

BL 17: The influential point of blood and the diaphragm shu, BL 17 treats disorders of the shen, primarily those caused by blood stagnation and/or heat in the blood (e.g., insomnia, tachycardia, etc.). As the diaphragm has a strong connection to the Liver and jueyin, it has a very calming effect on the mind and nervous system. It is also in the area of the "ring around the chest" discussed in more detail in the following chapter within the taiyang zonal divergent section. It has the capacity to open the chest and regulate qi and blood, and is said to even nourish blood.

> BL 46: Less commonly used, this point shares many attributes of its inner shu and can be used for calming the mind and nervous system.

BL 18: The back shu of the Liver, BL 18 is an effective point for calming the nervous system and harmonizing the emotions. It has a function of brightening the orifice it opens to, the eyes, and hence allowing for clearer perceptions/vision. BL 18 is also effective at eliminating wind and calming hyperactive wei qi, either by coursing the qi (release obstructions at the point), or anchoring (needling with tonification inwards towards the Du mai or down towards BL 23 and the Kidney back shu). It also deals with the inability to let go of the past (failures/traumas, etc.) and future (frustrations of what one cannot achieve).

> BL 47: The outer shu of the Liver, BL 47 gives access to and roots the hun/ethereal soul. As a wood element point, it helps to restore a sense of direction and vision towards one's destiny and purpose in life. Like its inner shu counterpart, BL 47 also courses the Liver and rectifies qi, strengthens the Spleen, and harmonizes the Stomach; it also regulates the bowels. Relating to DRRBF, the Wood phase mediates forward progress and growth with the ability to retreat and nourish reserves. In this regard, BL 47 can be used to project the hun into the external world (and theoretically beyond) as well as to anchor the hun and retreat into the blood for nourishment and quietude. It can also help to alleviate anger and frustration.

BL 19: The Gall Bladder's shu point, like its yin counterpart, has an influence over the diaphragm and eyes and can be used to regulate qi within the chest and reveal clarity of one's vision (internal as well as external). It can be used with BL 17, tapping into the energetics of the diaphragm, to nourish the blood, thus providing a more substantial grounded home for the hun. BL 19 can provide courage in shy, timid people and help them to express themselves and be decisive.

> BL 48: This point can strengthen yang deficiency and help to provide comfort and receive nourishment from others. It helps by breaking down one's armoring.

BL 20 and 21: The back shu of the Spleen and Stomach respectively, these points can strongly supplement the earth to promote groundedness and stability in the chaos resulting from trauma. Regulating the functions of the digestive organs, these points can also be effective where a NST condition overwhelms and insults the digestive system, creating an irritable bowel and nervous stomach from wei qi hyperactivity in the GI system.

BL 49 and 50: The outer shu points to the Earth phase, these points can further enhance the functions of the inner shu points as well as providing support to the yi, treating such symptoms as obsessive-compulsive disorders, difficulty concentrating and processing information, poor memory, etc. Combining these points with others on the earth channels, such as ST 40, SP 9, ST 8, and ST 1, can relieve the damp and phlegm obstructing the orifices to allow for proper separation of pure and impure, and thus more accurate perceptions, understanding, and contextualization of one's experiences and a healthier internal narrative. These points can also provide a sense of nurturing and contentment.

BL 22: As a representation of the Triple Burner, BL 22 is an important point for the restoration of the proper dissemination of yuan qi to the back shu points. Able to impact yang qi, BL 22 becomes an integral treatment for those stuck in the fight/flight/freeze response, able to unlock and invigorate frozen yang (especially with the use of moxibustion), or help ground hyperactive yang qi back to the Kidneys.

BL 51: The outer shu of the Triple Burner, BL 51 assists with harmonizing the Stomach and managing damp (and heat) accumulation and ensuring smooth functioning of the Triple Burner mechanism. As a fire element point, BL 51 also assists with promoting the circulation of qi to the Heart, warming Heart yang.

BL 23: As the back shu of the Kidneys, BL 23 is one of the more commonly used points in the treatment of Heart Shock. It strongly supplements the Kidney yin (source of the nervous system) and yang (and ming men), strengthens the bones and marrow (including the lower back and spine), brightens the eyes and sharpens hearing, nourishes jing-essence and blood, and anchors/grasps qi. Thus, this point's energetics has the ability to address a few of the Heart Shock treatment strategies.

BL 52: The outer shu for the Kidneys, BL 52 helps to strengthen one's willpower, often weakened post trauma. Tapping into the yang, it can help treat exhaustion, depression, hopelessness, and despair. Tapping into the yin, it can help one to internalize in service of discovering his potential and meaning in life.

Ba Liao points: The points on the lower back and sacral foramen are most often used in the context of trauma with pain and injuries, both to the lumbosacral area, as well as the pelvis and lower abdomen, regulating qi and blood within those areas. This includes sexual traumas, especially when issues of vulnerability don't allow direct needling to the lower jiao. BL 32 and 33 can treat cardiovascular problems and wind (excess wei qi) moving into the chest.

BL 36: The use of BL 36 within the context of this book tends to be as part of a luo and sinew channel treatment wherein pain or traumatic injury was sustained to the Bladder channel. In that case, as described in the preceding chapters, the Bladder luo point can be needled (either towards or away from the area of pain depending on the stage), followed by a point proximal to the he-sea point to regulate blood. Where the issue is in the lower back, sacrum, or gluteus area, BL 36 is my point of choice, then followed by a sinew treatment. Additionally, BL 36 lies within the BL DM pathway and, when needled from bottom to top, can be used to lift the qi-yang. As strengthening the earth is a treatment strategy within Heart Shock, BL 40, BL 10, BL 36, and BL 20–21 (and/or the respective outer shu points) can be used to raise sunken Spleen qi and assist with the transformation and transportation of qi and fluids, as well as assist the yi burdened by any dampness.

BL 39: As the lower he-sea of the Triple Burner, BL 39 can assist with moving obstructions within the lower jiao, freeing qi and fluids.

BL 40: As the he-sea point on the yang water channel, BL 40 allows for deeper access to the Bladder and Kidney organ systems. It helps to release the lower back, freeing up yang qi for proper dissemination. It is a major point in dermatology which can clear heat from the blood with rashes and skin disorders, and as all itchy painful rashes pertain to the Heart,[117] Heart Shock can be a major etiology. BL 40 is also the lower confluent to the BL/KI divergent meridians, giving it tremendous usage in the treatment of Heart Shock (discussed in the following chapter). As a sinew meridian knotting area, BL 40 helps to relax the sinews and has a strong impact on calming the nervous system.

BL 57: As a point on the calf, BL 57 lies on one of the more potent areas impacted by the fight/flight/freeze response and implicates the sinew channel with a direct impact on calming the nervous system and freeing up yang qi along the channel.

BL 58: The luo point, BL 58 is often used along with a sinew treatment for acute and chronic musculoskeletal traumas as discussed earlier, especially when blood stagnation is involved. It also has a function of strengthening the Kidneys.

BL 60: The jing-river and fire point, BL 60 has a strong influence on the lower back, strengthening it and the Kidney yang. It can soothe and relax the sinews for tightness due to nervous system tension and/or pain from trauma, and dispel taiyang channel pathogens/wind and cold. It can also regulate blood within the pelvis and uterus. Its name, Kun Lun, refers to the pure land, the entrance to which is at the foothills of the Himalayas. The name suggests that this point can guide one into and through the passage of life/death and can ease major transitions. It promotes a state of peace, allowing one to atone for sins to relieve guilt.

BL 61: As a point on the Yang Qiao mai, it can treat the individual who sees himself as a victim, helping him stand up to the world.

BL 62: The opening point for the Yang Qiao mai, BL 62 can open the portals (eyes and ears), and can treat wind and nervous system disorders (e.g., epilepsy, tics, etc.). It can assist with clearing EPFs, soothes the sinews and nervous system, and can calm the shen (e.g., insomnia and anxiety).

BL 63: The xi-cleft point, BL 63 is excellent for treating pain. It can soothe the sinews and open the portals, as well as quiet the spirit.

BL 64: The source point, BL 64 can free the channels, dissipate wind, and strengthen the back and Kidneys. It is also able to quiet the Heart and spirit, open the portals, and clear the brain.

BL 65: The shu-stream and sedation point, BL 65 can dispel wind and EPFs, clear heat and toxins, as well as sooth and relax the sinews.

BL 66: The ying-spring and water point, BL 66 has the capacity to settle fright (calm it within its nourishing water) and quiet the spirit.

BL 67: The jing-well and tonification point, BL 67 can clear wind and open the portals and brain, and clear the eyes, relaxing tension within the nervous system. It is commonly used within the context of a sinew channel treatment to release the wind and cold, as well as for its impact on the eyes and BL 1 with the registering of light and initiation of wei qi circulation. In terms of roots and terminations, BL 67 and BL 1 assist with proper reception of stimuli and capacity for clear perceptions.

Fire phase (take two)

After the polarity switch from Fire to Water (Heart to Kidneys), it returns back to Fire and the Pericardium/Triple Burner before moving to the Wood phase.

Pericardium channel functions

- Regulates the vessels and blood circulation.
- Assists the Heart in housing the mind and shen.
- Maintains flow of qi in the chest.
- Distributes qi to, and impacts the function of, the Stomach and diaphragm.
- Manages the Heart and Kidney communication.
- Protects the Heart (from external pathogens as well as from emotional trauma).

Pericardium channel continuum approach

At the Pericardium progression has begun to burn up the interior and cause degeneration, creating a strong motivation to clear the pathogen, with symptoms such as anxiety, frustration, irritability, chest bi, 5 center heat, panic disorder, running piglet qi, etc. as the upper and lower body begin to lose communication.

Triple Burner channel functions

- Integrates the qi of the whole body and integrates the function of the upper, middle, and lower jiaos.

- As a shaoyang channel it distributes qi to the head and face, regulates the qi on the sides of the body, and treats shaoyang disease.

- Regulates the body fluids' metabolism, including the water functions of the Lungs, Spleen, and Kidneys.

- Impacts the lymphatic and endocrine systems, via its management of the fluids.

- Disseminates yuan qi.

- Regulates temperature and the even distribution of warmth and manages the Heart–Kidney communication.

Triple Burner channel continuum approach

Degeneration continues at the Triple Burner, especially that of the sensory orifices. As the Pericardium loses its ability to manage the Heart and Kidneys (above and below), the middle jiao becomes stagnant and one's ability to digest, assimilate, and eliminate is compromised. Severe life-threatening illnesses can manifest at this stage (cancers with night sweats, etc.), as can the psychological manifestations of delirium and dementia.

DRRBF[118]

Building on the Fire phase information above, the following apply.

Pericardium

The Pericardium protects the Heart from pain, obtains nourishment for the spirit, and enables safe contact with other egos.

Pericardium yin deficiency

This individual is the emotional doormat who wears their heart on their sleeve. They impulsively fall in love and are poor judges of character, and have difficulty protecting themselves in relationships.

Pericardium yin excess

The opposite of the above, this person's Heart is closed. They are bitter, vengeful, and defensive without much capacity for true intimacy.

Pericardium yang deficiency

This person lacks the ability to effectively express themselves and communicate with others. Their timing and presentation are poorly integrated and they are generally not well received. They experience significant frustration.

Pericardium yang excess

This person is summarized as style over substance. They are so obsessed with being precise that they lack the capacity for spontaneity and flexibility and lose the forest for the trees.

Triple Burner

The Triple Burner is an organ system that in Chinese medicine we consider to be without "form." Its function is maintaining stability, harmony, and equilibrium, integrating the three brains as well as left and right brain functions, allowing for correct sensory and perceptual functioning, as well as the three burners. The Triple Burner controls the internal thermostat.

Triple Burner deficiency

This person has difficulty integrating and coordinating the various aspects of sensory and perceptual functioning and cannot reconcile inconsistencies. Verbal and performance skills are not balanced.

Fire acupuncture points for trauma

Pericardium

PC 1: A WOS point, PC 1 opens the chest, promotes the circulation of qi, diffuses the Lungs, and clears heat. An important point to treat betrayals, PC 1 creates a sense of safety and intimacy and affords one the ability to restore the Heart to its pre-trauma state.[119] PC 1 can be used when a patient is being bombarded with images and hallucinations and hot phlegm harassing the shen. Its jueyin relationship to the Liver and the breast assist with opening the chest and diaphragm. It can treat fears and phobias, anxiety, and manic behavior. It can help provide connection and foster deep spiritual love and warmth. Due to its location on the breast, PC 2 can be used as an alternate point.

PC 2: Similar in energetics to PC 1, PC 2 can treat feelings of vulnerability and return one to a place of innocence and guilelessness, allowing one to keep the Heart open.

It can also nourish Heart blood and treat issues with long-term memory, clear empty heat, and assist with mitral valve prolapses. It is an excellent point for treating patients lacking in love and security.

PC 3: The he-sea, water point, PC 3 clears heat and cools the blood, clears fire toxins, invigorates the blood and removes stasis, opens the orifices, and calms the mind and shen. One of my most commonly used primary channel points for Heart Shock, it treats palpitations, insomnia, irritability, restlessness, etc. as it can harmonize the communication between the Heart and Kidneys. PC 3 is also able to regulate the Stomach, and downbears counterflow qi.

PC 4: The xi-cleft point, PC 4 is considered the master of all the xi-cleft points and treats the varieties of emotional flare-ups and emergency conditions such as acute chest pains, bleeding, hysteria, etc. It can quiet the Heart and spirit, clear heat in the blood, relax the chest and diaphragm, and regulate qi and stop pain (emotional and physical).

PC 5: The jing-river, metal point, PC 5 nourishes the Heart and quiets the spirit, relaxes the chest and diaphragm, harmonizes the Stomach, soothes the sinews, clears phlegm fire from the Heart and orifices, and nourishes Heart blood and yin (borrowing it from the Kidneys).[120] PC 5 can also help tap into a patient's denial of certain aspects of his life via communicating Heart and Kidneys by bringing deeply held unconscious issues to the consciousness.[121] PC 5 can also treat volatility in the emotions, with laughter and/or crying for no reason, as well as tapping into the Bao mai, bringing circulation to the pelvis, and also treating running piglet qi. As a metal point, it can assist with letting go of old sadness and grief, and as its alternate name gui lu or ghost path reveals, it is useful in possession, lust, or the inability to let go of lost loves.[122]

PC 6: The luo point and confluent of the Yin Wei mai, PC 6 has been discussed in the luo vessel chapter. Briefly, it can clear heat and eliminate irritability, relax the chest and regulate qi throughout the diaphragm, harmonize the Stomach, and regulate Heart qi and invigorate blood. An excellent point for calming the mind and nervous system, PC 6 can treat insomnia, irritability, anxiety, chest stuffiness, pain, etc. A very useful point to release suppressed emotions, PC 6 can allow the patient to get something off his chest.

PC 7: The shu-stream, earth, source, and sedation point, PC 7 clears heat from the Heart, quiets the spirit, relaxes the chest, clears heat from the blood, and harmonizes the Stomach. Also a ghost point, PC 7 treats depression, possession, and obsession with the past, as well as phlegm harassing the Heart and its psycho-emotional symptoms, including muddled or scattered expressions.

PC 8: The ying-spring, fire point, PC 8 clears Heart fire, extinguishes wind, cools the blood, and quiets the spirit. A major energetic point used in qigong, PC 8 helps to communicate our cultivated self to the outside world. It helps to extend compassion and relieve judgment. When tonified, it can bring yang to awaken the Heart and rekindle joy; when sedated, it can release "excess joy" and desires, and treat restless organ syndrome and fidgetiness. Also harmonizing the Stomach, PC 8 can treat rebellious qi as well as mental disorders from heat harassing the shen.

PC 9: The jing-well, wood point, PC 9 brings a relationship to the Chong mai and, when tonified, brings blood to the middle burner and Liver. It can revive consciousness and open the portals, clear heat from the Heart, expel wind, and return yang to the Heart. Its connection to the Liver brings an influence over the eyes and one's vision of his true self and intuitive nature.

Triple Burner

SJ 1: The jing-well, metal point, SJ 1 gets fed from PC 8 and treats heat in the blood with underlying yin deficiency, trying to release fire toxins to the qi and wei level, often accompanied by irritability and restlessness, etc. As a jing-well point, it can resuscitate and open the portals. Through its name, guan chong, it has a relationship to the Chong mai and can also invigorate blood. According to Jarrett, it can be used for those who rush into relationships (fire), yet withdraw feeling vulnerable and exposed.[123]

SJ 2: The ying-spring, water point, SJ 2 strongly calms the shen and treats fright palpitations, fear, anxiety, etc. and strengthens the willpower. SJ 2 can also help strengthen communication between the Heart and Kidneys. It has a strong influence over the water/fluid dynamic and hormonal system. It also opens the portal of the ear and has an influence over the cervical spine and the area of Du 14, helping its function of calming the nervous system.

SJ 3: The shu-stream, wood point, SJ 3 clears heat from the head and influences the portals of the eyes and ears. It can strengthen the mind and regulate qi, as well as influencing the spine (when needled deeply, as it can communicate with SI 3 internally). According to Dr. Hammer, and used often by myself for this purpose, SJ 3 can open the internal duct of the Triple Burner, strongly influencing the Stomach, the separation of pure from impure, and regulating the qi dynamic.

SJ 4: The source point, SJ 4 can strengthen and invigorate Kidney yang and original qi, as well as tonifying the Chong and Ren mai. With SJ 14, SJ 4 can help release latent pathogens from the shoulder, neck, and scapula as it tries to hide in the divergent channels.[124] It is often bled for this purpose, followed by needling SJ 2 to protect the fluids. SJ 4 also relaxes the sinews and influences the Stomach, and fluid transformation.

SJ 5: The luo point, SJ 5 has been discussed in the previous chapter, and as the confluent of the Yang Wei mai, SJ 5 will be discussed in more detail in the following chapter. Briefly, it resolves wind and heat and can bring pathology out of latency, clears toxins, opens the portals of the ears and eyes, and subdues Liver yang and a hyperactive nervous system. As part of the Yang Wei (yang linking) channel, with SI 3, it can have a strong influence over the spine. SJ 5 can also be used to clear excess heat from the Heart and fire channels. As the external gate, with PC 6 (internal gate), these points can mediate internal and external relationships, setting boundaries for what external influences can reach the Heart, and what one chooses to share with the outside world.

SJ 6: The jing-river, fire point, SJ 6 affects the chest and voice, allowing one to vent suppression and release pent-up thoughts and emotions (and the shaoyang in general). It also releases the lower by downbearing counterflow and freeing the bowels. It can clear heat and expel wind and also opens the ears. Its alternate name, flying tiger, alludes to the metal element as SJ 6 can treat rapid breathing, chest pain, and diaphragmatic restriction (especially when combined with GB 34).[125]

SJ 7: The xi-cleft point, SJ 7 has a strong impact on the chest and can soothe the Liver and rectify qi. It opens the portals of the eyes and ears, can clear heat from the Triple Burner, and stops pain.

SJ 8: The 3 yang meeting point, SJ 8 can treat sudden loss of voice (a common symptom during trauma) by freeing up yang to the throat.

SJ 10: The he-sea, earth, and sedation point, SJ 10 is one of my commonly used points when using the primary channels. It has strong psychological functions for calming the shen and treating apprehensiveness, depression, sadness, anxiety, insomnia, and also palpitations (by either clearing heat with sedation, or nourishing/astringing yang qi back to the chest with tonification, depending on diagnosis). It can be combined with the outer shu points and luo points associated with the emotion and/or psychological presentation. It also transforms phlegm in the channels, courses fire, and relaxes the sinews and tendons (and nervous system).

SJ 12: Named dissolving happiness, SJ 12 can treat Heart fire and lack of communication between the Heart and Kidneys with symptoms such as excessive laughter, extreme excitement, hyperactivity in the nervous system with wind symptoms, and stiff neck (use with PC 6 for this latter symptom as this luo symptom derives from excess heat and wind rising to the head).[126] SJ 12 can also allow one to relax and unwind, especially during sexual intercourse (especially with difficulty orgasming), by restoring fluid circulation to the reproductive organs and/or warming yang.[127]

SJ 13: Classically, this point was bled for the treatment of madness, insanity, mania, dian kuang, and hot phlegm harassing the Heart symptoms. It can be combined with PC 5 for that purpose.[128]

SJ 14: As a point proximal to the he-sea, SJ 14 can invigorate blood and has an effect on the luo channel. As a main point regulating circulation in the arm, it can help those who cannot cope to get a better handle on life.[129]

SJ 16: A WOS point, SJ 16 is the master point of the WOS points and provides a window to the spirit and eye and opens all the portals, allowing for purer perceptions and understanding. SJ 16 can help provide warmth and alleviate depressions and fears. It helps to release the neck, affects the breasts, and clears fluids congesting the portals, helping to return hearing, smell, vision, etc. SJ 16 is also the upper confluent point of the SJ/PC DM, which will be further discussed in the following chapter.

SJ 17: The wind screen, SJ 17 can free the portals and sharpen hearing, relieve wind and pain, and discharge heat, including sudden emotional volatility from impact to the Heart. Also useful as a protection for people concerned about social appearances and what others think of them.[130]

SJ 18–23: While not points I use often, each have certain functions for opening the portals, settling the spirit, quieting shock, and brightening the eyes, including SJ 18 for fear, and SJ 19 for fright palpitations and Heart–Kidney communication.

Heart and Pericardium points to treat the nine Heart pains

A method of using and combining the Heart and Pericardium points, described by Jeffrey Yuen, can be used as a step-by-step process of reawakening from trauma and overcoming it. In this model, a point on the Heart channel is combined with a point on the Pericardium channel in a particular order, depending on the stage one finds the patient. Moving through nine stages, the first step is represented by HT 1 and PC 9, the second by HT 2 and PC 8, the third by HT 3 and PC 7, etc. Following is a very brief rationale and description of the method.

Step 1: HT 1 and PC 9

HT 1 represents the idea of courage, the ability to handle situations in life (treats cold/ numb extremities), and endless possibilities. PC 9 affects the tongue and speech and resuscitates yang. Together, these points allow one to recognize and take ownership of one's struggle, and to surrender to life (and potentially a higher power). HT 1 is treated with moxa, and PC 9 sedated to open the chest and free the shen. Kidney points to address and strengthen courage can be added to these points.

Step 2: HT 2 and PC 8

HT 2 represents the ling-soul, innocence, and the capacity to begin reflecting on, and purifying, the experiences of one's life. Its name, qing ling, arouses the idea of wood, which houses the ling-hun (collective experiences), and purifies the blood (memories stored in the blood). HT 2 is typically treated with moxa in this regard to bring warmth to the Heart and burn up the perversities. PC 8 clears heat from the Heart, especially when bled, and can allow for the letting go of traumas and deep wounds. Wood points can be combined with these points, especially ones which strengthen and access the hun.

Step 3: HT 3 and PC 7

HT 3, the water point, reflects an acknowledgment of the formative aspects of one's life and looking at one's traumas, recognizing the full extent of our pain and that we are but a small drop in the larger sea. It allows for the invigoration of blood, preventing one from becoming stuck in any experience. It can also treat hot phlegm and open the orifices and that which prevents one from seeing/perceiving differently. PC 7 furthers this acknowledgment, providing the ability to move and bury the past and pain, allowing forgiveness and the capacity to heal. Forgiveness and letting go are virtues of metal, thus one can combine metal points to strengthen this step, e.g., LU 1, LU 2, LU 7, LI 4, etc., to allow for release of tears and cathartic water to flush away the past.

The first trinity, steps 1 through 3, provides the courage to acknowledge one's pain, let go of guilt, and provide forgiveness. While one need not treat all nine steps in order, beginning with these three is important to provide context and initiate one into the healing process.

Step 4: HT 4 and PC 6

HT 4 provides a glimpse of one's path, now that one has gained awareness of, and the strength to overcome, the past. PC 6, the inner gate, allows one to see the things distorted perceptions of the past have prevented. It rids the worry and fear associated with the possibility of negative outcomes. PC 6 is reduced for anxiety, worry, and shen disturbances, especially that of falling back into old habits and triggering environments. Also a ghost point, it releases one from the bondage of old behaviors and pain.

Step 5: HT 5 and PC 5

HT 5, the luo point, provides the capacity to release and express one's pain, sorrow, grief, shame, etc. from the Heart, without having to suppress it, hide it, or be governed by it. These painful experiences no longer gain residence in the shen, but are free to move. PC 5 allows for a certain detachment from experiences, by simply bearing witness and acknowledging the divine presence in things. One is no longer the same person as the one who was traumatized, but rather one who has released the weight of the past off of his chest.

Step 6: HT 6 and PC 4

Both HT 6 and PC 4 are xi-cleft points that, when sedated, treat accumulations of yin and phlegm oppressing the Heart, weighing one down. HT 6, when tonified, can nourish HT yin, providing a deeper sense of comfort about who one is. PC 4 can treat acute pain relapsing from deep-seated wounds and blood stasis, keeping one's traumas from being fully released.

The second trinity, steps 4 through 6, is important for assisting patients through relapses and recurrences of symptoms through the healing process as they move along their lives and begin to partake in habitual behaviors and be exposed to past environments.

Step 7: HT 7 and PC 3

HT 7, the source point, allows one to see one's inner light and furthers the process of one's spiritual awakening, resurrecting one's spirit. PC 3 assists the patient in reshaping his identity, no longer influenced by outside influences. Small Intestine points can be added in to assist with separating out the pure from impure.

Step 8: HT 8 and PC 2

This step represents the manifestation of the spark and connection to heaven above and something larger than oneself. As one finds her path, and reshapes her identity, she becomes able to live more spontaneously with less desires and being less beholden to desires or needs. HT 8 reflects the saying "home is where the heart is." It can treat hypersensitivity of wei qi and the nervous system (e.g., allergies) and help someone be comfortable in all circumstances and environments. Liver points can be added to this step to assist with the free flow of one's qi and re-creation of identity.

Step 9: HT 9 and PC 1

In this step one attracts the positivity she has been cultivating, and regains her enthusiasm. Perceptions are clear, and there is no resistance to the flow of life. Consciousness has been restored, the curriculum learned, and one now becomes a guide and beacon to assist others on their journey. Triple Burner points can be added to this last step in terms of its capacity to disseminate one's light/yang/shen.

The third trinity, steps 7 through 9, is about peeling off the layers/obfuscations to the natural illumination of the shen.

Wood phase

Liver channel functions

- Promotes the free flow of qi throughout the entire body, smoothing the circulation of blood and body fluids.

- Regulates mental functions and the emotions.

- Impacts and balances the functions of the internal organs via managing the directionality and movement of qi.

- Impacts the endocrine system and functions in relationship with the pancreas, thyroid, adrenals, pituitary glands, and ovaries.

- Stores the blood, including housing the Hun, regulating sleep and detoxifying.

- Regulates wei qi and blood circulation to the muscles, sinews, ligaments, and tendons.

- Opens to the eyes.

- Manifests in the nails as an outward expression.

Liver channel continuum approach

At the Liver channel, we see strong wind symptoms as attempts to rid pathology or, when too deficient, spread pathology. Autointoxication takes place and organ systems break down. With the Liver's domain over the reproductive organs, one may see the challenges and pathology that have been unable to be dealt with in this incarnation prepare to be transferred to the next.

Gall Bladder channel functions

- Regulates qi and the sides of the body.

- Influences the bones and joints.

- Influences decision-making.

- Regulates the functions of the Gall Bladder.

Gall Bladder channel continuum approach

By the time the Gall Bladder channel is reached, the body struggles to adapt to the pathology, and when this is not possible, it provides a dramatic last-ditch resolution. Healing crises are common at this stage as the Gall Bladder, a curious organ with contact to the yuan level, tries to bring latent pathogens out of the constitution to discharge them. Its impact on the brain (via the channel pathway and as a curious bowel) can show up with psychological disorders, wind, and circulation disorders of the brain (e.g., strokes) and, via the blood vessels, heart attacks.

Five Phases

Traditionally, the Wood Phase is associated with the springtime and the energies required for birth and growth. Spring is a time for the blooming of new life after the quiet respite of winter. It is associated with creativity (birth of new ideas) and the unfolding of one's potential as its energies allow for the free flow of self-expression (the free flow of one's qi is unique to the individual). The emotion associated with the Wood phase is anger and also includes restlessness, irritability, and frustration. This is seen as the natural consequence of the inhibition of the Wood phase's natural drive to grow and experience a free flow towards its directed goal. Feeling blocked causes mental discomfort and irritation in one's inability to achieve. Stress taxes and overburdens the Liver and Gall Bladder demanding they divert their attention away from their innate development.

The Liver is the planner, equipped with a vision of the future. The Gall Bladder is the decision-maker. It is an important footnote that according to Chinese medicine decision-making must precede planning. This is reflected in the "Chinese clock" in which the body's energies circulate in the Gall Bladder prior to moving to the Liver. Decision-making, to be effective, must come from a clear intuitive understanding of what is best for oneself. Should decisions not be made first, an undue burden is placed on the Liver which does not know which contingency to plan for. This creates tremendous stress, frustration, irritability, and anger as the energy within the Liver stagnates, creating heat, nervous system tension, and eventual depletion of the Liver organ system. Anger is an emotion with an energetic direction; its vector is to move upwards and ascend.

The resulting stagnation creates heat, the natural byproduct of the struggle between the body's metabolic activity and the immoveable object (ongoing stress). Heat builds up in the body and eventually seeks an outlet. If the individual is strong enough, the heat will find its outlet in one of a few ways: (1) the skin; (2) the urine; (3) the stool; and (4) vomiting (more in acute cases). If the individual cannot move this heat out, it will remain in the body creating havoc in the most vulnerable areas and/or the blood. If one is vulnerable in the colon, we may see eventual signs like colitis, diverticulitis, etc. If the heat moves into the blood the eventual response will be the drying out of the moisture content of the blood, leading to "blood thick" in which the blood becomes more viscous. This impairs circulation further, creating more heat, and a vicious cycle ensues. Once the blood thickens sufficiently the vessel walls themselves, which require the moisture of the blood to maintain suppleness and elasticity, begin to dry out and harden, often revealed by a Ropy pulse (see Figure 6.1). This process of arteriosclerosis can take many years but is readily diagnosable on the pulse in all its varied stages from prediction (based on the pathogenesis just described and the precursors on the pulse), to mild, moderate, and then severe. As such, this process can be prevented if caught early enough, reversed if mild or moderate, and managed if severe. The long-term consequences of this condition are significant Heart diseases, strokes, etc.

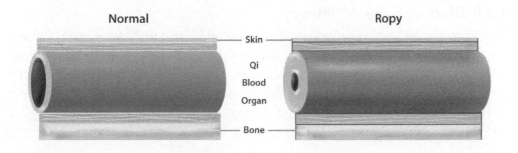

Figure 6.1: Ropy pulse
Reproduced with permission from Eastland Press

DRRBF[131]

From this perspective, the Wood phase is responsible for the drive to grow and evolve. Its major functions are for advancing (building/anabolism) and retreating (detoxification/catabolism), psychologically manifested in decisions about whether one should pursue growth and development or retreat in order to detoxify, rest, and replenish. A balance between the two is required, otherwise the constant advance exhausts one's reserves and results in collapse/exhaustion and a forced retreat.

From a DRRBF perspective there are certain vulnerable points in life, where factors beyond our control stunt the development of specific aspects of our growth/evolution and cause the bodymind to adapt in ways that allow for safe contact with those that we require for our health and well-being. For the wood personality, there are four patterns that develop.

Liver yin deficient

This individual, while not looking for a fight, does not have the ability to back down and retreat when challenged. His ego is always on the line and he fears humiliation. This person is generally resentful and is constantly vigilant in preparation for conflict; he is in a constant state of readiness and nervous system tension, and hence, frequent anxiety results. This person needs to feel in control, and his fear of being controlled leads to trouble with intimacy.

Liver yin excess

This is the proverbial pacifist in the extreme with a powerful fear of her own aggression. With this lack of assertiveness, this person does not put herself out and exchange ideas and is hence impeded on a cognitive level. She will avoid conflict and confrontation at all costs and as a result loses the opportunity for real intimacy.

Gall Bladder yang deficiency

This person grows up being emasculated, stunting his innate drive to assert, causing passive-aggressive, stubborn, spiteful, undermining, and passively resistant behavior. As a result, he learns adaptive behaviors to assert himself in the negative, becoming spiteful and eventually preoccupied with vengeance as a way of living out his anger that can have no external expression. Constant low-grade irritability and feelings of worthlessness pervade.

Gall Bladder yang excess

This is the unremittingly aggressive individual who tends to walk over others in pursuit of his own needs. His judgment and planning abilities are poor as everything gets sublimated with his current obsessive preoccupation.

All of the above personalities generally have a masochistic body structure in that their armoring has been turned inwards on themselves. They have a strong surface musculature but, because of their imbalances, the blood normally controlled by the Liver does not support and nourish their muscles, tendons, sinews, etc. and they are generally unable to sustain prolonged exertion.

Wood acupuncture points for trauma

Liver

LR 1: The jing-well, wood/horary point, LR 1 can open the portals, clear the spirit, and return yang. It promotes the smooth flow of qi and can soothe the sinews and relax the nervous system. As the most distal point, it impacts the entire channel and can regulate qi and blood in the pelvis, chest/diaphragm, as well as head. With the Liver's impact on the eyes, it can provide a vision of one's true self and provide self-esteem. As a jing-well point it helps to treat fullness in the region of the Heart and diaphragm. Its name, great pile, suggests its help in ridding the garbage/baggage/attachments impacting one's essence by detoxifying. Moxa is most commonly used for this point to burn up the trash.

LR 2: The ying-spring, fire, and sedation point, LR 2 can drain excessive Liver fire and cool blood heat resulting from hyperactivity of the nervous system. As such, it is a good point to treat agitation, restlessness, frustration, etc. with heat from stagnation harassing the spirit. It has an affinity to the eyes and helps to clarify perceptions for those who see things that aren't there (e.g., ghosts and/or clouded perceptions). It can also clear heat from the muscles as a result of nervous system tension, which causes hypertonicity/hyperactivity.

LR 3: The shu-stream, earth, and source point, LR 3 soothes the Liver and the nervous system. It moves the Liver blood, expels wind, restrains floating yang, strengthens qi, and calms the mind. It can be used when the nervous system overacts on the digestive system with hyperactive wei qi in the gut or the Liver overacting on the Spleen/Stomach. Iconic of the free and easy wanderer, LR 3 can assist with the freedom of movement in the sinews, as well as the emotions. Its name, tai chong, gives an association to the Chong mai, and its use in invigorating the blood, as well as shen disorders, from blood stagnation and rebellious qi. It also treats poor self-image/esteem, especially where created by life experiences and traumas. LR 3 can also treat fright wind and fear of change. With LI 4, it helps to synchronize to the present moment.

LR 4: The jing-river, metal point, LR 4 courses the channel and promotes the free flow of qi and blood with a strong influence over the chest. Drawing on the metal, it can bring a sense of spirituality and higher perspective to cut through suppressed grief and/or anger. As a jing-river point it can treat change of complexion, and can be used for when Heart Shock creates a blue-green hue. The metal point on the Liver channel (which assists all organs/channels with directionality of qi), LR 4 helps the Kidneys grasp Lung qi and influences ming men, especially in terms of the lower back, pelvis and genitalia, and ankles (which image and treat the reproductive organs).

LR 5: The luo point, LR 5 has an influence over the lower jiao and assisting with detoxification and chronic persistent emotions that have been nagging one repeatedly, much like a parasite causing self-destructive behavior and damaging one's essence. Its psycho-social functions have been detailed in Chapter 5. LR 5 can also relax the musculature of the genitalia which images the neck, creating a resonance to the WOS points and allowing it to treat pent-up emotions, deep-seated fears and traumas, etc.

LR 6: The xi-cleft point, LR 6 regulates qi and blood and can be used for acute pain, physical and/or emotional.

LR 8: The he-sea point, LR 8 nourishes Liver blood, pacifies Liver fire, soothes the sinews, and invigorates qi and blood in the channels. Through nourishing Liver blood, LR 8 assists in strengthening Heart qi, as well as regulating the hun and housing the spirit. It can nourish the eyes, providing blood to allow for clearer perceptions, nourishes and softens the muscles, and helps to quiet the spirit. The Liver also sends blood to the Kidneys to support essence, and LR 8, the water point, can support Kidney jing where nervous system tension and hyperactivity of the adrenals has left one depleted.

LR 9: Not as commonly used as the other points, LR 9 has an impact on softening and regulating the circulation in the lower jiao as well as impacting the Ren and Chong mai, making it a good choice where traumas to the pelvis and reproductive organs are involved, or when utilizing an 8x treatment.

LR 10 through LR 12: Like LR 9, these points have an impact on the lower abdomen and Ren and Chong mai and are used mostly for local pelvic and reproductive pathologies resulting from trauma.

LR 13: The front mu of the Spleen and the influential point of the zang organs, LR 13 courses the Liver and rectifies qi, quickens the blood, and benefits the Spleen and Stomach. It is a primary point for the nervous system overacting on the digestive system (the Liver overacting on the Spleen and/or the Stomach) and is a point on the GB/LR DM, used for repetitive traumas and those due to chronic stress (see the next chapter). Named "camphorwood gate" (a main material used for coffins), it allows one to bury the past and let go. Camphor opens the Heart and can vaporize phlegm, allowing one to see things that are no longer useful in one's life. With its relationship to the Spleen, LR 13 can be useful for shen disturbances, especially obsessive-compulsive disorder, and agitation from phlegm misting the orifices.

LR 14: The Liver's front mu, and point on the Yin Wei mai, LR 14 is also the last point on the Liver channel which moves internally to connect to the Lungs via the diaphragm. As such, it can move qi and blood and regulates the chest dynamic. Reflected in its name, complete gate, LR 14 reflects the end or completion of the circulation of qi and a new beginning wherein one can tap into the inspiration of the Lungs and metal to start anew. LR 14, especially with LU 1, helps to synchronize one to time and the present moment, as well as to one's environment, making one less sensitive and vulnerable. As a Yin Wei mai point, it can help treat Heart pain and assist with reconciling the disparate and traumatic events of one's life. Via the Yin Wei mai, LR 14 can act to invigorate blood and/or consolidate yin/blood/fluids to support one's jing-essence. It can also treat heat in the blood resulting in shen disturbance. Additionally, LR 14 dispels pathogens and heat from the blood chamber, harmonizes mid-stage pathogens, transforms phlegm, and disperses stasis; it can also calm the Liver and promote the smooth flow of Liver qi, and benefit the Stomach.

LR 14 alternate: 3 cun lateral to Ren 12 at the border of the ribcage, alternate LR 14 is a very important point and one frequently used by myself to strengthen and anchor the Liver, especially when the pulse at the left middle position is Empty.

Gall Bladder

GB 1: A major impact on brightening the eyes, GB 1 allows one to let go of habituated worldviews and see/experience things unadulterated/untainted/undistorted by negative experiences. It dispels wind and discharges heat, courses the channels and frees qi stagnation, and relieves pain.

GB 2, GB 3, and GB 4: These points all provide access to the ear portals, allowing for proper differentiation and interpretations of what one hears. They dispel wind, course the Liver and Gall Bladder, free the channel, settle fright, and relieve pain. GB 2, in particular, the auditory convergence, can also allow one to hear her inner thoughts and conscience, tapping into one's inner wisdom.

GB 5 through GB 9: These points clear heat from the Gall Bladder and settle and calm the spirit. GB 8 affects the brain, opens the diaphragm, and treats wind-phlegm, timidity, and shyness. It is one of the points in the gu treatment protocol (see Chapter 9). GB 9 calms the shen, and treats hysteria, mania, palpitations, and fear associated with the Gall Bladder.

GB 11: The head portal yin, GB 11 helps bring fluid/moisture/yin to the portals of the head to maintain their clarity of perception. When reduced, it can open the portals.

GB 12: Located near GB 20 and SJ 16, GB 12 has a strong influence on the brain and emotions, and unblocks stagnation in the head. It is said to rouse the brain and open the portals, dissipate wind, and clear heat.

GB 13: Ben Shen, the root spirit, is a major point, and one of my most commonly used points on the primary channels (and sinew channels) for settling and quieting the spirit. It treats all mental-emotional disorders (including mania, anxiety, panic, jealousy, and envy) as well as insomnia, dizziness, palpitations, etc. As a three yang of the arm sinew meeting point (ST 8/GB 13 area), it has a strong influence on the nervous system and relaxes the sinews, calms the Liver, and rids wind. It can treat the surging of yang into the brain affecting the shen, phlegm misting the Heart orifices, obsessive thoughts, etc. As its name suggests, it has an ability to root and ground an unstable spirit, also enabling communication between above and below. The spirit is manifest in the eyes, and GB 13 helps one to root and anchor one's vision and see one's path in life more clearly.

GB 14 through GB 16: Not used as commonly for me, these head points can brighten the eye portals.

GB 18: Another point on the head with an impact on the portals, GB 18 has an impact on the Metal phase and is useful for the patient who is constantly distracted, helping him to live more in the moment (assisting the po). It can diffuse and descend the Lung qi, assist with rectifying the chest and shallow breathing, and free the portals. The point is very centering and useful for shen disturbances, dementia, daydreaming, and the feeling that someone/something is sitting on the chest (possession: see Chapter 9).

GB 19: On the head, GB 19 can rouse the brain and free the portals, as well as soothe the sinews and release wind (twitching eyes, facial tics, etc.). Helping to "empty the brain," its name, nao kong, is consistent with the Buddhist notion of kong-emptiness, freeing oneself from an incessant internal dialogue and overactive mental activity.

GB 20: More commonly used than GB 18 or GB 19, GB 20 also courses wind and clears the head and brain, opens the portals, brightens the eyes, and sharpens hearing. It can free the channels, harmonize qi and blood, and subdue the Liver. An excellent point for calming the nervous system, GB 20 is often used to relieve stress and calm the shen, and is very useful for anxiety, insomnia, and hyperactivity. Between these three points, seeking the most tender areas can direct one to the best treatment point.

GB 21: The shoulder well, GB 21 can free the channels, especially opening up all the jing-well points of the hands (GB 30 does this for the feet); it is very useful for relaxing the sinew channels. As many shoulder points do, GB 21 treats phlegm, but also can open the portals and relax the nervous system. It also has an impact on opening the chest (freeing lactation).

GB 22: A major energetic point as the three yin meeting point of the arm sinew meridians, as well as the SI/HT divergent channel, GB 22 relaxes the chest and promotes qi circulation, soothes the sinews, and unlocks the wei qi circulation. Its name, yuan ye, signifies its use with the fluids/marrow/ye and hormonal system and it is useful in regulating the ye circulation in the brain (cerebrospinal fluid), pelvis (sexual fluids), and endocrine system as a whole. It is a major point for internalizing wei qi and assisting with bringing pathogens into latency. Also originally considered the great luo of the Spleen, GB 22 can treat psycho-social and emotional disorders via its management of the blood and ye (see SI/HT DM in the following chapter).

GB 24: The front mu of the Gall Bladder, GB 24 is a powerful point to open and release the chest, and can treat frustration, irritability, and tendency towards anger. Its name, sun and moon, signifies its capacity to harmonize yin and yang, eliminate black and white thinking, and reveal the unity behind all things. It also courses the Gall Bladder qi, promotes the functions of the Liver, and can harmonize the middle burner.

GB 25: The front mu of the Kidneys, GB 25 is an important point for strengthening and anchoring the Kidneys, warming cold and transforming fluids, relaxing the sinews, and anchoring yang back to its source. Where trauma has created paralysis and immobility, GB 25 can arouse the yang and promote movement.

GB 26 through GB 28: This trinity forms the lower trajectory of the Dai mai and can be used to consolidate or release pathogens from holding. They also have a strong impact on circulation through the pelvis and impact the Liver and Kidneys.

GB 29: A Yang Qiao mai point, GB 29 assists with helping one to stand up to the world, not buckling from pressure. It can treat pain in the hips and knees where one has difficulty feeling grounded.

GB 30: Like GB 21 did for the upper body, GB 30 opens the jing-well points of the legs/feet. It can activate wei qi circulation and is an important point on the sinew channels and relaxing the lower back and nervous system. Also a Yang Qiao point, it can provide motivation to face a hostile world and provide energy and resources/stamina to meet challenges.

GB 34: The influential point of the sinews, GB 34 is a primary point to relax the nervous system and treat a host of sinew disorders as it is also a binding area for the three leg yang sinew channels. It also impacts the diaphragm and opens the chest while promoting the smooth flow of Liver qi and treating rebellious qi.

GB 35: The xi-cleft point of the Yin Wei mai, GB 35 relaxes the Gall Bladder and quiets the spirit. It soothes the sinews, invigorates blood, and relieves pain (as a Yin Wei mai, one can extrapolate this to relieve the nine Heart pains).

GB 36: The xi-cleft point of the Gall Bladder, GB 36 can clear heat and toxins and remove obstructions from the channel. It can release the Liver and Gall Bladder and treat pain.

GB 37: The luo point, GB 37 has been detailed in the previous chapter. Briefly, it regulates the Liver, brightens the eyes, rids wind, clears heat, regulates the diaphragm, ribcage, and breasts, and treats a variety of shen disorders such as apprehensiveness, timidity and shyness, etc.

GB 38: The jing-river, fire/sedation point, GB 38 can treat bi-obstruction syndrome and soothe the Liver, resolve depression, stimulate courage, and help one to express themselves, as well as harmonizing the shaoyang. As the fire/sedation point, I often use GB 38 to treat hyperactivity in the nervous system, with fidgetiness (along with GB 34), anger, and frustration (along with GB 41 if the patient is suppressing tears).

GB 39: The influential point of marrow, GB 39 benefits the essence and nourishes the marrow, also clearing heat from the marrow (when there is a latent pathogen burning up the structure and depleting reserves). It can also clear heat and wind-damp from the Gall Bladder and eliminate wind from the channel, especially when there is an underlying Kidney yin deficiency at the root. Its name, the suspended bell, alludes to the bell which sounded when a person died, and GB 39 is said to treat and relieve a heavy Heart (depression, melancholy) when afflicted by grief and stagnant Lung qi.[132]

GB 40: The yuan-source point, GB 40 clears heat from the Liver and Gall Bladder, and promotes the smooth flow of Liver qi, treating shaoyang pathogens, inversion qi, and damp-heat. As a source point on a yang channel, it has an impact on Ren 17 and the qi of the chest. In its relationship to the curious bowels and yuan qi, GB 40 can also strengthen willpower and the mind, and assist with decision-making. As it taps into the source, it allows for a more inclusive vision and perspective on life, clearing habituated differentiations. An additional benefit to the Heart Shock patient, GB 40 is said to treat chronic non-healing wounds[133] (acupuncture analog to the resins in herbal medicine).

GB 41: The shu-stream, wood/horary, and confluent point of the Dai mai, GB 41 can open the belt vessel, clear fire and rid wind, open the portals of the eyes and ears, course the Liver and Gall Bladder, and transform phlegm obstructions. Its name is near to tears and GB 41 is useful for relieving frustration, irritability, and anger, allowing one to release her tears and cathartically clear her toxic emotions. As the confluent of the Dai mai, GB 41 can be used to access the Dai, either bringing pathogens out of latency, or storing them for a later time.

GB 42: Not as commonly used as GB 41, GB 42 can bring pathogens into a state of latency, clear Liver and Gall Bladder heat, open the portals of the eyes and ears, and anchor qi to the Kidneys.

GB 43: The ying-spring, water, and tonification point, GB 43 can clear excess heat in the Gall Bladder, extinguish wind and subdue Liver yang, open the ear portals, and relieve pain. It is a good point to course the Liver qi and treat the diaphragm and lateral costal region.

GB 44: The jing-well, metal point, GB 44 can open the portals (above and below) and treat loss of consciousness, tinnitus, and bowel stagnation, as well as fullness/distension under the Heart and ribcage. It clears heat and drains fire, extinguishes wind and courses the Liver, subdues Liver yang, and calms the mind and nervous system. According to Jarrett, it harmonizes the emotions and addresses timidity and fear preventing one from taking action, as well as pruning away unnecessary growth, allowing for a clearing of vision and more directed and successful movement towards one's goals.[134]

A note on the third trinity of primary channels

The third trinity of primary channels (PC/SJ/GB/LR) deals with perceptions and habituations: how people become accustomed to thinking, perceiving, and acting in particular ways, narrowing options in life and restricting experiences based on historical likes and dislikes. Knowing what one likes and dislikes, most of us tend to live lives that have become limited and routine, and when that routine has become something more restrictive than nourishing, disease processes can take hold. No longer allowing one's Liver qi to move freely (which of course is not some fixed one-size-fits-all pathway of circulation, but rather unique to the individual in expressing his curriculum), life becomes stagnant. Expecting to heal in such an environment is naïve at best, and as the famous quote goes, "Insanity is doing something over and over again and expecting a different result."

In treating patients who are stuck in their pathologies, as most Heart Shock patients are, trapped and haunted by their past and the destructive wake that it has left behind, it becomes imperative to rock the boat and encourage a new direction. I encourage my patients to eat differently, to try new foods, find a new route to work, engage in activities that are new, take up a new hobby, instrument, or language, frequent a new restaurant, reach out to a friend they haven't seen in a while, etc.

As wind is the cause of hundreds of diseases, we can understand wind to be a metaphor for change. The inability to change and adapt leaves us vulnerable. Health allows for all possibilities, and the less differentiated we are, the more likelihood and potential one has to remain healthy. Most people become increasingly habituated as they age, and the aging process can be seen as a restriction in the free flow of one's Liver qi. Flowing water never decays, thus one must allow for uninhibited spontaneous movement. Treating the third trinity of the primary channels provides a broadening of perceptions and an opening up of the narrow-funneled habituations at the root of disease. Many of these acupuncture points have the capacity for clearing the orifices and opening the portals of perception, allowing for the possibility of change to take place. New pathways open, new roads are traveled, new experiences widen the lens, and new possibilities for healing emerge.

More Classical acupuncture treatments

Ge Hong's 9 Flower treatment[135]

Another treatment useful in Heart Shock, and building on the idea of the nine Heart pains as differentiation/habituation as described above, is Ge Hong's 9 Flower treatment. The nine acupuncture needles are done in a particular order to open the chest and Heart and resurrect the shen. The protocol begins with needling right-side KI 21, the gate of mystery, to tap into the darkness. Next is right KI 23, which brings the energetics up to the chest, the spirit seal, and the light. As you peel off that which is blocking the shen, one's light can be revealed. This point also helps to diffuse the Lung and "let go." The third point, right ST 19, also assists in letting go by separating the pure from impure. The next needle is right KI 19 which gathers the jing, and brings it to the fifth point, Ren 14, the front mu point of the Heart. The points are then repeated on the left side, totaling nine needles in the shape of a flower. The flower symbolizes the opening of the Heart and letting go, its beauty revealed, but also never complaining as it reaches full maturity and decay as its petals fall, represented by the expression "falling flowers never complain."[136]

Ge Hong's 9 Flower Protocol

Right KI 21
Right KI 23
Right ST 19
Right KI 19
Ren 14
Left KI 21
Left KI 23
Left ST 19
Left KI 19

Windows of the Sky (WOS) points

As mentioned above, Windows of the Sky points are significant in that they provide actions towards clearing and opening the portals of perception, connecting us to the heavens above and grounding us in the earth. As these points have mostly been discussed in their associated primary channel point discussion section, below is simply a list of these powerful points.

LU 3

LI 18

BL 10

SI 16

SI 17

PC 1 (PC 2 is often substituted for women)

SJ 16

ST 9

Ren 22

Du 16

Herbal formulas for the treatment of Heart Shock
Shen-Hammer lineage
Sheng Mai San (modified)

Within the Shen-Hammer lineage, there are many herbal formulas which can and have been used to successfully treat Heart Shock and its sequelae. As the primary impact of Heart Shock is on Heart yin, the initial base formula should strongly focus on the strategy of nourishing and astringing the Heart's yin. As such, the Shen-Hammer lineage often begins the construction of a formula with a modified version of Sheng Mai San (hereinafter SMS). SMS contains Ren Shen, Mai Men Dong, and Wu Wei Zi. As a modification to focus more heavily on Heart yin, Xi Yang Shen is substituted for Ren Shen (or sometimes simply added to the formula depending on other diagnoses). While classically Ren Shen has a function of nourishing fluids, Xi Yang Shen is more nourishing to the yin and, as such, is prioritized in the formula base.

Interesting note on Mai Men Dong and Heart/Lung yin tonics: As discussed earlier, as pathology moves to the ying level, volition is involved to some degree with our emotions. Trauma is a very complex phenomenon, which incorporates elements of the ying level and our consciousness, but also our autonomic unconscious aspects (nervous system, wei qi dynamics), as well as impacting our core and yuan qi. As emotions have a willful component, and as trauma impacts the will and creates systemic chaos, patients can often spiral downhill unable to control their thoughts. When a patient is unable to exert one's will and shift her internal narrative about a trauma, the treatment strategy of promoting latency is warranted via calming the nervous system and nourishing yin and blood. Sun Si-miao recommended Mai Men Dong and Heart/Lung yin tonics for this process of forgetting one's trauma and stopping the obsessive thinking on it.[137]

Yunnan Bai Yao

Another main strategy is to invigorate the blood and also to astringe the bleeding (physical and emotional) that takes place post trauma. Many within the lineage use a particular protocol with Yunnan Bai Yao (hereinafter YNBY) in combination with SMS. The protocol is as follows: The little red pill is taken before bedtime, and the following day the orange capsules are begun, starting with 1 capsule 2x/day the first day, 1 capsule 3x/day the second day, 1 capsule 4x/day the third day, and then from day 4 until one finishes a total of 64 capsules, 2 capsules 4x/day. After the completion of this cycle, one waits a week to ten days to reassess if YNBY can be used for a second cycle.

Many practitioners do not like the use of YNBY due to the belief that all the ingredients have not been revealed by the Chinese government, creating an ethical dilemma on the appropriateness of prescribing the formula. To my knowledge, the ingredients have been released in total, hopefully eliminating this concern. The use of YNBY, however, need not be relied upon if one truly understands the treatment strategies that I have been detailing in the course of this book. My belief is that herbal formulas should be tailored to the individual who is being treated, not relying on any protocols whatsoever. While early in my career I used YNBY as above, I have not relied on it in over a decade, choosing instead to write personalized, tailor-made formulas where each ingredient is purposeful and relevant to the individual patient in question. Often, SMS is used as a beginning base formula, but not exclusively, as there are many occasions where it is inappropriate, or would simply be less effective than focusing on other herbs and strategies.

More on SMS and its modifications

The base formula of SMS is, however, an excellent beginning to the creation of a herbal formula and easily accommodated within a larger formula incorporating the other Heart Shock strategies. Its focus in the context of Heart Shock is on nourishing and stabilizing the Heart yin. Xi Yang Shen strongly nourishes the yin, as well as also strengthening Heart qi. Mai Men Dong assists in building the fluids, and Wu Wei Zi builds blood and also astringes the yin with its sour flavor consolidating yin and yang back into the vessels to communicate. Other herbs can be added or substituted to treat the Heart yin as appropriate. Some of my common choices include using Sheng Di Huang if there is concurrent blood deficiency, blood heat, or Heart fire; Bai He if there is Lung yin deficiency and/or unstable emotional patterns; Fu Xiao Mai for its impact on calming the spirit, especially with Da Zao and Zhi Gan Cao for unstable moods, or insomnia with sweating; Shu Di Huang if there is also blood deficiency; Suan Zao Ren which nourishes Heart yin and blood and with its sour nature helps to astringe qi and fluids in the Heart, making it one of the most important herbs for anxiety and insomnia; Bai Zi Ren which nourishes Heart yin and calms the spirit, also preserving and astringing Heart yin; E Jiao if blood deficiency or consumptive conditions; and Yu Zhu if there is also wind symptoms in the sinews like tics, tremors, spasms, etc., for diabetic patients, or for palpitations with slow heartbeats.

The other Heart Shock strategies include opening the orifices, invigorating blood, calming the nervous system, strengthening and anchoring the Kidney qi-yang, etc. To open the portals, there are a number of herbs that I often choose from, including Shi Chang Pu, Yuan Zhi, Yu Jin, Niu Huang, and Bo He. Shi Chang Pu and Yuan Zhi are often used together, and Yuan Zhi will also settle the spirit and descend, assisting with the communication between the Heart and Kidneys. Yu Jin is very good for opening the orifices and clearing the portals, but also rids damp and heat and treats phlegm misting the Heart orifices. In addition, it will also invigorate the blood and relax the Liver, assisting with other treatment strategies. Niu Huang is reserved for extreme cases with severe shen disturbances. Bo He can be useful to clear heat and irritation from the eyes and nose and calm the shen, while also relaxing the nervous system and calming the Liver.

Herbs to invigorate the blood include Yu Jin as mentioned, but also Dan Shen, Chuan Xiong, Si Gua Lou, Lu Lu Tong, Niu Xi, Chi Shao, Hu Po, Ji Xue Teng, Ye Jiao Teng, etc. Yu Jin also opens the portals and clears damp-heat from the Liver and Gall Bladder; Dan Shen will also clear heat from the chest and invigorate blood around the diaphragm; Chuan Xiong moves the blood (relies on Lung qi), treats wind, and relaxes the Liver and nervous system; Si Gua Lou opens the chest and gets rid of phlegm; Lu Lu Tong is a powerful herb for unblocking blood in the chest (Dr. Shen used Si Gua Lou and Lu Lu Tong often); Niu Xi invigorates the blood and has a downward action, helping descension; Chi Shao will also treat heat in the blood and disturbing the shen; Hu Po (amber resin) also treats parasitic conditions (we've discussed already and will in more detail the idea of trauma as a parasite), and as a heavy mineral settles palpitations and calms the Heart, while invigorating blood; and Ji Xue Teng and Ye Jiao Teng are also helpful in that they both strongly nourish the Heart blood simultaneously.

To strengthen and anchor qi-yang back to the Kidneys and stabilize the Triple Burner, I often choose from Du Zhong, Zi He Che, Yang Waishen, Rou Gui, Fu Zi, Ren Shen, etc. Du Zhong is very good at consolidating and anchoring yang to the Kidneys, as well as treating the lower back and knees (structure); Zi He Che is one of the most powerful, but difficult to find, herbs for strengthening the Kidneys and essence; Yang Waishen, a recently available alternative to Zi He Che, is the Kidneys and reproductive organs of the goat, very strong for strengthening the Kidneys and essence; Rou Gui strengthens the Kidney yang (and Heart) and also helps to invigorate the blood; Fu Zi strongly nourishes and descends/anchors Kidney yang to the lower dantian and ming men; Ren Shen nourishes Kidney and original qi (as well as Heart qi and tonifies the earth); and She Chuang Zi strengthens Kidney yang and also treats parasites.

To calm the nervous system, my most commonly used herbs include Dang Gui, which also nourishes and harmonizes the blood, extinguishes wind, and downbears; Bai Shao, which nourishes the blood, relieves pain, relaxes the muscles, preserves yin, and harmonizes the ying and wei; Yu Jin, which also opens the portals and clears phlegm and damp-heat; Xiang Fu, which opens the chest and also regulates qi through the Triple Burner; Ge Gen, which nourishes yin, clears heat and relaxes the muscles, and anchors ascendant yang; Qiang Huo, which guides to the taiyang and Du mai, expels wind-cold-damp, and relaxes the upper back, neck, and spine; Du Huo, which expels wind-damp, releases the exterior, and strengthens Kidney yang; Bo He, which frees constrained Liver qi and clears heat from the portals; Mu Xiang, which opens the chest, descends, and strengthens the earth; and Chuan Xiong, which moves blood, treats wind, and relaxes the Liver and nervous system.

For the secondary strategies of strengthening the Heart qi, opening the chest, regulating the Spleen and Stomach, etc., many of the herbs I use include:

Strengthen the Heart qi: Ren Shen nourishes Heart, original, and Kidney qi; Huang Qi strengthens the Heart and Kidneys, Liver, and Spleen/Stomach, and ascends the qi; Gui Zhi strengthens the Heart qi and promotes movement of qi and blood; Zhi Gan Cao strengthens Heart qi and moistens; Suan Zao Ren nourishes Liver blood to strengthen Heart qi; Gou Qi Zi nourishes Heart qi via Liver blood, benefits the essence, and brightens the eye portals, also enriching the yin; Sheng Di Huang nourishes Heart qi via Liver blood, clears Heart fire, and nourishes yin; and Shu Di Huang nourishes Heart qi via Liver blood and tonifies blood and essence.

Open and regulate qi in the chest: Gua Lou (most commonly Gua Lou Pi, but also Gua Lou Shi and Gua Lou Ren) opens the chest and transforms phlegm; Xiang Fu opens the chest and also regulates qi through the Triple Burner; Mu Xiang opens the chest, descends, and strengthens the earth; Jie Geng opens the chest and helps the Lung qi diffuse; and Xing Ren treats counterflow and can descend Lung qi as well as help diffuse.

Regulate the middle burner: Sheng Jiang strengthens and harmonizes the Spleen and Stomach; Da Zao tonifies qi and blood; Zhi Gan Cao (or Gan Cao as appropriate) harmonizes a formula while also strengthening the earth and nourishing Heart qi; Bai Zhu strengthens the earth and also stabilizes the exterior and stops sweating; and Huang Jing strengthens the earth, moistens the Lungs, and tonifies the Kidneys and essence.

The use of Tian Men Dong, Ling Zhi, and Mu Xiang is a trio that Jeffrey Yuen has taught in the past for different types of shen disturbances, used in the Daoist traditions, also good for treating parasitic types of issues (with which Heart Shock can have similarities). Tian Men Dong has a similar impact as Mai Men Dong in the SMS formula, its yin more strongly nourishing to the Kidneys; Ling Zhi nourishes the Kidney yang; and Mu Xiang helps to calm the nervous system, while also strengthening the Spleen and Stomach, and has a descending action. Other common herbs I use include Hu Po, which also invigorates the blood and calms and settles the Heart; and Bing Lang, which promotes qi circulation and reduces accumulations in the middle and lower burner. More information on parasites and ghosts can be found in Chapter 9.

Common primary strategy herbs used to modify SMS

Heart yin	Orifices	Invigorate	Anchor KI	NST
Xi Yang Shen	Yuan Zhi	Yu Jin	Du Zhong	Dang Gui
Mai Men Dong	Shi Chang Pu	Dan Shen	Ren Shen	Bai Shao
Wu Wei Zi	Yu Jin	Chuan Xiong	Fu Zi	Yu Jin

Heart yin	Orifices	Invigorate	Anchor KI	NST
Sheng Di	Niu Huang	Chi Shao	Zi He Che	Xiang Fu
Shu Di	Bo He	Ji Xue Teng	Rou Gui	Ge Gen
Fu Xiao Mai	Xi Xin	Yi Jiao Teng	Yang Waishen	Qiang Huo
Bai He		Niu Xi	She Chuang Zi	Du Huo
Suan Zao Ren		Lu Lu Tong		Bo He
Bai Zi Ren		Hu Po		Mu Xiang
E Jiao		Bie Jia		Chuan Xiong
Yu Zhu				Long Gu
				Mu Li
				Dai Zhe Shi

Common secondary strategy herbs used to modify SMS

Heart qi	Open chest	SP/ST	Parasites
Ren Shen	Gua Lou	Ren Shen	Tian Men Dong
Huang Qi	Mu Xiang	Huang Qi	Mu Xiang
Gui Zhi	Xiang Fu	Bai Zhu	Ling Zhi
Zhi Gan Cao	Jie Geng	Zhi Gan Cao	Hu Po
Sheng Di	Xing Ren	Huang Jing	She Chuang Zi
Shu Di	Lu Lu Tong	Sheng Jiang	Bing Lang
Gou Qi Zi	Si Gua Lou	Da Zao	
Suan Zao Ren			

Dr. Shen's formulas

Heart Tight[138]

Shi Chang Pu	2.4g
Chuan Xiong	4.5g
Mu Xiang	4.5g
Fu Shen	9g
Yuan Zhi	4.5g
Suan Zao Ren	9g

Yu Jin	9g
Gua Lou Pi	9g
Chen Pi	6g

Heart Tight is essentially a diagnosis of nervousness of the Heart with underlying Heart yin deficiency. Typically, it presents with a Hesitant pulse wave and a Tight quality in the left distal position. If caused by a recent trauma, the pulse will be slightly Rapid. The construction of the Heart Tight formula demonstrates the primary treatment strategies of calming the shen (Fu Shen, Yuan Zhi, Suan Zao Ren) and relaxing the nervous system (Chuan Xiong, Mu Xiang, Yu Jin), as well as strengthening Heart yin and blood (Suan Zao Ren), while opening the chest (Chuan Xiong, Mu Xiang, Yuan Zhi, Gua Lou Pi), invigorating qi and blood (Chuan Xiong, Yu Jin, Mu Xiang), anchoring to the Kidneys (Yuan Zhi), and strengthening the Spleen and Stomach (Chen Pi and Fu Shen).

Heart Closed: Essentially the same formula as Heart Tight, Heart Closed refers to a qi stagnation condition; Gua Lou Pi and Chen Pi are removed and substituted with Huang Lian (to treat the heat from stagnation) and Chen Xiang (to aromatically open the Heart and disperse Heart qi stagnation).

Heart Small: More of a Heart blood stagnation condition, Ding Xiang is added to the Heart Tight formula to warm and aromatically open the Heart.

Heart Vibration: A progression of the Heart Tight scenario, Heart Vibration is characterized by increasing worry and the heat that is generated from it. Deng Xin Cao is added to the Heart Tight formula to treat it.

Qi Wild

Dang Shen	10g
Huang Qi	10g
Sang Ji Sheng	12g
Si Gua Lou	6g
Yuan Zhi	6g
Wu Wei Zi	2g
Mai Men Dong	10g
Duan Long Gu	18g
Duan Mu Li	18g

Dr. Shen's Qi Wild formula, while not specifically related to the Heart, treats another systemic issue from separation of yin and yang. This formula contains heavy calm spirit herbs along with astringents to nourish and especially anchor the qi, yin, and yang. Without being locked into any ingredients, the formula represents these strategies, which are also useful for Heart Shock, another systemic instability requiring calming, anchoring, and astringing. As with all of Dr. Shen's formulas, directionality is always a key component and reflects his specific choices of herbs. In the Qi Wild formula, a big focus is on the earth; Dang Shen and Huang Qi strengthen the Lung, Spleen, and Stomach and the earth element as a whole, and it provides a degree of stability. While these two provide the qi for the earth, Mai Men Dong provides the yin and substance. Huang Qi also strengthens the Kidneys, and is used a lot in the Shen-Hammer lineage for its ability to strengthen the Liver. Yuan Zhi opens the orifices and spirit, and guides the yang back towards the yin, helping communicate Heart to Kidney. Sang Ji Sheng strengthens the Liver and Kidney yin, and the formula is anchored by Long Gu and Mu Li which have been charred to further protect leakage. Si Gua Luo helps to open the chest, allowing the unobstructed movement between the burners, and Wu Wei Zi helps to astringe. From the vantage of a Heart Shock formula, switching Xi Yang Shen for Dang Shen gives the SMS formula, and the other Heart Shock strategies are already present as Si Gua Lou unblocks the channels and collaterals providing the necessary movement. Of course, additional blood invigorators can be added as needed.

Dr. Hammer's formulas

Hyperactivity in a five-year-old with birth trauma

Shi Chang Pu	3g
Chuan Xiong	3g
Chao Jing Jie	5g
Hei Fang Feng	5g
Mu Xiang	3g
Zhu Fu Shen	10g
Chao Suan Zao Ren	12g
Long Chi	25g
Ci Shi	25g
Huang Qin	3g
Jiao Gu Ya	12g
Jiao Mai Ya	12g
(Zhu sha) Deng Xin Cao	3 bundles

The above formula was prescribed by Dr. Hammer for a five-year-old boy with hyperactivity rooted in Heart Shock from trauma at birth. Many of the herbs that I have highlighted above are included here with the purpose of stabilizing and calming the Heart, nourishing Heart blood and astringing Heart yin, and anchoring to the Kidney, while relaxing the nervous system tension and hyperactivity. Jing Jie and Fang Feng are useful for releasing the hyperactivity and wind, but also important is that they protect the exterior from additional stresses from being internalized. The Long Chi anchors, calms, and astringes, the Ci Shi anchors and calms the Liver, the Huang Qin and Deng Xin Cao clear heat from the chest, and the Gu Ya/Mai Ya help digest the minerals, preventing stagnation.

ADD in a teenage boy

Dang Gui	6g
Chuan Xiong	4.5g
Bai Zhi	4.5g
Sang Ji Sheng	9g
Fu Shen	9g
Yuan Zhi	6g
Sheng Di Huang	9g
Tu Si Zi	9g
Long Chi	15g
Ci Shi	15g
Shan Zhu Yu	9g
Shen Qu	9g
Deng Xin Cao	3 bundles
Xi Yang Shen	4.5g
Ren Shen	4.5g
Zi He Che	4.5g

This next formula by Dr. Hammer uses similar strategies, with a stronger focus on nourishing Heart yin than the previous one. Sheng Di Huang and Xi Yang Shen nourish yin and clear heat from the Heart, and regulate the Liver. Dang Gui and Chuan Xiong nourish blood and invigorate the Liver, and open the chest. Bai Zhi helps to open the orifices and provides a connection to the interior and yangming. Sang Ji Sheng helps strengthen the Kidney and release the sinews. Fu Shen and Yuan Zhi calm the spirit and open the orifices. Tu Si Zi and Shan Zhu Yu strengthen the Kidneys and, along with Long Chi and Ci Shi, stabilize and astringe to the lower burner. Deng Xin Cao helps to clear heat that's harassing the Heart. Ren Shen strengthens the original qi and with Zi He Che boosts the Kidneys. Shen Qu helps to digest the cloying herbs and minerals.

Heart Shock causing arrhythmia

Xi Yang Ren	9g
Ren Shen	9g
Mai Men Dong	9g
Wu Wei Zi	6g
Hong Ren Shen	4.5g
Rou Gui	3g
Fu Zi	0.25g
Shi Chang Pu	9g
Ye Jiao Teng	6g
Zi He Che	2g
He Huan Pi	8g
Long Chi	9g
Yu Jin	5g
Suan Zao Ren	9g
He Shou Wu	9g
Bai Zi Ren	3g
Dan Shen	6g
Gan Cao	3g
Gan Jiang	3g
Fu Xiao Mai	20g

This next formula of Dr. Hammer's is quite large, and I don't recommend the inclusion of so many herbs generally. Dr. Hammer came from a Kampo herbal background and tended to combine formulas together, but my experience is that a formula this large is unnecessary and can dilute its impact. Nevertheless, it is helpful as a teaching tool to understand the strategies being employed. Heart yin is being nourished and astringed with Xi Yang Shen, Mai Men Dong, Wu Wei Zi (Sheng Mai San), Suan Zao Ren, and Fu Xiao Mai; blood is being invigorated with Dan Shen, Rou Gui, Yu Jin, and Ye Jiao Teng; the portals are being opened with Shi Chang Pu and Yu Jin; the Kidneys are being strengthened and anchored by Zi He Che, Ren Shen, Rou Gui, Fu Zi,[139] and Long Chi; the nervous system is relaxed by Ye Jiao Teng, He Huan Pi, Yu Jin, and Long Chi; and the Spleen and Stomach are being influenced by Ren Shen, Rou Gui, Gan Jiang, and Gan Cao. Additional herbs such as He Shou Wu and Bai Zi Ren serve to strengthen the Heart qi and blood in order to provide sufficient residence to calm the arrhythmia.

Heart separation of yin and yang

Xi Yang Ren	4.5g
Hong Ren Shen	4.5g
Fu Zi	0.25g
Zi He Che	4.5g
Bai Zi Ren	4.5g
Long Yan Rou	6g
Suan Zao Ren	6g
Yu Jin	6g
Shu Di Huang	9g
Ye Jiao Teng	9g
Yuan Zhi	9g
Sha Ren	1.5g
Fo Shou	3g
Dan Shen	9g
Mai Men Dong	6g
Chang Pu	6g
Gan Cao	3g
Chuan Xiong	4g
Long Gu	5g

Another formula by Dr. Hammer, this was used to treat the separation of yin and yang of the Heart. Fairly similar to the other formulas, one can see the use of SMS without Wu Wei Zi, using the sour astringent Suan Zao Ren instead, plus a number of herbs to strengthen Heart qi and blood (Long Yan Rou, Bai Zi Ren). Ren Shen, Zi He Che, and Fu Zi are used to strengthen and anchor the Heart and Kidney yang; blood is invigorated and the chest is opened with Dan Shen, Chuan Xiong, and Yu Jin; the portals are opened with Shi Chang Pu and Yuan Zhi; the nervous system is calmed with Long Gu and Ye Jiao Teng (which also nourishes and invigorates the blood); the earth is nourished and protected from dampness with Sha Ren and Fo Shou (which also regulates the Liver); and it is harmonized with Gan Cao (which also nourishes the earth).

Classical and traditional formulas and Heart Shock

Below are short discussions on a wide variety of herbal formulas that can be used to treat Heart Shock and trauma. By no means an exhaustive list, the representative formulas below can demonstrate the strategies employed and/or the modifications necessary to treat the gamut and complexity of Heart Shock within one's patients.

Fu Shen Tang

Fu Shen	9g
Ren Shen	6g
Yuan Zhi	9g
Fang Feng	4.5g
Rou Gui	3g
Du Huo	6g
Long Gu	15g
Xi Xin	1.5g
Gan Cao	3g
Bai Zhu	6g
Gan Jiang	3g
Suan Zao Ren	9g

Fu Shen Tang is a useful formula for Heart Shock with concurrent consumption/ taxation and the inability to express the emotions. It incorporates a number of the Heart Shock strategies, including calming the shen (Fu Shen, Yuan Zhi, Long Gu, Suan Zao Ren); settling the will (Rou Gui, Xi Xin, Yuan Zhi); protecting the exterior (Fang Feng, Xi Xin, Bai Zhu); opening ming men (Du Huo, Rou Gui); scattering cold to rectify the Triple Burner dissemination (Rou Gui, Du Huo, Xi Xin, Gan Jiang); invigorating blood (Rou Gui); strengthening original qi and releasing to the exterior (Ren Shen, Fang Feng, Du Huo, Bai Zhu); and strengthening wei/Lung qi responsible for smooth contraction (Ren Shen, Bai Zhu, Gan Jiang). One can modify this to increase the blood-invigorating aspect as needed, either by increasing the small dose of Rou Gui, or adding additional herbs.

Gui Zhi Gan Cao Tang

Gui Zhi	30g
Zhi Gan Cao	15g

A Classical Shang Han Lun formula for Heart qi deficiency, Gui Zhi Gan Cao Tang treats palpitations with the cardinal symptom of desire to keep the hands pressing on one's chest and epigastric area, often accompanied by a tendancy towards fear, nightmares (lack of wei protective qi in the chest), etc. The dynamic of Gui Zhi and Zhi Gan Cao helps to bring yang back to the Heart, promote movement of Heart qi, and also strengthen the middle burner and fluids. While not by itself sufficient to treat the typical complexity of Heart Shock, it is a building block useful in the construction of Heart Shock formulas. For example, adding Long Gu and Mu Li create Gui Zhi Gan Cao Long Gu Mu Li Tang which can also anchor and astringe floating Heart yang.

Zhi Gan Cao Tang (Honey Fried Licorice Decoction)

Zhi Gan Cao	12g
Ren Shen	6g
Da Zao	30pcs
Sheng Di Huang	48g
E Jiao	6g
Mai Men Dong	9g
Huo Ma Ren	9g
Gui Zhi	9g
Sheng Jiang	9g
Rice Wine	

Zhi Gan Cao Tang is a popular formula that treats palpitations, fatigue, anxiety, restlessness, irritability, insomnia, emaciation, constipation, cough, night sweats, fright, etc. in patients presenting with deficient and irregular pulse configurations (typically irregular pulses have their roots in trauma prior to the age of maturation). Its focus is on strengthening Heart qi, yin, and blood, but from the perspective of our Heart Shock strategies, one can find that it also strengthens the Kidney yang (Ren Shen, Zhi Gan Cao), nourishes the earth (Ren Shen, Da Zao, Sheng Jiang), and mildly invigorates the blood (Rice Wine). The previous formula, Gui Zhi Gan Cao Tang, is included within this larger formula, and additional herbs can be added to further invigorate blood as well as calming the nervous system (one can argue that Rice Wine accomplishes this, and such a large dosage of Sheng Di will calm the nervous system and clear heat and agitation from the Heart and Liver), and opening the portals (Rice Wine as a spirit may have some small action here).

Gui Pi Tang (Restore the Spleen Decoction)

Suan Zao Ren	30g
Zhi Yuan Zhi	30g
Long Yan Rou	30g
Dang Gui	30g
Fu Ling	30g
Bai Zhu	30g
Huang Qi	30g
Ren Shen	15g
Mu Xiang	15g
Zhi Gan Cao	7.5g

Powder and take 12g with 5 pieces of Sheng Jiang and 1 piece of Da Zao infusion

Gui Pi Tang treats Heart blood and Spleen qi deficiency with symptoms such as excessive worrying, obsessiveness, memory loss and forgetfulness, depression, palpitations, anxiety, phobias, insomnia, fear and panic attacks, fatigue, etc. with Thin and Reduced pulses. Applicable to Heart Shock where the Heart blood deficiency is more pronounced than the Heart yin, it can also be easily modified. Heart yin and blood are nourished by Suan Zao Ren, Long Yan Rou, and Dang Gui; blood is invigorated by Dang Gui; Heart qi is nourished by Huang Qi, Ren Shen, and Zhi Gan Cao; the Kidneys are tonified with Ren Shen and Huang Qi; the portals are opened by Yuan Zhi; and the Spleen and Stomach are supplemented with Ren Shen, Fu Ling, Bai Zhu, Huang Qi, Mu Xiang, and Zhi Gan Cao, plus Sheng Jiang and Da Zao. Additional herbs to invigorate the blood and tonify Heart yin are easily added to Gui Pi Tang as needed.

Bai Zi Yang Xin Wan (Biota Seeds to Nourish the Heart Pill)

Bai Zi Ren	120g
Gou Qi Zi	90g
Shu Di Huang	60g
Xuan Shen	60g
Mai Men Dong	30g
Dang Gui	30g
Fu Shen	30g
Shi Chang Pu	30g
Zhi Gan Cao	15g

Powdered into pills and taken with honey

Bai Zi Yang Xin Wan is a formula known to treat emotional distress, insomnia, amnesia, palpitations due to fright, and nightmares. It nourishes the Heart by tonifying yin and blood (Bai Zi Ren, Gou Qi Zi, Shu Di Huang, Mai Men Dong), cools the blood (Xuan Shen), and calms the shen (Fu Shen, Shi Chang Pu). Blood invigoration is handled by Dang Gui, though additional herbs can easily be included to augment this strategy. While it doesn't nourish Kidney yang or assist with the Triple Burner dissemination, it does nourish essence (Shu Di Huang, Gou Qi Zi). The portals are opened by Shi Chang Pu, which treats any phlegm misting the Heart, and Gou Qi Zi nourishes and brightens the eyes. The middle burner is nourished by Fu Shen and Zhi Gan Cao. Additional herbs to relax a hyperactive nervous system can be added, e.g., Bai Shao, Xiang Fu, etc., as well as herbs to strengthen and anchor Kidney yang if necessary from the clinical picture.

Yang Xin Tang (Nourish the Heart Decoction)

Suan Zao Ren	12g
Bai Zi Ren	6g
Ren Shen	12g
Fu Shen	9g
Mai Men Dong	12g
Shu Di Huang	9g
Sheng Di Huang	9g
Dang Gui	9g
Wu Wei Zi	6g
Lian Zi	6g
Deng Xin Cao	6g
Zhi Gan Cao	3g

Yang Xin Tang is another formula which nourishes the Heart and calms the shen, often with a backdrop of blood deficiency and a weak constitution. The presentation is typically palpitations with anxiety, insomnia, forgetfulness, low-grade fever, withered complexion, slightly red tongue, and Reduced pulse qualities. As a Heart Shock formula, it contains SMS (using Ren Shen instead of Xi Yang Shen) and further nourishes the Heart yin and blood with Suan Zao Ren, Bai Zi Ren, Sheng Di Huang, and Shu Di Huang; it invigorates the blood with Dang Gui; it calms and/or clears heat from the shen with Suan Zao Ren, Bai Zi Ren, Fu Shen, Lian Zi, and Deng Xin Cao (Dr. Shen used this in his Heart Tight formulas above); it nourishes Kidney yang (Ren Shen); and it strengthens the Spleen and Stomach with Zhi Gan Cao. Herbs to open the portals such as Yuan Zhi or Yu Jin (which will also calm the nervous system) should be added, as well as a herb to increase the blood-invigorating aspect.

Gan Mai Da Zao Tang (Licorice, Wheat, and Jujube Decoction)

Fu Xiao Mai	9–15g
Gan Cao	9g
Da Zao	10pcs

A Jin Gui Yao Lue formula for Heart blood deficiency and Liver qi stagnation causing restless organ disorder, Gan Mai Da Zao Tang nourishes the Heart, calms the shen, strengthens the earth, moves the Liver, and calms the nervous system. Fu Xiao Mai strengthens the Heart and calms the spirit and treats palpitations, insomnia, irritability, and emotional instability (labile emotions), Gan Cao strengthens and nourishes the middle and all the organs, and Da Zao nourishes blood, calms the spirit, and supplements the earth. A simple formula, any of the three herbs can have their dosage altered to prioritize any of these strategies. And while it does not satisfy all the Heart Shock strategies, it can serve as a base formula to be modified accordingly. For example, He Huan Pi can be added to calm the spirit, as can Yuan Zhi to settle the will and anchor to the Kidneys, and other herbs to invigorate the blood.

Tian Wang Bu Xin Dan (Heavenly Emperor's Tonify the Heart Formula)

Sheng Di Huang	120g
Dan Shen	15g
Dang Gui	30g
Bai Zi Ren	30g
Yuan Zhi	15g
Ren Shen	15g
Fu Ling	15g
Tian Men Dong	30g
Mai Men Dong	30g
Xuan Shen	15g
Wu Wei Zi	30g
Suan Zao Ren	30g
Jie Geng	15g
Zhu Sha	15g

Tian Wang Bu Xin Dan (a modified version) was the formula I used in my very first Heart Shock patient while still an intern in medical school. The patient, a 28-year-old female, had been amenorrheic for 12 years. She had been coming regularly to the Pacific College of Oriental Medicine (PCOM) clinic for six years, being treated with the same old TCM strategies and acupuncture points and herbal formulas to no avail. When I first met her I recognized Heart Shock as the primary insult. As I pitched this to my supervisor, I was surprised to be met with great resistance, only to be told that Heart Shock and Heart/Kidney not communicating was not a valid TCM diagnosis for amenorrhea. I persisted in my arguments and eventually tired out my supervisor, who reluctantly agreed to let me pursue the Heart Shock strategy. Acupuncture was performed based on communicating Heart and Kidneys, and Tian Wang Bu Xin Dan was prescribed in modification. Within six weeks the patient had her first period in 12 years, and she has received her menstruation monthly ever since, now the mother of two children.

Tian Wang Bu Xin Dan contains SMS (Ren Shen instead of Xi Yang Shen) and strongly nourishes Heart yin with additional herbs such as Sheng Di Huang, Bai Zi Ren, and Suan Zao Ren. It strengthens the Kidneys with Ren Shen (yang), Tian Men Dong, and Xuan Shen (yin), regulates qi in the chest (Jie Geng), invigorates blood (Dan Shen, Dang Gui), opens the portals (Yuan Zhi and the no-longer-used Zhu Sha), calms the nervous system (Suan Zao Ren, Bai Zi Ren, Yuan Zhi, Dan Shen, Zhu Sha), and strengthens the earth (Ren Shen, Fu Ling, Mai Men Dong). It treats palpitations, anxiety, insomnia, fatigue, night sweats, restlessness, inability to concentrate, etc.

Niu Huang Qing Xin Wan (Ox Gallstone Clear the Heart Pill)

Huang Lian	15g
Huang Qin	9g
Zhi Zhi	9g
Yu Jin	6g
Zhu Sha	4.5g
Niu Huang	0.75g

Powder and make into pill with honey

Niu Huang Qing Xin Wan is a powerful formula for clearing Heart fire, phlegm-fire harassing the Heart, and opening the portals for acute and severe shen disturbances with delirium, seizures, mania, etc. When I have given this formula in the past, I have always used it in conjunction with another formula accommodating the Heart Shock strategies, and often combining it with a similar formula to the ones discussed above. A very difficult formula to source these days due to the last two ingredients, substitutions are necessary (examples might include Hu Po and/or Dai Zhe Shi to replace Zhu Sha, and, if necessary, herbs to replace Niu Huang can include She Xiang, Su He Xiang, Shi Chang Pu, etc.).

Wen Dan Tang (Warm the Gall Bladder Decoction)

Ban Xia	6g
Chen Pi	9g
Sheng Jiang	12g
Da Zao	3pcs
Zhu Ru	6g
Zhi Shi	6g
Gan Cao	3g

A Sun Si-miao formula, Wen Dan Tang can be used after a major illness or trauma wherein the person experiences emotional upset, irritability, restlessness, insomnia, sadness, fear (Classical symptom of cold in the Gall Bladder), and an inability to move past experiences/traumas/illnesses. Liver-wood is about growth, and the Lungs-metal about letting go and living in the moment. Wen Dan Tang works with the strategy of reorienting the hun and po for someone stuck in her trauma, unable to move forward, be in the moment, and continue to grow and mature to the next stage of life. The dynamic of the formula warms and incites the Gall Bladder to engender qi and move on from the past, and removes obstructions to its growth (phlegm blocking the po) in the present. As wood becomes stagnant, not able to be fed by water-Kidneys, hot phlegm can eventually be produced, causing more explosive unstable emotions and psychological presentations, as well as neurological symptoms. The formula addresses this manifestation as well. The dosages are small to allow a slow and gradual shift in one's experiences, perceptions, and judgments (i.e., opening the portals gradually).

While not satisfying much of the Heart Shock formula strategies as set forth above, Wen Dan Tang can be used as part of the overall strategy. It is not always necessary to incorporate every Heart Shock strategy into each formula; certain strategies can be prioritized for periods of time as the clinical presentation warrants. Typically, when I use this formula as part of my strategy, I will alternate Wen Dan Tang with another Heart Shock formula, doing Wen Dan Tang on days 1, 3, 5, etc. and the other formula on the even days.

Gui Zhi Jia Gui Tang (Cinnamon Twig plus Cinnamon Decoction)

Gui Zhi	18g
Bai Shao	9g
Sheng Jiang	9g
Da Zao	4pcs
Zhi Gan Cao	6g

Gui Zhi Jia Gui Tang is the same formula as Gui Zhi Tang with a doubling of the Gui Zhi dosage. This one shift in the formula alters its dynamic to strengthening and unblocking the Heart yang and opening the chest. It is used to treat fear, fright, running piglet disorder, palpitations, shortness of breath, cold limbs, cyanosis, chest pain, etc. While not a formula I use in isolation (as the extra dose of Gui Zhi can further aggravate the separation of yin and yang of the Heart), it can be used very successfully within the framework of the Heart Shock strategies, especially when sufficient Heart yin and blood herbs are included.

Ling Gui Cao Zao/Fu Ling Gui Zhi Gan Cao Da Zao Tang
(Poria, Cinnamon, Licorice and Red Dates Decoction)

Fu Ling	25g
Gui Zhi	12g
Gan Cao	6g
Da Zao	15pcs

Ling Gui Cao Zao is another formula that treats palpitations, along with fatigue, water beneath the Heart, shortness of breath, cold limbs, etc. Again, not to be used by itself for the treatment of shock, it can be incorporated into a larger strategy where the transformative actions of the Spleen are compromised, creating damp assailing the chest.

Bentun Tang

Gan Cao	6g
Chuan Xiong	9g
Dang Gui	9g
Ban Xia	12g
Huang Qin	9g
Ge Gen	15g
Bai Shao	9g
Sheng Jiang	12g
(Gan) Ligen Bai Pi	9g (Sang Bai Pi usually substituted)

From the Jin Gui Yao Lue, Bentun Tang is another formula that treats running piglet qi, its onset brought about by fright and terror[140] which disturbs the Kidneys and/or Liver, and affects the Heart via the Chong mai. The formula as written above demonstrates a primary strategy of regulating the Liver and calming an overactive nervous system, clearing ascendant heat, and anchoring its qi. It also nourishes the blood and regulates/downbears Stomach qi. Other Heart Shock strategies include invigorating the blood (Dang Gui and Chuan Xiong). Modifications as appropriate to build back Heart yin, strengthen and anchor Kidney yang, and open the portals can be included to round out the strategies.

Essential oil treatments for shen disturbances and the emotions

Like the other modalities discussed, essential oils can be used to satisfy all the Heart Shock strategies. Below, I will list (with a short commentary for some) the most common essential oils I use in my practice for the above strategies, plus options for using oils based on common psychological presentations. Most of these have been informed by my studies with Jeffrey Yuen, and used in my clinical practice often. Besides the particular oils, however, is the way in which they are used, e.g., diffusion, application to acupoints, baths, perfumes, etc. Essential oils, much like herbs, have multiple functions associated with them; they have channel affinities, tastes, natures, directionality, etc. A full discussion of this information and its methods is beyond the scope of this text and the reader is referred to the teachings of Jeffrey Yuen for more information. The information provided is restricted to that which is most relevant for treating Heart Shock.

Nourish Heart and calm the spirit

Geranium	Nourishes Heart yin and blood, communicates Heart and Kidneys, invigorates blood
Angelica	Nourishes the Heart, invigorates blood, strengthens the Lungs and Spleen, treats ghost/gui
Clary Sage	Yin nourishing and anchoring to the Heart and Kidneys, clears heat and treats anxiety, OCD, mania, insomnia, etc.
Benzoin	Astringes Heart qi and yin, diffuses Lung qi, strengthens the Lungs and Spleen
Jasmine	Nourishes yin, relaxes nervous system
Rose	Nourishes yin, clears heat, regulates the Liver

Invigorate blood

Geranium	See above
Angelica	See above
Frankincense	Also opens diaphragm, treats non-healing wounds/traumas
Myrrh	Also opens diaphragm, clears heat in the Stomach, treats non-healing wounds/traumas
Lavender	Also relaxes nervous system and releases exterior, opens the chest, moves Liver qi
Ginger	Strengthens the Spleen and Stomach

HT/KI communication

Yin	Geranium	See above
	Clary Sage	See above
	Ylang Ylang	Also clears heat
Yang	Fennel	Nourishes Heart and Kidney yang, strengthens Liver qi
	Cypress	Very astringent oil. Cypresses are the trees that line the cemeteries; they are very good for grief as they resonate with the po to overcome sadness; they anchor qi back to the chest and down into the Kidneys

Open orifices

Most oils can open the orifices, especially top notes for a quicker action.

Rosemary (all chemotypes)	Verbenome treats more phlegm, Camphor strengthens Heart qi
Peppermint	Also clears heat, regulates Liver qi
Citrus	Most also clear heat and relax the nervous system, Oranges clear Heart fire, Lemon/Lime more Liver affinity
Eucalyptus (all chemotypes)	Radiata impacts the orifices and is safest, Citriadora clears heat, Globulus treats wind-cold, Polybractea treats damp-cold, Smithii treats damp-heat, Dives treats phlegm-damp
Cinnamon Leaf	Activates taiyang
Camphor	Opens the orifices, treats parasites, relaxes the nervous system and muscles
Basil	Impacts Bladder channel and fight/flight/freeze-type responses (one of the oils for BL/KI DM), opens orifices of the nose, entryway to yangming

Calm the nervous system

Lavender	Regulates the Liver qi, relaxes the nervous system and mind
Lime	Soothes the Liver and relaxes the muscles
Basil	Impacts Bladder channel and fight/flight/freeze-type responses (one of the oils for BL/KI DM), opens orifices of the nose, entryway to yangming
Sandalwood	Opens the Heart, clears heat, opens the orifices
Vetiver	Nourishes blood, calms and anchors the Liver, communicates Heart and Kidneys, tones the sinews, invigorates the blood
Spikenard	Clears Heart fire and treats tachycardia, insomnia, anxiety, etc. Subdues Liver wind
German Chamomile	Relaxes the Liver, subdues wind, calms the shen, treats NST overacting on DSW

Clear heat in the Heart

Melissa	Clears heat in the blood, relaxes and opens the chest, treats Liver blood stasis and rebellious Stomach qi
Neroli	Also tonifies the Spleen
Orange	Clears Heart fire and treats arrhythmia, palpitations, tachycardia. Can be used for wind heat too
Valerian	Also subdues internal wind

Regulate qi in the chest/open diaphragm

Lavender	See above
Frankincense	See above
Benzoin	See above
Angelica	See above
Sandalwood	See above
Geranium	See above
German Chamomile	See above

Excitement/anxiety/agitation/vexation

Orange	Clears Heart fire and treats arrhythmia, palpitations, tachycardia. Can be used for wind heat too
Neroli	Treats Heart fire and severe trauma and shock to the Heart. Soothes and relaxes muscles and hyperactive wei qi, including atrial fibrillation, chest pain, etc., and hysteria
Frankincense	As a resin, treats non-healing wounds. Good for the patient who exaggerates his suffering, and has anxiety. Opens the diaphragm, and regulates the Liver qi and blood
Melissa	See above
Sandalwood	Opens chest, clears heat
Myrrh	As a resin, treats non-healing wounds, PTSD, etc. Treats and clears Stomach fire, e.g., plum pit throat, hyperthyroidism, tooth decay, tachycardia, racing mind, etc.

Nervousness: Heart affecting the Lung with volatility, trembling, etc.

Cedarwood (Himalayan)	Provides a sense of protection (wood law of signature); clears Lung heat and helps those who feel inadequate or judged. Treats hot phlegm and wind
Roman Chamomile	Increases white blood cells, immunity, and sense of feeling protected
Palmarosa	Protects those easily influenced (infected) by others' negative energy (thoughts, feelings), treats allergies and wei qi sensitivity/hyper-reactivity, including what others think of you. Clears pestilent qi, wind-heat, and infections

Irritability/agitation: Fan: non-voluntary movement (brain and muscles), insomnia

Sandalwood	See above
Roman Chamomile	See above
Cistus	Regulates Liver qi
Melissa	See above

Restlessness/vexation: Zao: mental-brain, insomnia

Vetiver	Antispasmodic. Good for restless legs, too
Lavender	See above
Lemon	Treats cramps, gout, etc. Clears Stomach and Liver fire
Clary Sage	Deals with Liver wind, spasms, tremors
Carrot Seed	Nourishes Liver blood
Sweet Marjoram	Treats Liver fire and high blood pressure, breaks hot phlegm, descends Stomach qi

Joy

Extreme joy manifests as mania, desires, and lack of satisfaction. Also for those who require a lot of effort to experience happiness.

Spikenard	Anchors the Heart and treats Heart fire, anchors Liver wind
Neroli	See above
Lemon Verbena	Top note which treats Heart and Liver fire
Fennel	Strengthens Heart and Kidney yang to animate, awakens the Liver
Cinnamon Bark	Opens ming men, strengthens Heart/Kidney yang

Grief/sorrow

Eucalyptus	Helps to let go, to expectorate and diffuse the Lungs, radiata to open sensory orifices, globulus, polybractea, dives if chronic with phlegm
Spikenard	Penetrates into the water and depths of one's sadness, bringing Liver blood to provide comfort. Calms the Liver's impact on the Lungs
Cypress	Evergreen oil that affects Lungs, it is astringent, providing comfort and a path back to the Kidneys and constitution to allow for reflection and regrowth
Nutmeg	Astringes the Kidneys, helps to move yang upwards and disseminate, promotes appetite (interest in life)
Palmarosa	Good for one who is distraught and anxious, very soothing oil

Difficulty in expression

Vetiver	Goes deep to access the Kidneys and the root of one's fear and sadness, nourishes the blood and provides comfort
Pine	Descends and warms the Kidneys, providing ability to support oneself
Mimosa	An oil for those who feel guilt and remorse, clears blood heat and fire toxins, calms the shen and promotes relaxation
Bay Laurel	Breaks phlegm

Bereavement: period of isolation and not wanting to come out; depression

Cypress	Breaks phlegm; descends Lung qi and promotes urination (bodily tears)
Benzoin	Diffuses Lung qi as astringes/protects the Heart
Patchouli	Affects Chong mai and the blueprint, allows for renewal, rebirth. Extracted from dead, dried-up fermented leaves, it represents resurrection. Also useful to treat parasites, ghosts, and for those who cry a lot
Atlas Cedar	Mucolytic, regulates the Liver qi, impacts the luo vessels, and draws out latency
Camphor	Awakens the yang and opens the portals, treats sudden shock

Tendency to cry a lot

Ylang Ylang	See above
Patchouli	See above
Geranium	See above

Worry: earth/metal: overthinking about loss, grief, sadness

Bergamot	Uplifting, good for generalized anxiety disorder (constant negative narrative) and vulnerability, brings wei qi up, relaxes the nervous system and returns to internal ying level
Fir (Silver, Balsamic, Douglas)	Tonifies and diffuses Lung qi. Helps one feel less vulnerable
Clary Sage	For those who always blame themselves and take on too much responsibility, causing damage to the Kidney yin. Nourishes yin, treats panic attacks, phobias, running piglet qi, and Liver fire causing wind
Sage	Treats Stomach fire and obsessiveness
Myrrh	Treats those who worry based on previous traumas/wounds that won't heal

Fear

Generally florals are combined with spice oils. Spices manage the thought processes (ying level) that help overcome fear. Flowers manage the portals and the Liver and Heart. Fear is a lack of communication between the Heart and Kidneys preventing water (KI) from displacing jing-essence and qi to the respective organs. For the fear aspect, one must consider what the fear is of, and how water/Kidneys are displacing it.

Spices: narrative	Anise	Clears Stomach and Liver fire, and treats trapped emotions causing insomnia and irritability, etc.
	Fennel	See above
	Caraway	Rids phlegm-damp and clears the thought processes, tonifies the Spleen, downbears the Stomach
	Coriander	Rids dampness and damp-bi, tonifies the Spleen
	Cardamom	Harmonizes the Spleen and Stomach, treats damp and fermentation/dysbiosis, summerheat, parasites, etc.
	Nutmeg	See above
	Black Pepper	Warms the interior, unfreezes yang, increases immunity, oxygenation, circulation, and digestion
Florals: fear		
Wood: failure, change	Melissa	See above
	Lavender	See above
Fire: love, appropriateness; fear of relationships	Orange Blossom	See above
	Rose	See above
Earth: gossip, attention, fear of being noticed	Roman Chamomile	See above
Metal: judgment, vulnerability, fear of getting hurt, and letting go	Ylang Ylang	See above
Water: self, sexuality	Rose	See above
	Jasmine	Nourishes yin, promotes comfort, trust, and faith, descends Liver yang
	Narcissus	Nourishes yin, promotes acceptance, harmonizes the Heart and Kidneys, calms the shen

Shock/fright: need to resuscitate yang

Black Pepper	See above
Basil	See above
Peppermint	Helps with acute resuscitation and restoring yang
Fennel	HT/KI communication, unfreezes yang qi
Vetiver	Descends to the water and fear and settles fright

Cynicism/bitterness

Mimosa	See above
Yarrow	I Jing stalks, helps with wind and change, relaxes muscles, releases wind and heat, breaks hot phlegm, ascends Spleen qi, and regulates the Liver
Pennyroyal	A toxic oil in the mint family, it stimulates bile/courage to persevere

Insomnia

Sandalwood	Opens chest, allows one to increase breathing capacity to allow for sleepiness
Valerian	Clears Heart fire, cools the blood, treats restlessness, anxiety, tossing and turning, etc.
Cistus	Astringes, deepens breath
Hops	Spicy, sweet, cooling, establishes HT/KI communication, relaxes chest, improves concentration and meditation
Rosemary	Small amount to protect wei qi during sleep state

Anti-depressant/stress management

For stress and tension building up. Use top notes for acute issues, and base notes for chronic ones.

Chamomile	See above
Orange	See above
Tangerine	Opens chest, allows one to let go and receive joy
Lavender	See above
Melissa	See above
Neroli	See above

cont.

Petitgrain	Leaf of mandarin orange, wei qi oil, good for anxiety, rebellious ST qi (helps with descension) and ST qi stagnation
Rose	See above
Sandalwood	See above
Valerian	See above

Tranquilizing (for anxiety)

Chamomile	See above
Fir	Warming
Orange	See above
Petitgrain	See above
Rose	See above
Geranium	See above
Marjoram	See above
Juniper	Warms the blood, treats joints and wind-damp-cold bi-syndrome, analgesic
Nutmeg	Warming, astringent, analgesic

Nightmares (fear)

Also see oils above for fear.

Citronella	Especially for kids who hear voices at night or see things. Wards off insects, ghosts, etc.
Mandarin	See above
Orange	See above
Neroli	See above
Angelica Seed	Archangel: summons the angels to protect
Rosemary	Strengthens wei qi to protect during sleep state

cont.

Emotional extremes

Mania/hysteria/ aggression	Clary Sage	See above
	Sandalwood	See above
	Atlas Cedar/ Cedarwood	See above

	Vetiver	See above
	Neroli	See above
	German Chamomile	See above
	Yarrow	See above
Delirium	Valerian	See above

Withdrawal/isolation/bipolar/obsessive-compulsive disorder (OCD)/depression

Withdrawal	Jasmine	Low self-esteem, suicidal
	Ylang Ylang	Addresses the inadequacy we feel
	Bergamot	Brings the yang up, opening up the shades of one's life, to see further into life, see illumination, it's an invitation
	Grapefruit	Breaks up accumulations, its outside help
	Mimosa	For those who feel burnt out, treats fire toxins
Isolation	Narcissus + Bergamot	Narcissus is the water immortal, only needs water to grow in; as long as you give a little water it'll grow, just like loneliness
Bipolar	Cedarwood	See above
	Ginger	See above
	Ho Leaf	Opens orifices, treats phlegm, harmonizes the Spleen and Stomach
	Rosewood	Similar to Ho Leaf
	Camphor	Diffuse
OCD	Clary Sage	See above
	Sage	See above
	Cedarwood	See above
	Sandalwood	See above
Depression	Basil	Stimulates the Lungs and wei qi for depression
	Bergamot	See above
	Pine	See above
	Fir	See above
	Spruce	Strengthens Kidney yang (good for endogenous depression), analgesic, communicates Lungs and Kidneys, stimulating, and can pull latency out of deeper levels

CHAPTER 7

Divergent Meridians

As we have already discussed, the three types of qi, much like the three major depths they reflect on the pulse, are wei qi, ying qi, and yuan qi. The domain of the sinew channels is primarily wei qi, that of the luo vessels, ying qi, and the primary channels deal both with ying and wei. The divergent channels, the subject of this chapter, are a conduit of, and have their primary influence over, the relationship between wei qi and yuan qi. The divergent meridians (DMs) do not relate to ying qi, thus have less of an impact on internal reflection, thought processes, and emotions. As discussed in Chapter 5, ying qi is impacted by society and influences one's psycho-social development.

As a review, wei qi regulates one's reflexes and instinctual responses (e.g. sweating when overheated, and getting chills when exposed to cold).[141] It is called to action when we feel the need to protect ourselves, whether physically or emotionally, and can often manifest through our sinews via armoring. As we learned in Chapter 4, wei qi circulates in the exterior (skin, sinews) and interior (smooth muscle contractions).

Yuan qi is concerned with the constitution and genetics, and influences the skeletal system, bones, and marrow. It is conveyed by the divergent meridians (which also influence wei qi) as well as the 8x meridians.

Both wei and yuan have a role in managing and maintaining one's structure: wei qi deals with muscles, sinews, and tendons, and yuan qi manages the bones and marrow. Together, they make up the musculoskeletal system's energetics. As function dictates form, wei qi stagnation and the creation of tension and armoring can have a major impact over the bones. And yuan qi's role over structural/skeletal integrity allows for the ranges in which muscles can move.

The divergent channels mediate the outside (world – wei qi) and the inside (constitution – yuan qi).[142] They have a major role in managing exposure to external toxins (which include EPFs, radiation,[143] traumas, etc.) which can often become retained pathogens within, and how these toxins can be externalized when a patient has sufficient resources or the right opportunity arises (e.g., fetal toxins being expressed with infectious diseases). From a psychological vantage, the divergents can mediate personal conflicts or differing worldviews with others that are an assault to one's internally held beliefs and values. It also helps us express our deepest selves to the world. As wei qi and the sinew channels mediate mood, and the luo vessels deal with emotions and psycho-social development, the divergent channels reflect the manifestation of one's deepest self in terms of one's temperament/nature.

The divergent meridians can be tapped as either zonal pairs (wei qi) or elemental pairs (yuan qi) as follows:

Elemental DM	Zonal DM
BL/KI	Taiyang: Bladder/Small Intestine
GB/LR	Shaoyang: Gall Bladder/Triple Burner
ST/SP	Yangming: Stomach/Large Intestine
SI/HT	Taiyin: Spleen/Lung
SJ/PC	Shaoyin: Kidneys/Heart
LI/LU	Jueyin: Liver/Pericardium

The zonal divergents

The zonal divergents prioritize wei qi and deal with chronic musculoskeletal, eye, ear, nose, and throat (EENT), and/or skin problems.[144] The ordering of the zonal DMs is different than with the sinew channels, being that the hand and foot channels are paired (in contrast to the sinew channels where all the leg yang channels are traversed prior to moving to the arm yang channels). Thus, the movement of wei qi in the zonal divergents goes from taiyang (BL-SI) to shaoyang (GB-SJ) to yangming (ST-LI) to taiyin (LU-SP) to shaoyin (HT-KI) to jueyin (LR-PC). Another clinical difference is the sinew channels generally are called upon to deal with acute problems, while the zonal divergent channels address more chronic ones.

The zones also have areas of influence wherein they hold pathogens in a state of latency and that can be released via needling or gua sha. These zonal "rings" and regions are:

- Taiyang: The zonal taiyang governs the "ring around the chest," and encompasses the area of the upper Bladder shu points roughly equivalent to the BL 15–17 area, wrapping all around the body and meeting up in the chest in the area of Ren 15–17. The taiyang has its relationship to wind-cold, and this pathogen often goes latent and internal in the area of SI 12, which can also be needled, gua sha'd, or cupped to release latent cold.

- Shaoyang: The zonal shaoyang manages the "ring around the pelvis," roughly corresponding to the Dai mai, in particular the area from LR 13 to GB 29. In those too sensitive or modest to have this area palpated and released, as an alternative one can utilize the area surrounding the mastoid (GB 12–20 to SJ 16 area). The shaoyang corresponds to wind-damp and this area tends to show up in the area of the upper thoracic and/or the trapezius muscle.

- Yangming: The zonal yangming is released via the "ring around the collar," which includes the area of Du 14, LI 15, GB 21, ST 12, and Ren 22, and wrapping around the neck. Its correspondence is to wind-heat, and latency is often found in the area of LI 15 and the ST 5 area.

- Taiyin: The zonal taiyin's area of influence picks up where yangming ends, and where it internalizes, i.e., the throat. Its region is that of the ST 9 and LI 18 area.

- Shaoyin: The zonal shaoyin has its influence over the area of its termination point, Ren 23.

- Jueyin: The zonal jueyin manages the area of the chest at PC 1.

The elemental divergents

As the zonal divergents are used more commonly with chronic wei qi disorders, the elemental divergent channels tend to be used more for internal and chronic degenerative ones.[145] The zonal divergents can always be used in conjunction with the elemental divergents, often assisting in opening blockages, making the elemental treatments more effective.[146] The elemental pairings resonate more strongly with yuan qi, and their circulation follows a progressive order and utilization of a particular resource. The elemental pairs, of which there are six, represent a "confluence." These confluences are:

First Confluence: BL/KI

Second Confluence: GB/LR

Third Confluence: ST/SP

Fourth Confluence: SI/HT

Fifth Confluence: SJ/PC

Sixth Confluence: LI/LU

Divergent meridian physiology

The divergent meridians function by trying to prevent EPFs that have gained access to the interior (and IPFs) from entering the organs themselves.[147] This is done by diverting the pathogenic factor to the joints (yin of yang)[148] using jing-essence to contain it. This process of latency can reveal itself with symptoms of bi-syndrome, i.e., joint pain, as the body tries to protect against developing an organic condition. This is a type of "disease nemesis theory" wherein the development of arthritic pains, for example, reflects a safer alternative to inflammation in the organs themselves.[149]

When there are sufficient resources to contain the pathogen, no symptoms would even present, until such time as the resources have been consumed, and the damage the pathogen created revealed.

This disease nemesis theory functions as a preventative ecological, rather than strictly pathological, response. When confronted by a pathogen, if the wei qi is sufficient, it will expel it. If not strong enough to expel, but strong enough to prevent it from entering the zang fu, then the EPF is diverted to the joints via the divergents.[150] The divergents are the sun luo (grandchild luo) as they are two steps away from the sinews (if the sinew channels can't deal with an EPF it can go inward to the longitudinal luo, then potentially to the transverse luo reaching the source (yuan level)). If one has blood and/or fluid deficiency, or the pathogen is very strong, it can bypass the luo vessels and directly penetrate towards the organs, relying on the divergent channels to intervene. Using the antique points of the primary channel to further understand this progression, if a taiyang pathogen is not stopped at the Bladder channel via sweat, and if it goes unchallenged at the luo point, it will continue to the he-sea point where it can internalize to the organs (note that the he-sea point of the Bladder channel is BL 40, its divergent meridian confluent point). As the pathogenic factor moves inwards, it becomes embroiled and wrapped up with wei qi and deposited into the joints, assisted and maintained by jing-essence. How long it can remain here is dependent on the quantity of resources to maintain it in latency.

For a pathogen to be kept in latency, it requires a resource to maintain it, e.g., jing, blood, jin, ye, qi, and yang. As a pathogen enters the interior, it becomes internal heat, especially as wei qi which is warming is now embroiled with it, calling on yin to cool it off or make it latent. This constant expenditure of yin depletes reserves of essence, blood, and/or fluids (depending on which divergent confluent is maintaining it).

A retained pathogenic factor can manifest as latent heat or latent cold. Latent heat generally shows itself via a Slippery and/or Rapid pulse picture, and in the Shen-Hammer lineage often with Robust Pounding at the Blood of Organ and Substance of Organ depths. If the zonal divergents are involved, and the pathogen is also being held on the wei level, one might see a Slippery and/or Tight pulse at 3 beans of pressure. Latent cold is held at the level of essence and the body depletes its jing to hold the pathogen there, eventually causing Kidney yang deficiency and revealing cold-bi signs and symptoms in the joints.

When latency is lost, a Triple Burner pulse (Classical pulse diagnosis) may appear as well as varying degrees and locations of Empty pulses (Shen-Hammer pulse diagnosis, described in Chapter 2). A Triple Burner pulse involves a Robust Pounding pulse which is found in the moderate and superficial aspects of the right proximal position, up to the 3 beans of pressure. A method to determine the Triple Burner pulse involves placing all three fingers at 9 beans of pressure, then pressing on the proximal position down to 12–15 beans, pumping the cun position, then the guan position, to 12–15 beans, and slowly releasing the proximal. A positive

Triple Burner pulse is one in which the pulse forcefully pounds and lifts one's finger to the wei level. This reflects the heat/inflammation/toxicity that is no longer being maintained in dormancy.

Latency also involves trapped wei qi along with the pathogen, and the heat from the internal pathogen and wei qi struggle slowly diminishes the essence. This creates deterioration in the joints and bones (and other structures on the divergent meridian pathway), burns up the structure, and results in chronic degenerative disease.[151]

When to use the divergent meridians

The uses of the divergent channels are extremely diverse, and the specific uses of each of the elemental channels will be detailed below. However, some of the more common categories of ailments one would look to the divergent channels include:

- intermittent signs and symptoms
- signs and symptoms that switch sides, including symptoms on one side that have their origin on the other
- bone and joint pain
- chronic EENT and skin disorders
- autoimmune disorders
- hyperactivity of wei qi, with underlying deficiency of yuan qi or jing-essence.

Progression of divergent channels

As the divergent channels become activated in response to a strong pathogen, yin resources become diverted to assist the wei qi, and translocate the pathogen. In the first confluence (BL/KI), jing-essence is used to blanket, cool, and dampen the pathogen. If that strategy fails, either because the pathogen has been able to overcome or consume the jing, or because jing was insufficient from the start, the body will try to use the blood to hold the pathogen at the second confluence (GB/LR). When that blood is diminished or insufficient, the thin bodily fluids, the jin, are used to keep the pathogen latent at the third confluence (ST/SP). As the jin becomes consumed, the ye (thick fluids, including the hormones) are tapped into at the fourth confluence (SI/HT). By this time, with the yin resources having been depleted, the next response is the utilization of yuan qi to attempt to slow down the pathogen at the fifth confluence (SJ/PC). By the time the sixth confluence (LI/LU) is called upon, most reserves have been consumed, leaving only yang qi to hold the pathogen and maintain stability.

This model can be very helpful in working with Heart Shock patients, especially to promote dormancy when the patient is suffering from debilitating anxiety, panic, etc. One can look to see what form of yin may still be available to temporarily suppress the symptoms and slow down the process, while helping build up the patient's resources, buying time to release it in the future when the patient is stronger. One can assess the status of the patient's resources via the pulse, choosing the confluence associated with the most abundant one (e.g., GB/LR for blood, ST/SP for thin fluids, etc.). If all the forms of yin are deficient, one must choose the SJ/PC or the LI/LU divergent meridians and use either yuan qi or yang qi to contain the pathology.

Each of the six confluences has its distinct personality and nature, as well as resources it manages within the context of the divergent channels. They are detailed below.

First confluence

Channels associated: BL/KI

Resource: jing-essence

Confluent points: BL 10, BL 40

Yang lower confluent: BL 40

Yin lower confluent: KI 10

BLADDER DIVERGENT CHANNEL PATHWAY[152]

The BL DM begins at BL 40, travels to BL 36 and BL 35, to Po Men (anus), and up the spine/Du mai to connect with the Kidney organ at Du 4 and BL 23. It goes from Du 4 to Ren 4 (front mu point for its zonal pair, Small Intestine), to Ren 3 (its own front mu), to the Bladder organ itself. (This Du 4 to Ren 4 pathway is Dai mai.) From the lower back it continues up the BL channel (or Hua Tou Jia Ji points depending on source), exiting the spine to go from BL 32 to BL 28, and up to BL 17 (influential point of blood), where it circles to the front, crossing GB 22 to connect with Ren 17 and entering the Heart. It continues up the back to BL 11 (influential point of the bones), to BL 10, where it meets the KI divergent channel, going internally into the brain at Du 20 (influence on the shen).[153]

INDICATIONS FOR THE BLADDER DIVERGENT CHANNEL[154]

The BL DM is often used in the context of treating chronic pain. As part of the disease nemesis theory explained earlier in this chapter, as latency is compromised from the translocation of the pathogen, bi-syndrome results with musculoskeletal pain along the trajectory, including headaches, back pain, knee pain, etc. As it traverses the sacrum/pelvis and occiput, it creates a strong resonance between these two areas. And as the DM plays a major role in jing and fluid regulation, it reinforces influence over the reproductive areas by its ability to treat hormonal disorders.

The trajectory also encompasses the lower two yin, and inflammatory issues from stagnations here can also result and be treated by the DM. This connection to the lower yin and the ascending trajectory also assists with lifting Spleen yang for treating prolapses, hemorrhoids, etc.

A major component is the utilization of the back shu points, especially the Heart and Kidneys, and the BL DM can assist with helping communicate these two essential systems in providing overall stability. It is the yang aspect communicated in the BL DM, and the yin aspect with the KI DM. Along these lines, the BL DM communicates with the Great Wrap (Da Ba), already discussed in Chapter 5. Here the relationship with the Bao mai and Dai mai provide further linkage.

BLADDER DIVERGENT PERSONALITY[155]

As a Water phase channel, the Bladder represents the capacity for survival and ability to adapt for that sake. Bladder constitutions tend to be more spirit-oriented and, from a physiognomy perspective, have round faces. As the yang aspect, those of this personality have strong feelings (wei qi), but as a water type, tend not to express it. The Bladder divergent taiyang zone helps people to express (i.e., ring around the chest). This personality type tends to take charge and take risks, and appreciate the opportunity to move through challenging obstacles. They are confident in their actions, strong willed, and like to dominate, but are not very intellectual or creative. They compensate for, and hide, their intellectual weakness by making sure they overcome obstacles and obtain credentials. They are action-oriented, and like being in charge and taking on responsibilities. As a taiyang personality, these people tend to go to extremes (and can even become bipolar).

The Bladder is about mobilization of jing and being able to convey to the outside world (wei) one's intrinsic nature (Kidney). When unable to express oneself, one may develop tightness and tension in the throat, chin, neck and vocal cords, jaw, sinuses, paravertebral muscles, etc. with frustration, anger, and chronic tension. And as the Bladder divergent channel makes a connection to the Dai mai, stagnation can impact the yuan level and the curious organs with repressed sexual tension and stagnation of jing in the pelvis (including cysts, fibroids, prostatitis, etc.).

As the Bladder innately needs to express and convey the essence of our being, it represents from the divergent perspective our ability to convey and embrace life. Anything that compromises this ability and suppresses wei and yang qi, e.g., shock, traumas, and fears that impact our capacity for action, can have far-reaching impact on the Bladder divergent channel and all that it maintains. Additionally, some traumas create exuberant wei qi and can manifest with seizures, hypersensitivity/hyperactivity, etc. In this regard, we see the wei qi component of the Bladder sinew meridian impacting the Bladder divergent channel. To treat, one opens the Bladder divergent channel (BL 10, BL 40) and addresses the taiyang zonal meeting points (ring around the chest and SI 12 area), plus one adds in the Bladder sinew, the three yang confluent points, and its jing-well (BL 67). One can further address the structure via the scapula and the Small Intestine sinew to strengthen one's ability to reach out and extend into life.

KIDNEY DIVERGENT CHANNEL PATHWAY

The Kidney DM begins at KI 10, goes to BL 40, and meets the Bladder DM traveling with it to BL 23, where the Kidney DM meets with (and possibly creates) the Dai mai, encircling the waist region at GB 26, SP 15, ST 25, and KI 16 (original Dai mai). From BL 23, it enters the Kidney and Bladder organs, travels up the Kidney primary meridian to the root of the tongue (via Ren 23), then loops around to the back to connect with BL 10, the upper confluent point.

INDICATIONS FOR THE KIDNEY DIVERGENT CHANNEL

The Kidney divergent channel has a relationship with the Dai mai. It is able to pull pathology (both physical and emotional) out of Dai mai when it gets too full and can no longer maintain latency, and dump its own pathology into Dai mai to free up room in its own channel and areas of influence. It traverses through the nape of the neck for treating occipital headaches and stiff necks, including chronic whiplash. It also travels to the throat and can treat tension and restricted movement, pain, or swellings in this area.

The KI DM influences the brain and spinal cord, connecting intimately to the marrow and the mind.[156] It connects to the tongue via Ren 23, and hence communicates with Yin Wei mai. With the BL DM it connects the uterus, bladder, and spine to the Kidney channel and hence the chest, and can use Kidney yin to assert latency for these areas. Communicating to the chest, it utilizes the dynamics of the Kidney front-shu points, which treat various types of yin stasis (the Bladder back-shu points treat qi deficiency, while the Kidney front-shu points treat yin stagnation).

Together, the KI and BL DMs connect with five of the 8x channels: Dai mai (BL 23, GB 26 to KI 16 (and the Bao mai)); Chong mai (Ren 4 and Ren 3); Ren mai (Ren 4 and Ren 3); Yin Wei mai (Ren 23); and Du mai (Du 1 and Du 4).

KIDNEY DIVERGENT PERSONALITY

The Kidney divergent person is highly sensitive and vulnerable. They are easily affected by what others say and often require protection from their own vulnerabilities and fears, needing to seek an inner sanctuary. As they feel exposed when in crowds and public, they seek solace in being alone and often tend towards spiritual paths as they find comfort in going inwards. With little interest or enthusiasm for external things, they crave the mysterious. Opposite to its Bladder counterpart, the Kidney divergent personality is a seeker, but, as a pessimist, has little confidence of finding answers. Less robust than the Bladder taiyang, the Kidneys have a far greater sensitivity to EPFs, epidemics, and pestilent qi. Their morphology is a round face with more fleshiness (fluid) than with the Bladder (which is bonier as a yang energetic).

Second confluence

Channels associated: GB/LR

Resource: blood

Confluent points: GB 1, Ren 2

Yang lower confluent: GB 30

Yin lower confluent: LR 5

GALL BLADDER DIVERGENT CHANNEL PATHWAY

Beginning at GB 30, it goes to the inside of the hip and the pelvis to the border of the pubic hair at Ren 2 (lower confluent and connection to Chong mai), where it meets with the Liver DM. From here it ascends to the floating ribs, GB 25 (Kidney front mu) and LR 13 (Spleen front mu). From there, it enters the Gall Bladder organ via GB 24, and the Liver organ via LR 14. The Gall Bladder divergent channel then goes into the chest and Heart via either Ren 17 or Ren 14. It then travels to ST 12, Ren 22, and Ren 23, up along the jaw to ST 5, reaching GB 1, its upper confluent point.

A second trajectory is described in the Lei Jing, providing a relationship to the ears. In this trajectory, the GB DM diverges at GB 22, going internal to Ren 17, then traveling up to ST 12, climbing behind the ear to SJ 16 and SJ 17 to the extra point Taiyang, and then into Du 20 to communicate with the brain. The pathway comes back out of the brain to go to GB 1 and crosses over to the opposite side to LI 20. Shima and Chace say that on its way up to the head, before it gets up to the outer canthus of the eye, it goes to Eye Tie, the optic nerve.[157]

INDICATIONS FOR THE GALL BLADDER DIVERGENT CHANNEL

Like all DMs, the Gall Bladder DM treats chronic pain along its trajectory, e.g., chronic hip, sciatica, and rib pain, etc. It has a strong relationship to the sinews and joints. Classically, it relates to the bones, and with the Liver assists in moving blood to the sinews. In the context of the divergent mechanism, the GB DM mobilizes blood to the bones/joints to maintain latency.

The GB DM impacts the mu points and can treat stagnations in these areas, including an enlarged Liver or Spleen, and remove obstructions causing palpitations, chest pain, etc.

It has an influence on the neck, throat, esophagus, and Heart via its pathway and can treat the vocal cords and other neck/throat symptoms, hiatal hernias, angina, bitter taste in mouth, palpitations and being easily frightened, timidity, etc.

The Gall Bladder DM goes to the eyes and ears and treats symptoms related to the head, e.g., dizziness, heavy head, hypertension, migraines, etc.

The Gall Bladder DM also relates to the Dai mai and the external genitalia and is used for lower burner symptoms, especially damp-heat, and mediates latency in this area.

GALL BLADDER DIVERGENT PERSONALITY

The Gall Bladder as a wood yang element is idealistic, creative, and goal-oriented. The morphology of one with a Gall Bladder personality is a pointed, angular jaw. The Gall Bladder divergent personality is ambitious and likes to lead, but is mindful of recognition and making sure others notice their achievements. Generally of a strong constitution, they have good stamina and are rarely sick when young. As their ambitions grow and accumulate, frustration around achieving goals escalates and tension arises around the muscles and sinews, creating an inability to relax. As a shaoyang, the Gall Bladder divergent person can be easily swayed. But they are enthusiastic and optimistic people who believe there is always more that can be accomplished, but can become over-extended (remember the DRRBF Wood phase of advance and retreat balance). They are good motivators, but when they can't complete everything they desire, can get angry. Swaying to extremes, they are sometimes hot, sometimes cold, physically and emotionally.

Energetically, the Gall Bladder divergent channel is responsible for activation of the hips and pelvis, mobilizing blood to support jing. It travels along the mu-accumulation points of the Kidneys, Spleen, Gall Bladder, Liver, and Heart/chest as well as influencing the neck, throat, and eyes. The Gall Bladder is about engagement and decision-making in terms of where to expend one's resources and what direction to move in life. When overwhelmed, the Gall Bladder divergent person becomes wishy/washy and indecisive. This even reflects itself with pain and other symptoms that are intermittent and change locations. Its influence over the throat provides an ability to clear one's throat and express oneself. If this is blocked, energetically this person holds her lips tight, grinds the jaw, and may even vomit to expel that which she doesn't want. Thus, the Gall Bladder regulates the gag reflex and retching, the ability to release something recently ingested and regurgitate what is unwanted back out. This is part of its decision-making aspect. Patients who constantly need to clear their throat reflect this indecisiveness of what they want to digest and make a part of themselves, creating turbidity and phlegm. Not only does this show up in the throat and abdomen, but also in the upper portals of the eyes and ears with difficulty digesting emotions and indecisive internal narratives. When blockages occur, the Gall Bladder divergent person holds stagnation in her chest, smooth muscles of the abdomen (peristalsis), throat, and eyes.

LIVER DIVERGENT CHANNEL PATHWAY

The Liver divergent pathway begins at the dorsum of the foot[158] (ST 42, where the GB luo ends), ascends to LR 5, and travels to Ren 2 and Ren 3, where it meets the GB DM and travels with it.

INDICATIONS FOR THE LIVER DIVERGENT CHANNEL

One of the main uses of the LR DM is due to its influence over the pelvis and genitalia. Its confluent point, LR 5, is also the Liver luo point, thus it can manage gynecological and reproductive organ problems from wei qi stagnation and/or hyperactivity (heat and inflammation), damp-heat, as well as blood stasis.

The Liver and Gall Bladder divergents affect the "ancestral sinews," i.e., the genitalia (though some say they relate to the diaphragm or the abdominal rectus).[159] They play a role in sexual arousal, and like the Liver luo, they can be used to treat abnormal sexual arousal as well as infertility and impotence. In this case, the Liver divergent can be used to reduce excess wei qi in the area, or allow more blood to convert to, and nourish, jing.

While for the primary channels the Spleen manages the blood, in terms of divergent philosophy, it is the Liver divergent channel that holds the blood, preventing leakage.

LIVER DIVERGENT PERSONALITY

The Liver divergent person is highly temperamental and is likely to deal with high blood pressure as they are nervous, fidgety, bite their nails, and are moody. Unpredictable and, as a result, often entertaining, they have unrealistic visions of the future and tend towards blood stasis. Like the Gall Bladder divergent personality, they crave attention and change, and can become irritable when it's prevented. They are pioneers in their related fields (with far-reaching visions), but can suffer difficulty in organization (i.e., their visions often lack metal's ability to organize a step-by-step process to achieve).

Third confluence

> Channels associated: ST/SP
>
> Resource: jin (thin fluids)
>
> Confluent points: BL 1, ST 30
>
> Yang lower confluent: ST 30
>
> Yin lower confluent: SP 12

STOMACH DIVERGENT CHANNEL PATHWAY

The Stomach divergent pathway begins at ST 30, goes deep into the abdomen, where it enters the Stomach organ at Ren 12 and the Spleen organ at LR 13, then goes to the Heart organ at Ren 17 or Ren 14. It goes through the throat to Ren 22, up to ST 9 and Ren 23, and into the mouth. The pathway emerges out at the corner of the mouth (ST 4), travels to the nose (LI 20), goes to ST 1 (meets Ren mai), and then on to BL 1, where it meets the Spleen DM at its upper confluent point. BL 1 is said to activate ST 42.[160]

INDICATIONS FOR THE STOMACH DIVERGENT CHANNEL

Because much of the fluids have been consumed by this time, pathologies are often chronic at the ST DM. As it has a strong influence over the abdomen, and further communicates with the Spleen, the ST DM is often used for insufficient Spleen qi and a host of gastrointestinal disorders with hyperactive wei qi, such as colitis, gastritis, and other inflammatory conditions with deficient yin underlying.

Its trajectory provides a greater influence over the face, including the eyes, mouth, and nose, the pure yang of the Stomach nourishing them with yin. Sinusitis and inflammatory eye disorders are common here. As heat from the yin deficiency ensues, jing can become damaged and tooth decay, polyps, and loss of vision can result.

Like the other two confluences before it, the ST DM has relationships with the 8x meridians, namely the Chong mai (ST 30), where heat and inflammation can enter and damage the blueprint causing self-destructive behavior, and the Qiao mai (BL 1), which can create aggressive behaviors, both towards oneself and the outside world.[161]

STOMACH DIVERGENT PERSONALITY

The Stomach divergent person is strong-willed with conviction. She appreciates power, but is not concerned with achieving goals. Her morphology is a squarish chin. The Stomach divergent person likes to be engaged with others and create connections, and is also mindful of boundaries. She makes an excellent liaison and mediator, though can be dominating, domineering, and overpowering at times. As an earth person, she seeks security and stability, values groundedness, and has a knack for blending in. The Stomach divergent person is generally quick to learn and absorb new things and discard what is not needed (separates pure from impure).

The Stomach divergent person embodies one's intrinsic right to demand. They want satisfied what their senses crave; to bring things in, store it, and make it a part of them. Those with needs that cannot be filled are experiencing Stomach divergent issues. People who look but cannot touch and feel that their needs cannot be filled have weakness in the Stomach divergent channel. They tend to never demand anything or ask of others. One with an overactive Stomach divergent channel will be overly demanding, compulsive, and obsessive. Tensions tend to be held in their abdomen (rectus muscles) and their mouths, sinuses, and the medial parts of eyes (BL 1/ST 1 area), often with wrinkles around the extra point taiyang.

SPLEEN DIVERGENT CHANNEL PATHWAY

The Spleen divergent meridian begins at SP 12, goes to ST 30, where it meets the ST DM at its lower confluent point, flowing with it up to Ren 22, ST 9, and Ren 23, where it branches off to the middle of the tongue, exiting through LI 20, to ST 1, ending at BL 1, the upper confluent point.

INDICATIONS FOR THE SPLEEN DIVERGENT CHANNEL

Like all the channels before (and after), the SP DM treats pain along its trajectory such as inner thigh and pelvic pain, and abdominal and esophageal pain. Its connection to the throat also allows it to treat thyroid disorders. Its relationship to the Stomach allows for treatment of all GI disorders, especially those with inflammation and underlying yin deficiency (e.g., wasting and thirsting, gastritis, etc.), and rebellious qi (e.g., nausea and retching).

It communicates with the Heart, and can treat mental-emotional symptoms, and with its connection to the Chong mai, furthers this impact. With the Chong, it can also treat issues revolving around blood (deficiency with stirring of wind, as well as stasis), and further strengthens the impact to treat abdominal and GI disorders.

The Spleen DM communicates to the mouth and tongue and can treat mouth ulcers, stiffness of the tongue, and unclear speech, and as it assists bringing yin to the upper orifices can also treat wind symptoms such as tics and spasms, and other deficient yin symptoms of the upper body like dizziness, dry mouth, etc.

SPLEEN DIVERGENT PERSONALITY

As yin earth, the Spleen divergent person is highly accommodating (and not demanding like her Stomach counterpart), believing that life unfolds on its own accord. She is more maternal, concerned with the needs of others, and can be found comforting, crying, and laughing with others as needed. She tends to be self-critical with a stocky body and squarish chin.

Fourth confluence

Channels associated: SI/HT

Resource: ye (thick fluids) and blood

Confluent points: BL 1, GB 22

Yang lower confluent: SI 10

Yin lower confluent: HT 1

SMALL INTESTINE DIVERGENT CHANNEL PATHWAY

The SI DM diverges at the shoulder (SI 10), descends and enters HT 1, moving to GB 22. It then goes to the Heart, via Ren 17, descending through the diaphragm to communicate with the Small Intestine organ. From SI 10 a branch goes into the scapula, then to ST 12, the throat, SI 18, and ending at BL 1.

INDICATIONS FOR THE SMALL INTESTINE DIVERGENT CHANNEL

The SI DM has a strong impact on the sinews. It can treat pain along the pathway, such as axillary pain with swollen lymph nodes, but because of its connection to GB 22 and SI 18, it also includes an influence over the sinews as a whole. Via these two major sinew channel meeting points, it can internalize wei qi from the yang and yin sinews. GB 22 provides access to the chest and furthers the Small Intestine's communication to the Heart. And like its sinew meridian counterpart, it can also treat the symptoms of Heart fire, including insomnia, restlessness, anxiety, chest pains, etc. This connection to the sinew channels allows it to treat the smooth muscles of the Heart (influencing rate and rhythm), as well as the digestive system (peristaltic and motility problems, IBS, food stagnation, nausea, vomiting, reflux, irritated mucosal lining, etc.).

Via GB 22, the SI DM also has a strong impact on blood issues (original great luo), as well as the hormones (Yuan Ye and relationship to the thick fluids). Through its upper confluent, BL 1, it communicates with the Qiao vessels and brain, impacting blood flow and fluids throughout, including an impact on memory and one's mental faculties.

The SI DM also has a strong influence on the digestive system as a whole, managing symptoms along the entire GI tract. As the ST/SP DMs precede it, they both also share BL 1 as the upper confluent, creating a further linkage.

SMALL INTESTINE DIVERGENT PERSONALITY

As a fire element, the Small Intestine divergent person is volatile, restless, people-oriented, extroverted, and highly intellectual. They believe their curriculum/destiny in life is a noble one and are up to the challenges to see it through and accomplish it. The Small Intestine provides our ability to resist demands on us from the outside and prevent those from manipulating our Heart. When life is not going according to plan and this person's demands are not being met, he can become tense and resistant, even defiant with a hardened expression. Frustration and the resultant tightness, especially in the pectoralis muscles and ribs where he holds his tension, can lead to lethargy.

The Small Intestine divergent channel has a major dynamic over the chest and thoracic cavity. Developmentally, it allows one to open his Heart and let others in. With traumas, the chest becomes highly armored, and shoulders become tense with arms held tightly to the body, not swinging naturally when one walks. Eventual fatigue in the limbs results from this unwillingness to open the Heart and engage in life, as defiance compensates for fear of being hurt. Tension in axillary lymph nodes can also develop from this armoring, often with autoimmune complications later in life, including digestive issues and chronic fatigue syndrome. The Small Intestine also has a major impact over the eyes and the movement of the ye into the brain. Post trauma, one sees fear and frightening experiences everywhere based on one's past.

HEART DIVERGENT CHANNEL PATHWAY

The Heart divergent meridian begins at HT 1, descends to GB 22, and enters the Heart organ via Ren 17, then descends to communicate with the Small Intestine organ. From the chest it travels internally to Ren 23, then to the tip of the tongue, where it diffuses into the face converging at BL 1. Jeffrey Yuen has also taught a descending trajectory from Ren 17 to Ren 8, similar to the Heart sinew channel and Bao mai, and also furthering its influence over the entire abdomen and GI tract.

INDICATIONS FOR THE HEART DIVERGENT CHANNEL

As the Heart is known for influencing peripheral circulation, it can provide circulation to all areas of its pathway. It makes a strong connection to the chest, the throat, and the eyes/brain. As such it can treat chest pains, difficulty speaking, stuttering, etc., blood and wei qi stagnation in the face, eyes, and brain, also making it influential in the treatment of memory disorders. Its action of diffusing wei qi in the face makes it an important choice in treating allergies. It circulates wei qi and blood to the extremities and can treat Raynaud's syndrome (moxa on HT 1 is very effective for this), wei atrophy disorder, etc.

The HT DM also influences the entire GI tract, making it important for the treatment of bowel disorders, including malabsorption, Small Intestine bacterial overgrowth (SIBO), and other hot/inflammatory conditions of the bowels. It can also treat heat from the Heart being vented via the Small Intestine to the Bladder, creating lin syndrome.

And as the Heart, it can treat psycho-emotional disorders of all varieties due to its impact on the blood and shen, and via its connection to GB 22 (dynamics of the chest, but also for blood as the great luo), as well as the brain.

HEART DIVERGENT PERSONALITY

The Heart divergent person is moved by a sense of honor and integrity. She'll decline a leadership role unless convinced by others it's for a noble cause. When hurt, betrayed, or traumatized, she will retreat to her inner sanctuary and disengage from social engagements and other people.

Fifth confluence

Channels associated: SJ/PC

Resource: qi

Confluent points: SJ 16, Ren 12

Yang lower confluent: Du 20

Yin lower confluent: GB 22

TRIPLE BURNER DIVERGENT CHANNEL PATHWAY

The Triple Burner DM starts at Du 20, descends laterally to the ears (SJ 16), then to ST 12, internalizing to communicate with the three burners, and spreading out at Ren 17, Ren 12, and the Ren 4–6 area.

An alternative pathway begins at GB 22, then enters the diaphragm and the chest. One branch goes down to the three burners, the other to Ren 12 and to SJ 16, then to the GB 12/BL 10 area where it communicates to the BL DM, before ascending to Du 20 and the brain.

INDICATIONS FOR THE TRIPLE BURNER DIVERGENT CHANNEL

At the Triple Burner DM, most resources have been used, resulting in a loss of structure and marrow. The body begins to use distorted responses such as creating dampness to reassert latency. The SJ DM can also come into play with healing crises, to help release pathology. It can be used for pain along its trajectory, especially from damp-heat. Chronic shaoyang pathogens in the sinews and joints manifest with fibromyalgia, rheumatoid arthritis, wei atrophy, etc.

It has a strong influence over the neck and vertex, and ensuring that the WOS points remain open is an important element in the success of its treatments. Symptoms such as dizziness, vertigo, etc. are common in this confluence. This channel communicates with all three burners and can also assist in raising yang qi, including the spirit, and can treat depression, prolapses, etc., as well as disorders of the chest (e.g., anxiety, palpitations, asthma, suffocating sensations).[162]

The Triple Burner also maintains the fluid system, and this DM can treat hormonal disorders, problems with nodules and swellings, etc.

TRIPLE BURNER DIVERGENT PERSONALITY

The Triple Burner divergent person is emotional, highly intuitive, and creative, and can even be psychic. She has a tendency towards labile emotions and can suffer from bipolar disorder. As a fire personality, she has a strong conviction towards noble causes, and can lead with her emotions to the point of becoming a martyr. She is highly expressive (verbally, physically, and emotionally), and can tend towards high blood pressure, high fevers, and hysteria. The Triple Burner involves the ability to control. Loss of latency brings loss of control, and Triple Burner excess people can become highly manipulative to reassert themselves and often instill fear to accomplish this. Eventually, with deficiency, depression and despair set in as control has been lost. The Triple Burner manages the dissemination of qi. When overwhelmed and latency has been lost, the individual may suffer fatigue, lack of groundedness, and being out of control. Rebellious qi symptoms such as vomiting, diarrhea, and dizziness can occur.

PERICARDIUM DIVERGENT CHANNEL PATHWAY

The Pericardium divergent channel begins at GB 22, moves into the chest to PC 1, to Ren 17, and descending to the middle and lower burners. A branch from Ren 17 goes to ST 12, to Ren 23, and then to SJ 16, ending at GB 12.

Indications for the Pericardium divergent channel

The PC DM treats pain throughout its channel, including chest, axillary, and hypochondriac pain. Its connection to the nape/GB 12 helps explain its use for neck pain and stiffness as well as ear/mastoid disorders. Its connection to the throat provides further use for vocal problems and plum-pit qi (often associated with its jueyin pair, the Liver).

It has a strong relationship with the SJ DM and fluid metabolism, especially in the treatment of damp-heat and blood heat. It helps to manage reckless movement of blood, as well as shen disturbances resulting from heat in the blood and heat harassing the Heart and shen.

Pericardium divergent personality

The Pericardium divergent person is energetic, romantic, and, like his fire counterparts, emotional. He is expressively pessimistic and sarcastic (bitter), reflecting that he has been burned before. As a result, he is afraid of failure and suffering hurt again.

Sixth confluence

Channels associated: LI/LU

Resource: yang

Confluent points: LI 18, ST 12

Yang lower confluent: LI 15

Yin lower confluent: LU 1

Large Intestine divergent channel pathway

The LI DM begins at LI 15, where it has two branches. One goes to Du 14 and then to ST 12. The second goes to the axilla and crosses the chest horizontally in line with the nipple. Here, one branch goes up to ST 12 and then LI 18, the other to the LI organ, possibly via ST 25.

Indications for the Large Intestine divergent channel

The LI DM treats pain throughout its channel's influence, including chest and throat pain as well as abdominal pain, joint pain, tendonitis, etc. Its connection to Du 14 provides access to the upper back, as well as all the yang primary channels which converge here, and via ST 12 access to the yin channels. It can treat inflammatory problems in the bowels (e.g., colitis, intestinal polyps), throat (e.g., sore throat, goiter), chest (e.g., costochondritis), and breasts (e.g., mastitis, breast cancer, insufficient lactation).

The Large Intestine DM treats Lung symptoms, including distension, fullness or congestion in the chest, asthma, wheezing, etc. It also impacts growth patterns in the upper burner (e.g., breast development) as well as hair (e.g., alopecia from heat burning the hair follicles).[163]

LARGE INTESTINE DIVERGENT PERSONALITY

As metal, the Large Intestine divergent personality is meticulous and image oriented. Concerned with how they are perceived, they seek to project an image of grace and beauty, controlling and rehearsing their movements and mannerisms. The Large Intestine is about establishing priorities and ordering the qi; those with this personality type value precision and strive to live up to ideals. They are composed and thoughtful in their response and demonstrations of emotion, and exhibit few extremes.

By the time one reaches the Large Intestine divergent channel there has been a loss of yang, autointoxication, and overall collapse. One is constipated with toxic thoughts and feelings and senses an impending doom. This uptight, anal personality cannot let go and surrender and creates stagnation and armoring around the chest, abdomen, pelvis, gluteus, and psoas region.

LUNG DIVERGENT CHANNEL PATHWAY

The LU DM emerges at LU 1 and goes to GB 22 and the chest, where it spreads to taiyang[164] and to the breasts. From the Lung, one branch goes to the Large Intestine organ, the other emerges at ST 12 and travels to the throat at LI 18.

INDICATIONS FOR THE LUNG DIVERGENT CHANNEL

The Lung DM overlaps with the Lung primary meridian, treating many of the same issues, including shortness of breath, asthma, chest pain, etc. It is the last DM within the sequence and the first of the primary channels, distributing wei qi to the Lung primary channel. This relationship also allows one to pull pathology out of the primary channels into the DM for latency.

As it governs wei qi, it treats wind-cold invasions, but different from the primary channel, here it treats chronic invasions from insufficient wei qi and low immunity. As the last DM, immunity is severely compromised and pathogens are running unchecked. It is not uncommon to find a host of late-stage cancers and autoimmune disorders by the LU DM.

Like the LI DM, the LU DM also has an impact on the breast, being able to treat its disorders by releasing stagnant wei qi in the chest. It also impacts the throat and can be used for tonsillitis, laryngitis, and thyroid disorders.

LUNG DIVERGENT PERSONALITY

The Lung divergent person is keen on setting priorities and detailed planning in service of maintaining order and breathing easy. He dislikes chaos, distractions, and being overly busy, which makes him fatigued; he requires fresh air and open spaces. Sensitive to demands on his energy, he needs a lot of sleep, otherwise he can become irritable. He is self-critical and vulnerable to how others perceive him, though he has a strong sense of justice and is willing to debate to prove others wrong. He appreciates solitude, and can be introverted, needing to make life a little simpler.

Needling technique and strategies for the divergent meridians

The needling technique for the divergent meridians depends on one's intention, i.e., whether one is trying to promote clearing by releasing the pathogen, or trying to promote latency. Both scenarios involve three-time needling, but the order differs depending on the strategy.

To promote latency, the three-time needling is Deep-Superficial-Deep (hereinafter DSD). To perform DSD, the needle is inserted and quickly moved to the deep yuan level where it is slowly vibrated to stir up yuan qi. It is then brought back to the superficial wei level to gather wei qi with circular needling, then needled back to the yuan level to assert latency. To accomplish this for a particular elemental divergent, one needles the confluent points associated with the channels from top to bottom with DSD, then one can choose appropriate points along the trajectory. Other points can be added to these treatments that relate to either wei or yuan qi (e.g., he-sea points, source points, 8x meridian points, etc.).

To promote clearing, the three-time needling is Superficial-Deep-Superficial (hereinafter SDS). To perform SDS, the needle is inserted into the wei level and a circular technique is performed, brought to the yuan level with a rapid vibrating technique to stir up yuan qi, and then lifted back to the wei level performing circular needling to release the pathogen to this domain. To clear a pathogen from an elemental divergent, one needles the confluent points of the said divergent channel from bottom to top with SDS, then chooses appropriate points along its trajectory. Other points related to wei or yuan can be needled, as well as any ashi points followed by the jing-well point to the associated nature of the pathogen (e.g., yangming for heat). Prior to the needling, one can also gua sha the zonal divergent related to the nature of the pathogen in question (this can be done for promoting latency as well).

Clearing blockages

When seeking to release a pathogen from the elemental divergent it is important to make sure the pathogen has a clear route to the exterior, lest it become stuck on its way out. Below is a list of a few points helpful in assuring an easy release. They should be checked and needled if blocked. As the pathogen will come out to the yang zones, the taiyang, shaoyang, and yangming areas should be opened. One can assess and needle the SI 10–12 area (taiyang), GB 12–SJ 16 (shaoyang), and ST 12–LI 15 (yangming). To ensure pathogens are released from the yin zones, one can also check and release holding at the yin sinew meeting areas, Ren 3 and GB 22.

Divergent channel treatment strategies

1. Promote latency: DSD needling
   a. needle the confluent points
   b. then needle the trajectory points
   c. follow with needling points related to wei or yuan qi
   d. can first release zones and blockages.
2. Release pathogen: SDS needling
   a. gua sha the affected zone
   b. clear blockages and holding areas
   c. needle the confluent points
   d. then needle the chosen trajectory points
   e. follow with needling ashi points
   f. end with the appropriate jing-well point.

Pulse diagnosis for the divergent meridians

Pulses for the divergent meridians will rely on the wei and yuan levels, assessing stagnations and holdings in these energetic layers. The ying level will also be assessed in order to determine available resources at one's disposal for either encouraging or maintaining remission, or providing sufficient fluids to dispel/expel a pathogen.

There are a few aspects to assessing the divergent meridians via the pulse. The first is to see if there is room to create latency in the yuan level. To do this, one presses to 15 beans and lifts pressure slightly off the bone (14 beans) and assesses the quality. Then one pushes back down to 15 beans. If the pulse disappears, this is deemed a Hidden pulse, suggesting that the body has the capacity to hide a pathogen and divert it. In the next chapter on the 8x meridians, if something is present at this depth, it will suggest activity of the second and third trinities of 8x meridians.

To find the presence of an elemental divergent pulse, the 14 beans of pressure will demonstrate a pulse of holding/stagnation, typically a Tight pulse. A zonal divergent pulse is seen when the pulse at the wei level matches the quality felt at the yuan level. The 15 beans of pressure should also empty/hide to confirm divergent activity. As the divergent channels emerge and relate to the zang fu, their reflexology follows that of the primary channels.

Elemental divergent channel pulse reflexology	
Left cun: SI/HT	Right cun: LI/LU
Left guan: GB/LR	Right guan: ST/SP
Left chi: BL/KI	Right chi: SJ/PC

The zonal divergent deals with the wei level, and these pulses follow the sinew meridian correlations, e.g., cun taiyang, guan shaoyang, chi yangming. From the divergent perspective, however, when looking at the wei level pulses, they are interpreted as being released from the interior domain, not internalizing as with the sinew meridians. Thus, their reflexology is different when found on the 6 beans of pressure than the yin sinews.

Pathology internalizing	Pathology externalizing
3 beans → 6 beans	6 beans → 3 beans
Taiyang → Shaoyin	Jueyin → Taiyang
Shaoyang → Jueyin	Taiyin → Yangming
Yangming → Taiyin	Shaoyin → Shaoyang

One way to distinguish whether this is emanating from the divergent channels and releasing from the interior rather than internalizing is that the 6 beans pulses manifest more medially (whereas yin sinews internalizing tend to be more lateral). It can also show up as a loss of latency whereby the Triple Burner pulse at the right proximal position is Rapid and Floating. In this latter scenario, there would be the presence of a Floating pulse in the yangming chi position with fullness and strength as one increased pressure. This would help define a zonal divergent issue. A Triple Burner pulse is indicative that the body is trying to rid pathology if the pulse is not Weak/Thin, demonstrating there is still integrity as it releases something toxic.

Divergent meridians' relationship to Heart Shock

The divergent channels have tremendous usefulness in the treatment of Heart Shock as they modulate the relationship between the wei and yuan qi, thus impacting the symptoms as well as root of nervous system energetics, as well as the dissemination of the body's resources. Each of the confluences has its unique signature that can impact various aspects of the Heart Shock strategies via the resource it manages, its channel trajectory, orifices traversed, 8x channel it connects with, etc.

One can also look at the confluences based on trinities, with the first three confluences representing one trinity, and the second three the next trinity. While any of the six confluences can be used to promote latency or clearing, utilizing the theory of progression through the elemental confluences, the first three confluences are best used to promote clearing as there are still yin resources available to flush out a pathogen. The second trinity is often used to promote remission/latency, while buying time to build resources and move it back to an earlier confluence.

Specifically in terms of trauma, one can further generally differentiate the first trinity by the types of trauma one is trying to manage and treat. The BL/KI divergent, as it deals with jing-essence, our deepest resource, can be utilized for traumas that were life-threatening. These traumas will have a dramatic and rapid impact on, and alteration of the dissemination of, one's jing, and manifest with deep-seated fears. The GB/LR divergent deals with the ying-blood level and our day-to-day consciousness and manages traumas that arise from an acute or chronic stress-induced event(s). An original stressful traumatic event can often recur with heightened responses when the individual is under a great stress. The ST/SP divergent manages the jin-fluids and at this confluent we are managing chronic long-term traumas that have damaged the fluids and the nervous system in trying to maintain the latency (dehydration). Nervous twitches, tics, and spasms are common, especially when the patient is nervous.

Bladder divergent

The Bladder divergent manages the relationship of the Heart and Kidneys in terms of how Heart and Kidney yang are supporting each other. The Bladder divergent pathway rises from BL 40 through the Bladder shu/Hua Tou points, wrapping around the waist and also the mid back around BL 15–17, moving through the GB 22 area, where it communicates the back to the front, specifically at the energetics of the Heart at the Ren 15–17 area. This strong communication between the Bladder, Kidneys, and Heart brings yang to the chest and assists in the Heart/Kidney communication. Thus, it can be used to activate yang or anchor it back to the Kidneys as BL 10 also has a Classical function of descending and anchoring excessive yang qi in the head.

Its relationship to BL 17, the influential point of blood, as well as the chest at Ren 15–17, provides a strong argument for utilizing this channel to treat psycho-emotional and shen disturbances, including anxiety and panic disorders. And as part of the Bladder divergent's relationship in mediating communication between the Heart and Kidneys via GB 22 (where the channel passes through to allow communication from BL 17 to Ren 17), it activates a relationship to the Da Bao and Bao mai (when combined with the Kidney divergent), further strengthening it as a treatment option for running piglet qi and a host of emotional imbalances as well as pelvic and reproductive disorders. This is further enhanced by the BL DM's association with the Dai mai.

Its relationship to GB 22, at the hamstrings, paravertebrals, and Hua Tou points, activates a strong influence over the fight/flight/freeze response and the nervous system as a whole. The nervous system is related to taiyang and shaoyin (as discussed in Part I), and this divergent channel can be tapped in order to relax the sinews and nerves in hypervigilant patients. Alternatively, it can be nourished and strengthened to assist with the Triple Burner's dissemination of yang qi along Du mai and the Bladder channel into its respective shu points. In this regard, when using the Bladder divergent, one can also needle the Bladder shu points of whichever organ system one is trying to impact as these points also deal with yuan qi.

BL 10 is a WOS point and as such has a profound impact on the portals. As mentioned above, it can descend excessive yang qi rising, but its impact on the portals is also enabled by the pathway moving from BL 10 into the brain at Du 20, then traversing back to taiyang, which some believe to associate with BL 1. Earlier in Part I, I discussed the relationship of the eyes and hypervigilance, constantly trying to search and look out for danger and perceived threats causing tension around the eyes and distorted perceptions. The BL DM is an excellent way of managing a nervous system tense condition as well as clearing obfuscations from this orifice.

The Bladder divergent person after trauma can present in a number of different ways. When wei qi becomes hypoactive, he will have a difficult time expressing himself and vocalizing his feelings. Unable to be who he is in the world, he will become tense and irritable. Freeing up wei qi with SDS needling would be appropriate here. Excessive wei qi will make his nervous system hyperactive, with potential yang-rising symptoms such as seizures, etc. He may also engage in risky behaviors, constantly seeking bigger and bigger thrills and excitement in life. Here, one seeks to anchor with DSD needling.

Kidney divergent

The KI DM runs up the midline of the body, sharing points along the Kidney primary channel into the chest and the Kidney shu points. Here, we see a major dynamic on the chest, specifically relating to trapped qi and yin stasis. This can impact the Heart, creating palpitations as well as rhythm and rate issues. The Bladder divergent created a relationship to the Heart and Kidneys by mediating yang qi, and the Kidney divergent creates a Heart/Kidney relationship via its communication with their yin component. Typical signs and symptoms of Heart and Kidney not communicating, with Kidney yin deficiency being unable to quell and contain Heart fire, can be seen and treated with this channel. Symptoms are tachycardia, insomnia, irregular heartbeat, nervousness and anxiety, red tongue tip with petechia, sweating, hot palms (including luo vessel understanding of this symptom, including fidgetiness, desiring stimulation, etc.), etc.

The Kidney divergent makes connections to a number of the 8x meridians, including the Yin Wei mai, Du mai, Dai mai, and the Chong mai, as well as the

Bao mai. I've already discussed the applications of Du mai to the nervous system and the dissemination of yang, as well as Bao mai associations with the Bladder divergent. The Chong mai relationship further strengthens the impact on the Heart and blood (and its management over the shen) with the upper shu points of the chest. The Kidneys and Chong mai both have a strong influence over the yuan qi and jing-essence, and also one's blueprint/constitution and personality (personality disorders were discussed in Chapter 5). The Yin Wei mai also creates a strong dynamic over the chest as well as blood circulation in the chest and pelvis. In addition, Yin Wei mai, as the linking channel, deals a lot with linking the most influential memories and aspects of one's lives. Traumas can be the most prominent of these, altering the course of one's life, which can be addressed with tapping Yin Wei mai and releasing via the divergent system. More will be discussed in the following chapter regarding these 8x channels.

The Kidney divergent also traverses the throat and neck (where it connects with Yin Wei mai) and allows one to assert and vocalize one's inner thoughts, needs, traumas, etc. by purging them from the Heart. Loss of voice, goiters, thyroid issues, etc. can reflect one's inability to express oneself post trauma, and releasing the throat with the Kidney divergent can be quite useful in treating these symptoms and stagnation from the Heart.

The Kidney divergent person tends to be sensitive and vulnerable to external influences, including EPFs, but also social interactions and other stimulations. For a nervous system weak individual, this DM, as well as using Dr. Shen's formulas below, can be very helpful.

Treating the BL/KI DMs can be done as individual channel treatments or together as a unit. When needling just the Bladder divergent, BL 10 and BL 40 are needled to gain access to the channel. When also utilizing the yin pair (and this goes for all the confluences), the yin pair's lower confluent should also be needled, in this case KI 10. Doing so unlocks access to the Kidney's channel and opens up the dynamics mentioned in the preceding paragraphs. The combinations of points and areas influenced can be extremely varied. For instance, to treat a female patient with Heart Shock post a life-threatening car accident manifesting with chief complaints including back pain, anxiety and panic disorder, fibroids, and insomnia, one may choose to needle BL 10 and BL 40, KI 10, right GB 41 (to open Dai mai), Du 4 (local point for pain and also a Dai mai point as it wraps around), Hua Tou, and Bladder shu points on areas of tension/tightness or which associate with specific functions, e.g., BL 23 (for low back pain as well as to impact reproductive organs), BL 15 (for anxiety and where channel wraps around to front), GB 22 (to impact chest), Ren 17 (for anxiety and insomnia), and Kidney channel ashi on lower abdomen (for fibroids and to anchor running piglet qi), as well as Kidney shu points such as KI 25 (for anxiety and insomnia) and Ren 23 (Yin Wei mai point as well as termination point for shaoyin, which also nourishes yin and can release the throat to allow for proper expression and release of one's trauma). In terms of needling technique, I may decide to needle the divergent channel confluent points with DSD needling to anchor and strengthen the patient, while using a more sedating vibrating technique on GB 41 to move qi and blood in the pelvis and using SDS needling on BL 15, GB 22, and Ren 17 to release any trapped and pent-up heat from stagnation that is harassing the shen and causing nervous system tension.

Gall Bladder divergent

The GB DM has a major usefulness in Heart Shock as it impacts the mu-accumulation points as well as the chest. Its alternate trajectory has it beginning at GB 22 and then entering the chest at Ren 17, giving it a strong relationship to the Heart and the treatment of shen disorders. As mentioned earlier, the Gall Bladder divergent is best used for traumas of a repetitive nature and/or traumas that are exacerbated by stressful conditions and when the personality tends to be one of nervous system tense. It traverses the front mu points of the Pericardium, Liver, Gall Bladder, Spleen, and Kidneys (and Bladder if one considers Ren 3 instead of Ren 2 as the confluent), enabling it to address a variety of disorders within those systems. For example, a patient suffering from Heart Shock from repeated disciplinary beatings as a child who presents with anxiety causing abdominal cramping and diarrhea when under stress can be treated with GB 1 and Ren 2 to open the GB DM, plus the addition of LR 14 and GB 24 with SDS to reduce stress and tension within the Liver and Gall Bladder, and LR 13 with DSD needling to strengthen and calm the Spleen and Stomach. Adding in GB 22 and using Ren 3 instead of Ren 2 as the lower confluent can address the wei qi impact on the smooth muscles of the gut to further calm the overactivity of the Liver on the Spleen and Stomach.

As the Gall Bladder divergent moves through the chest to the ribs and abdomen, one also sees an influence over the diaphragm (traditionally ascribed to the Liver's domain) which also regulates the movement of blood. With its relationship to GB 22 and the great luo of the Spleen, there is enhanced impact over the blood as well as a pronounced impact on wei qi. From a primary meridian perspective, the Gall Bladder (with the Liver) controls the muscles and sinews, making the GB DM very effective in the treatment of pain, especially where there is insufficient blood being shunted to the sinews. GB 22 and the great luo also treat pain all over the body. Thus, a trauma patient presenting with pain/heaviness/achiness (wind-damp) from a traumatic injury with a background of stress and anxiety aggravating said pain can be treated with the GB DM with SDS needling, then adding in GB 22 to impact wei qi while combining a sinew meridian treatment to release the musculoskeletal pain. The treatment would include Ren 2 and GB 1 SDS, Ren 17, LR 14, and GB 24 to manage and relieve stress, plus GB 22, local ashi points, and GB 44 to release the wind-damp bi.

This impact from GB 22 over wei qi in the chest also creates a regulatory component over the smooth muscle contractions of the Heart and as such can be very effective in regulating rate and rhythm issues.

Additional components of this divergent in terms of our Heart Shock strategies are that it, like the KI DM, traverses the neck and vocal cords and can be used to release the throat for expressing what is in one's Heart. It also has an ability to release the upper orifices, especially the eyes and ears, and can be important in helping a patient change their internal voice.

The Gall Bladder divergent also has a relationship to the Dai mai and is often used to either assist in pulling pathology out of the yuan level to be released via an SDS GB DM treatment, or to make additional room within the GB DM by reallocating its pathology to the Dai mai.

Liver divergent

The Liver divergent shares many of the same indications and uses as the Gall Bladder as it shares the Gall Bladder trajectory from the abdomen. The uniqueness of the Liver divergent is its stronger impact on the pelvis due to its connection to the Liver luo whose pathway is identical from LR 5 to the genitalia. Thus, it treats traumas to the pelvis/genitalia, most prominently sexual traumas as well as the sequelae of suppressed emotions/anger, repressed sexuality, lack of sexual interest and libido, inability to relax during sexual intercourse, STDs resulting from stagnation, etc. As it also reflects wei and yuan, the Liver divergent can be used for when stagnant wei and blood become trapped with the jing, creating symptoms such as cysts and fibroids, etc.

The Liver divergent person in general is nervous and fidgety and prone to being impacted by stress. She can be classified under Dr. Shen's nervous system tense/ nervous system weak and is hence quite vulnerable, especially when under stress or experiencing any circumstances which may be taxing to the qi and blood. Some very useful formulas by Dr. Shen are discussed below in the herbal section.

Stomach divergent

With the ST DM all the sensory organs are influenced, making it an excellent choice for clearing the portals in a Heart Shock patient with sensory issues and distorted perceptions which have impacted their internal narrative. The Bladder reached the neck/throat/jaw, the Gall Bladder the eyes and ears, and now the Stomach unites the rest of the senses to allow for a fuller capacity and picture of what one is sensing/ feeling. It can be used for patients who witnessed something horrible early in life (tension in eyes) and are perhaps afraid that it will happen again (worry lines around eyes). Or patients who tend to avoid looking at particularly painful aspects of their lives and tend to always see/hear things from only one perspective.

As we are also looking at a depletion of jing, blood, and jin at this confluent, the portals tend to manifest with dryness. The ST DM is about the fluids, and the fluids are necessary to flush pathogens out of the body. At this divergent one sees a fundamental inability to let go, especially of the way one sees and perceives. The ST DM can help one to understand that seeing is not necessarily believing, and only believing what one sees is a pathology that can be treated with the ST DM.

As the ST DM manages the fluids and we have already depleted the GB/LR divergent and its management of blood and the BL/KI dissemination of jing, typically one may see patients suffering from fluid and blood volume insufficiencies. Over recent years, I have experienced a number of younger patients (typically teenagers with histories of Heart Shock) with symptoms associated with POTS (Postural Orthostatic Tachycardia Syndrome), especially dizziness, fainting, weakness, palpitations, anxiety, and rate and rhythm issues. From a zang fu perspective and the Shen-Hammer pulse, I find significant dehydration and Heart yin and blood deficiency, often with the heart rate increasing 35, 40, or even more beats with exertion. Nourishing the fluids and blood with the ST DM is very helpful in correcting these symptoms. One may also include the SI/HT divergents (as they also share the same upper confluent point and manage blood and have a strong impact on the chest and head).

Another common use for the ST DM is for those patients who suffer from anxiety and nervousness with abdominal and GI symptoms such as pain, cramping, and diarrhea when nervous or upset, even such symptoms as gastritis, IBS, colitis, etc. This divergent can regulate smooth muscle movement in the abdomen and calm wei qi hyperactivity. These symptoms equate to a nervous system tense condition overacting on the digestive system.

The ST DM can be used to treat the person who is overly demanding, obsessive-compulsive, and can't seem to ever be satisfied (treat SDS to release), or those who have been beaten down and don't feel they can ever demand anything of others (treat DSD to strengthen). With its connection to Chong mai, one can also treat the person whose pathologies have corrupted his blueprint, causing him to self-harm. In this case, one should needle ST 30 with SDS to release it from the Chong and add in ST 45.

Spleen divergent

The SP DM accesses the middle of the tongue so is able to assist with trauma patients who recite the same narratives, incessantly promoting their distorted perceptions to the world. This divergent can use the Spleen's capacity to transform/transport and discharge phlegm that has been clouding the orifices and see new options and possibilities. It allows one to break free from habituated responses, choices, and points of view, and allows for release of the sensory orifices, causing watering eyes, nose, etc.

Its association with Chong mai makes it an excellent choice where there have been traumas that have impacted one's blueprint, causing a loss of self and direction in one's life. Sexual traumas, symptoms of stagnation in the pelvis post surgeries (trauma to the body), or other injuries with pronounced scar tissue can also be treated via the SP DM, as can problems with ovulation and reproductive functioning. Its association the Earth phase as well as the Sea of Blood and gu qi make it a good choice for overall nourishment in individuals who have been depleted from traumas with blood and/or fluid loss (even a diminished intrinsic factor and resultant anemia), especially if that has caused the stirring of wind. The SP DM treats wind in the upper orifices as well, with tics, spasms, etc. from nervous system tension and Liver wind, rooted in deficient fluids (which make up a large percentage of blood volume).

The SP DM person is highly accommodating, to the point of letting others take advantage of him. When taxed or depleted, he can be highly self-critical as well as suffer from symptoms of rebellious qi, especially in the chest and abdomen. Nervous system tension overacting on the digestive system is common in this Heart Shock patient when under stress or taxed and can present with a lot of irritation (yin-fluid deficiency) in the Stomach and/or bowels with a diminished intrinsic factor and thinning of the mucosal lining.

Small Intestine divergent

As we progress along the divergent continuum, one has now depleted jing-essence, blood, and the thin fluids, making it more difficult to maintain latency with resultant pronounced anxieties, panic, palpitations, etc. so common in the Heart Shock patient population. As we move into the next trinity, establishing latency becomes more prioritized. The reason being is that the depletion of these resources over time makes it difficult to release a pathogen/stress/trauma without some fluid source to discharge it (e.g., sweating, crying, etc.) for a proper resolution. At the SI DM, we seek the support of the thick fluids and blood to gain the upper hand and quiet the symptoms and manifestations of trauma while building resources and biding time for a future release.

The SI DM regulates the movement of wei qi into the Heart via GB 22 as well as blood and thick fluids (hormonal fluids). As wei qi becomes hyperactive and the ye becomes depleted, one begins to see signs of Heart fire in the Heart Shock patient. Anxiety, palpitations, and rapid heartbeat with arrhythmias (smooth muscle excitation), insomnia and nightmares (wei qi not protecting during sleep), and a cracked tongue that is red and peeling are commonly seen. As with some of the other confluences, the resonance with GB 22 and the great luo of the Spleen and Da Bao provides additional influence over psycho-emotional symptoms and blood/shen disorders without having to tap into the luo vessels. And as mentioned in Chapter 4, with the Small Intestine's regulation of the shoulders and ability to extend the arms via the scapula, the shoulders can become very tight with the chin jutting forward with other Heart fire signs and symptoms. Additionally, with this channel's impact on the chest, traumas and betrayals create armoring and tightness (Dr. Shen's Heart

Full and Heart Closed), as well as tense shoulders held tightly to the body, not swinging naturally when one walks. Eventually, fatigue sets in and the Heart remains closed to prevent being hurt further. These Heart Shock patients may present with ribside tension, axillary lymph swellings, chronic fatigue syndrome, etc. as they are constantly on guard seeing fear and frightening experiences everywhere.

With the major energetic provided by GB 22 and SI 18, both meeting points for the sinew channels, as well as the Heart's ability to regulate peripheral circulation (the Heart is its paired channel), the SI DM exerts a powerful impact on post-traumatic musculoskeletal disorders and pain. With its connection to GB 22, wei qi, the great luo, etc., this channel can also be used to treat the nine Heart pains, along with appropriate points as discussed in the preceding chapter.

The gastrointestinal system is another area where the SI DM shines. This channel has a broader influence on the GI than the ST DM, as it treats the entire digestive tract. It can nourish the thicker fluids, moisten the Stomach and intestines, clear inflammation, etc. and can be used for such symptoms as ulcers, nervous Stomach (nervous system tense overacting on digestive system), colitis, Crohn's disease, IBS, diverticulitis, esophagitis and Barrett's esophagus, tongue and canker sores, etc. When treating the Heart Shock patient for digestive issues secondary to trauma, one can very easily combine the SI/HT and ST/SP divergent channels as they share BL 1 as the upper confluent point. Thus, to nourish the thick and thin fluids to promote latency, one can needle BL 1, ST 30, and GB 22, plus choose appropriate points from each of these divergent channels along with other points of interest.

GB 22 is a major point to regulate the hormonal system, and the SI DM channel can be used to regulate dysfunction in many of the glands secondary to trauma. For instance, it is very common to see overactivity in the adrenals causing adrenal insufficiency and hypothyroidism. In such cases, one can tap the SI/HT DMs plus add in points related to the specific gland in question, e.g., Ren 22 and LU 1 for the thyroid, GB 25 for the adrenals (with Ren 4, front mu of Small Intestine), etc.

Patients with Heart Shock can often suffer memory problems, many even blacking out traumatic events too painful to remember. The SI/HT DMs impact the brain and Qiao vessels, assisting in day-to-day memory and short-term recollection. With their capacity to regulate blood circulation they can also be used to encourage blood flow in the head for those suffering from post-stroke (including speech issues) and concussion syndromes.

Heart divergent

The HT DM, as mentioned above, is a key channel to consider with issues of peripheral circulation, including the sequelae of traumatic injuries and attendant pain, symptoms related to brain/head/face/limb circulation, etc.

The HT DM person, when he is betrayed or suffers other trauma, tends to retreat inwards, becomes shy, and disengages from social interactions. He may even find it hard to look one in the eye and speak his mind/truth. The HT DM channel can be used to free up the tongue and speech, releasing trapped wei qi from the chest and throat, allowing one to re-engage with life.

And of course, the HT DM can be used for the gamut of psycho-emotional disorders, ranging from depression (especially hysterical and cyclothymic types),[165] anxiety, irritability, bipolar disorder, grief, betrayal, heaviness of the Heart, excitability, etc.

Triple Burner divergent

With the SJ/PC DMs, damp-heat, heat in the blood, and floating yang become predominant as severe yin deficiency asserts itself and is unable to control yang/fire which goes unchecked. A typical presentation of a Heart Shock patient at this level is one who is emotionally volatile, riding a roller coaster of emotions and spiraling out of control. Her life is typically in chaos and her pulse often reveals an Empty pulse in at least one of the principal positions. Needling DSD to promote latency and anchor/consolidate the qi is the most common protocol at this divergent to buffer the heat/irritation and inflammation that often presents.

One can also use the SJ DM to further release a pathogen during a healing crisis and allow for a more full resolution of the pathogen. A Triple Burner pulse will be present in these circumstances, and the divergent can be used to release the yangming heat from the interior and prepare it for release. Yangming sinew channels are often combined in this regard. At times, when patients present with strong emotional symptoms, the Triple Burner can be needled for a treatment or two with SDS to release the acute presentations, followed by DSD in subsequent treatments to put the person back into latency while one builds up resources for a future release. Oftentimes the SDS can prepare the body for a future DSD treatment (yang transforming to yin). Gua sha can also be implemented at the ring around the neck to assist with the release, as can ST 45 and LI 1. The use of neck and WOS points also exert a major influence in assisting the SJ DM, as discussed earlier.

A common theme with chronic Heart Shock patients is pain that eventually manifests, either from long-term unresolved injuries, or from the taxation on the Heart over time. This stagnation breeds heat, which eventually leads to a breakdown of structure and compensatory dampness and the resultant wei atrophy. Symptoms such as rheumatoid arthritis and fibromyalgia are common in this population, as is chronic fatigue syndrome. The SJ DM is a major player in treating these disorders.

The Triple Burner is in charge of fluid metabolism, disseminating it to all three burners. This includes the thin as well as thick fluids, and thus also has an impact on the hormones. At this point of the continuum, with the severe yin deficiency that presents, often turbid dampness is retained as compensation and one may begin to find cysts and other forms of yin stasis.

The Triple Burner with its regulation of the three jiaos, and in particular with its downward trajectory, is also implicated in rebellious qi symptoms. As a shaoyang channel, one often sees nausea, vomiting, dizziness, bitter taste, chest and rib distension, etc. as heat and dampness accumulate. This should be differentiated from a shaoyang external pathogen which will not demonstrate the history and signs/symptoms of a chronic degenerative process, including severe yin deficiency.

The SJ DM person under the circumstances of Heart Shock can feel out of control and lost. Compensation often comes in the form of manipulation of others to get what he needs or desires. When this cannot be accomplished, he becomes extremely depressed and despair sets in. In these circumstances, depending on the resources available, one can utilize DSD needling to anchor and astringe qi back to the middle jiao and the earth to provide some stability or, alternatively, use SDS to release obstructions of damp and heat weighing down the spirit and mobilize the shen. One can also use a combination of both DSD and SDS, e.g., needling the confluent points with DSD to astringe qi to the middle jiao, but needle Ren 17 and Du 20 with SDS to release the chest and lift the qi. Often with patients who experience despair, one will find Empty pulses in the Liver (left middle position) and/or Kidneys (left or right proximal positions) demonstrating a loss of control and chaos in those organ systems. I also often find a Sinking pulse in these same positions reflecting this lack of root and bottoming out of one's shen and spirit. (A Sinking pulse has the sensation of drawing one's finger down into the pulse rather than feeling the pulse strike up to the finger. Essentially, this is one feeling the diastole over the systole and feels like a vacuum sucking your finger inwards.)

Pericardium divergent

The PC DM will be singled out for treatment with the occurrence of blood heat patterns. Regulating the fire–water balance, the presentation at this divergent is heat in the blood causing significant shen disturbances such as severe intractable anxiety and panic disorder, mania, bipolar disorder, agitation, vexation of the chest, etc. With heat in the blood and no yin left to buffer, patients at this stage also show acute and chronic bleeding disorders. Symptoms may range from the less severe nosebleeds, rashes, and skin disorders to coughing blood and even the possibility of strokes.

The PC DM person often presents as one who has been betrayed in the past and traumatized by another. He is the bitter pessimist who is afraid to fail and be hurt again. Dr. Shen's Heart Small pattern fits this personality well.

Large Intestine divergent

By the time we reach the LI/LU divergents, jing, blood, jin, ye, and qi have become compromised and the body creates a last-ditch effort to summon yang to anchor and regain control.

In its relationship to Heart Shock, the LI DM has a strong influence over the chest and breasts. As stagnation persists in the chest from long-term holdings (grief and sadness being a major one) and closing of one's Heart, lumps, cysts, chest congestion and fullness (potentially, congestive heart failure), etc. begin to manifest. The heat from long-term stagnation may create wei qi hyperactivity with rapid heartbeat and breathing, reflecting the urgency of the situation at hand. The Large Intestine is about letting go, and the inability to do so by this time of the progression through the divergent continuum creates a scenario wherein the patient's choice, or inability to do so, creates potential life-threatening illnesses, forcing the patient's hand.

This divergent pair has a major influence over the breasts, and one of the more common cancers to afflict women is breast cancer. My experience over the years has confirmed that this disease has a major component of the inability to let go of suppressed emotions leading to intense buried frustrations and irritability. Of significant interest is a particular signature that I find on the pulse of breast cancer patients, namely a Restricted quality in the Special Lung Position (SLP) and an Empty quality in the Liver (left middle position). Often the affected area will also be Muffled. When these qualities are found together, breast cancer will be present on the opposite side of the SLP finding. What is interesting to note is that the SLP is found on a branch of the radial artery called the superficial palmar artery. As a branch to the radial artery, this position can be seen to "diverge" from the radial artery, creating a very strong correlation to the concept of a divergent channel diverging from the primary channel. The relationship to the Lungs and chest gives us the direct link to the LI/LU divergent channels, implicating their usage in acupuncture treatments of this condition. There are also intermediary stages to these qualities that can clue one in to a future breast cancer diagnosis, allowing one some time to treat and prevent its occurrence. In this scenario, one will find a Reduced Substance quality in the center of the SLP. Should that be allowed to progress, eventually the Reduced Substance advances to a point wherein it "pinches off" and separates, bifurcating the pulse, one side becoming Restricted. This process, in my opinion, reflects the formation of a tumor and eventual blockage of circulation to the tissues. I have had the unfortunate opportunity to diagnose this early stage and predict future breast cancers in a few patients who did not continue treatments, only to find out years later that it had in fact developed. Additionally, one may see early stages of Empty pulses in the left middle position manifesting as Reduced Substance at the organ depth. Attention should be paid to these signs, and treatments geared towards correcting them.

The LI DM brings connection to the Du mai at Du 14, and hence can be useful in regulating yang qi and hyperactivity of the nervous system. Needling with SDS can be used to release heat here, and DSD can be used to anchor yang qi. As all the yang primary channels converge at Du 14, it also allows access to the primary channel system and often one will choose yuan qi points such as he-sea, source, etc. Thus, for Heart Shock with a patient demonstrating anxiety, tension in her upper back, and chest fullness, the LI DM can be needled, adding in Du 14, BL 15 with a reducing technique (for the upper back tension as well as to treat the anxiety), and HT 3 (he-sea point which treats anxiety).

The LI DM person is a typical metal type who is meticulous and image-oriented. When suffering from Heart Shock, he tends to become constipated, uptight, angry, and anal, having a difficult time going with the flow and unable to accept his past and present circumstances. Treating the LI DM assists with letting go of preconceptions and allowing one to live in the present moment.

Lung divergent

The LU DM shares many of the applications of the LI DM, especially in terms of its influence over the chest and breast. The LU DM utilizes the energetics of GB 22 and LU 1, thus making it effective for treating wei qi circulation through the chest and treating heart rate and rhythm issues in the Heart Shock patient. For elevated rates, SDS is performed; for slow heart rates, DSD is utilized to bring yang into the chest.

The LU DM person is highly organized, and prioritizes her tasks by assigning appropriate value to things. When taxed from trauma and chronic illnesses, she becomes fatigued and exhausted by the demands on her time, causing her much-valued organization skills to crumble. Becoming tense and rigid, she seeks justice and proving others wrong to feel better. Releasing the LU DM when overwhelmed and nourishing it when deficient can ameliorate these qualities.

Herbal treatments for the divergent meridians

Herbal formulas that resonate with and treat issues within the divergent channels have multiple strategies to accommodate the wei and yuan levels, as well as freeing up blockages that may prevent release of the pathogen, or enough space to hold it in latency. The main strategies[166] are the following:

1. Resonate with the divergent meridians with herbs that impact the wei and yuan levels with Di Gu Pi, Xuan Shen, Bie Jia, Zi He Che, E Jiao, and other animal products such as Gui Ban, etc.

2. Use sinew herbs to open blockages and release the portals, like Gao Ben, Qiang Huo, Bai Zhi, Gui Zhi, Fang Feng, and Chuan Xiong.

   a. For wind-cold, add Gui Zhi; for wind-heat Bai Ji Li, Cang Er Zi, Bo He, etc.

3. Descend essence to the Kidneys/constitution with herbs such as Du Zhong, Xu Duan, Gou Ji, etc.

4. Release bi-syndrome with Du Huo, Qiang Huo, Niu Xi, Qin Jiao, etc.

5. Remove congestion and any nodules along channels with herbs like Hai Zao, Bie Jia, and Zhe Bei Mu. These also drain the lymph (of which the

DM regulate via all their channel pathways impacting the thoracic duct) and release toxins from jing.

6. Open the chest: BL/KI (Qiang Huo); GB/LR (Li Zhe He, Xiang Fu); ST/SP (Shan Zha); SI/HT (Dan Shen, Tan Xiang); SJ/PC (Dan Shen); LI/LU (Jie Geng, Ban Xia).

7. Use herbs that clear heat from qi stasis and damage to yin (e.g., steaming bone), including Hu Huang Lian, Yin Chai Hu, Qing Hao, etc.

8. If a healing crisis promotes excess discomfort, astringe and calm the shen with Shan Zhu Yu and Wu Wei Zi and/or use sea salt baths to relax the nervous system.

9. Calm the shen and strengthen the will: Yuan Zhi.

10. Release trapped wei qi from the lower jiao and protect jing and yuan with herbs like Sang Ji Sheng, Nu Zhen Zi, Wu Jia Pi, Gou Ji, etc.

11. Clear toxins from interior with herbs such as Pu Gong Ying, Bai Tou Weng, Ban Zhi Lian, Bai Hua She She Cao, Xia Ku Cao, etc.

One can see a resonance to many of our Heart Shock strategies embedded within the DM herbal priorities: opening the portals, strengthening and anchoring the Kidneys, calming the shen and nervous system, and opening and releasing the chest. Astringent herbs such as Wu Wei Zi and Shan Zhu Yu are also included to buffer healing crises, similar to the use of Wu Wei Zi in Sheng Mai San to astringe the Heart yin and calm the shen. There are also herbs that resonate more towards the zonal DM and those that resonate towards the elemental DM. They are listed below.

Herbs that resonate with the yang zonal divergent meridians

BL/SI: Ring around the chest with bi-syndrome, neck and back pain, allergies, etc.:

Gou Ji

Du Huo

Qiang Huo

Gao Ben

Mu Tong

Qu Mai

Dong Gua Ren

Ze Xie

Xiang Fu

Zhe Bei Mu

Bai Mao Gen

Gui Zhi

Fang Feng

Bai Ji Li

GB/SJ: Ring around the pelvis (and mastoid) with qi stagnation in the neck/chest/diaphragm/pelvis with tightness, and resultant heat/damp-heat, congealed blood, wind, etc.:

Fang Feng

Chuan Xiong

Ge Gen

Jiang Huang

Xiang Fu

Bei Mu

Niu Xi

ST/LI: Ring around the neck with inflammation, hyperthyroid, dry mouth and throat, bleeding gums, sinusitis, chronic fatigue, etc.:

Sheng Ma

Ge Gen

Xuan Shen

Mang Xiao

Dong Gua Ren

Huang Lian

Bai Mao Gen

Lu Gen

Herbs that resonate with the elemental divergent meridians

BL/KI:

    Ze Xie

    Che Qian Zi

    Qiang Huo

    Du Huo

    Gao Ben

    Gou Ji

GB/LR:

    Long Dan Cao

    Qin Jiao

    Xia Ku Cao

    Qing Pi

    Suan Zao Ren

    Chai Hu

    Tao Ren

    Wu Ling Zhi

    Xiang Fu

    Li Zhi He

ST/SP:

    Ge Gen

    Shan Zha

    Huo Xiang

    Zhi Shi

    Sha Ren

    Jiang Huang

SI/HT:

    Mu Tong

    Chi Xiao

    Ban Bian Lian

    Dan Shen

    Tan Xiang

SJ/PC:

    Chuan Xiong

    Xiang Fu

    Dan Shen

    Yu Jin

    Zi Cao

    Mu Dan Pi

    Chi Shao

LI/LU:

    Pang Da Hai

    Dong Chong Xia Cao

    Ling Zhi

    Jie Geng

    Ban Xia

Dr. Shen's nervous system relationship to divergent channels and formulas

In terms of the DM and the nervous system, the Bladder and Kidney DM represents the jing/structure and the wei/qi circulation. The NST condition typically shows up with a more robust individual reflecting more of the wei qi aspect. Dr. Shen's NST formula was discussed in Chapter 4. With a NSW condition, one often sees jing-level insults related to constitution and/or early life traumatic events. Below are a few of Dr. Shen's formulas[167] that implicate the nervous system, NSW in particular, and demonstrate an approach that I believe to be consistent with divergent meridian energetics. My analysis of these formulas is different than in the above referenced text by Dr. Hammer and Mr. Rotte, and is based upon my studies of Classical Chinese herbal medicine, of which Dr. Shen was expertly trained. I believe that seeking to understand these formulas through a Classical lens yields additional rich information and understanding of the herbal dynamics, vectors of movement, and overall level of pathology looking to be treated.

Nervous System Weak—original formula

Chuan Xiong	4.5g
Yu Jin	4.5g
Jing Jie	3g
Bai Shao	6g
Xiang Fu	4.5g
Yan Hu Suo	9g
Bai Zhu	6g
Huang Qi	9g
Shan Yao	9g
Gan Cao	4.5g

The difference between the Nervous System Tense formula (see Chapter 4) and this one is the addition of tonics, with Bai Zhu, Huang Qi, Shan Yao, and Gan Cao. There is a recognition that we still need to soften the Liver and move qi to release armoring and tension but, as the patient is deficient, tonification must take place to prevent further damage to the constitution. This formula, however, in my opinion, focuses more on the symptomatic presentation of a tense nervous system, while trying to protect the deficient root. Later in Dr. Shen's career this formula was modified, making it a much more suitable formula for the truly deficient NSW individual, and also resonating to the DM.

Nervous System Weak—recent/menopause, nervous tension, and weak body formula

Ren Shen	4.5g
Fu Ling	9g
Da Zao	9g
Bie Jia	12g
Yuan Zhi	6g
Bai Shao	6g
Nu Dao Gen Xu	30g
Chai Hu	3g
Di Gu Pi	9g

The above formula is instructive in that Dr. Shen uses it when there is tension in the nervous system with weakness underlying. As a nervous system formula, it creates a relationship between the lighter faster-moving energies (wei qi) and the denser yuan qi energetic. He also used it for menopause which typically presents symptomatically with floating yang (hyperactivity of the adrenals and wei qi activity) from underlying yin and/or yang deficiency. This is a common theme within the DM energetics. One of the first things to notice about this formula is the inclusion of the DM signature herbs to make the connection between the wei and the yuan levels, Di Gu Pi and Bie Jia. Di Gu Pi resonates to the Lung and Liver (wei qi), and Kidneys (yuan qi), and its energetic vector is that it moves wei qi inwards to the yuan level only to return back to the wei level, often to release pathology manifesting from yin deficiency or heat in the chest, abdomen, or blood. Bie Jia, which is heavy and yin tonifying, also breaks up and moves blood and yin stasis in the Liver, Spleen, and Kidneys (and pelvis).

The nervous system has its roots in the yin-essence of the Kidneys and the marrow, but it also relies on the Bladder channel pair, taiyang, for movement. Taiyang is related to wei qi, shaoyin to the yuan level. The mediator between the yuan and the wei is the shaoyang, associated with the Liver-Gall Bladder. From an herbal zang fu perspective, the Liver is seen as influencing the peripheral nervous system via its connection to the wei qi and its dominion over the muscles. Synthesizing these ideas, the above formula assists with communicating the wei and yuan levels with Di Gu Pi and Bie Jia, and taps into the level of the DM. To strengthen the root in a weak body Ren Shen is used, and because there is a warming quality to it, Bie Jia and Di Gu Pi can anchor any flaring yang by cooling any pent-up internal heat and nourishing Liver and Kidney yin. To mediate this, Chai Hu and Bai Shao regulate the Liver while nourishing fluids, with Bai Shao protecting against the drying nature of Chai Hu. Herbs are used to strengthen post-natal qi, e.g., Fu Ling, Da Zao, and glutinous rice (Nu Dao Gen Xu). Fu Ling also deals with any damp from the yin tonics. Yuan Zhi further assists the anchoring and communication of wei and yuan and settles the spirit, communicating Heart and Kidney. It is important to note that menopausal symptoms are often associated with hyperactivity of adrenal functioning as women in our day, not able to slow down at this rite of passage and internalize their resources, require the adrenals to work extra hard. As that heat/adrenaline gets metabolized in the blood/Liver, the result is often a flaring of yang with underlying yin and yang deficiency (from overworking of the adrenals). In this formula, Dr. Shen artfully addresses all these concepts, while using the directionality to tap into the divergent channels.

As a Heart Shock formula, this meets a number of the strategies set forth in Part I, but focuses primarily on the nervous system component. It can be modified, however, to accommodate more of the Heart Shock strategies quite easily. First, while Ren Shen does have some capacity to nourish the fluids classically, it can be replaced with Xi Yang Shen to provide a stronger yin nourishing quality. Or as we still need to strengthen Kidney yang, it can simply be added to the formula. The formula already includes strategies for calming the shen (Yuan Zhi), nourishing the earth (Ren Shen, Da Zao, Fu Ling, glutinous rice), calming the nervous system (Chai Hu, Bai Shao), invigorating the blood (Bie Jia), and clearing the portals (Yuan Zhi).

Nervous System Tense and Yin-Deficient Heat, February 2000

Zhi Bie Jia	12g
Chai Hu	3g
Qing Hao	9g
Di Gu Pi	9g
Fu Ling	9g
Yuan Zhi	4.5g
Long Chi	18g
Mu Li	12g
Yu Jin	9g
Chao Bai Shao	9g
Lu Lu Tong	12g

The Nervous System Tense and Yin-Deficient Heat formula contains many of the same herbs as the prior formula for NSW and menopause. The DM signature herbs (Di Gu Pi and Bie Jia) create a relationship between the wei and yuan level, also breaking up any turbid yin stasis, while clearing heat and anchoring and tonifying yin. Herbs to regulate the Liver (Chai Hu, Bai Shao, Yu Jin, Lu Lu Tong) are included and also herbs for heat from yin deficiency (Qing Hao, Di Gu Pi). Fu Ling helps to deal with damp, often a response to a yin deficiency. Yuan Zhi further assists the anchoring and communication of wei and yuan qi while also settling the spirit. Long Chi and Mu Li further assist with anchoring and astringing the yin while calming the shen. For the Heart Shock strategies, one needs to further strengthen Heart yin with herbs such as Bai He, Xi Yang Shen, etc., and if this pattern includes sweating, that herb can also be an astringent such as Suan Zao Ren, Bai Zi Ren, or Wu Wei Zi (Bie Jia also treats sweating). Adding in a herb or two to address Kidney yang would round out the last of the Heart Shock strategies as there are herbs to invigorate blood (Yu Jin and Lu Lu Tong), calm the shen (Yuan Zhi, Bai Shao, Long Chi, and Mu Li), regulate qi in the chest (Chai Hu, Yu Jin, and Lu Lu Tong), and open the orifices (Yu Jin and Yuan Zhi).

Additional Divergent meridian formula

Qing Gu San (Cool the Bones Powder)

Yin Chai Hu
Zhi Mu
Hu Huang
Lian
Di Gu Pi
Qing Hao
Qin Jiao
Bie Jia
Gan Cao

Qing Gu San is a formula traditionally used for steaming bone syndrome and yin deficiency of the Liver and Kidneys, which has such symptoms as sensation of heat in the bones, low-grade fever, irritability, insomnia, emaciation, thirst, dry throat, etc. with a Thin Rapid pulse and red tongue with little coat. Its primary focus is on clearing the deficiency heat, rather than strongly nourishing yin. It's a formula, however, that can be illustrative of the divergent meridian energetics as it taps into the DM using the signature herbs of Di Gu Pi and Bie Jia, and the pathology is such that a pathogen has penetrated deep into the bones and marrow. And while not a Heart Shock formula per se, it can definitely be modified to accommodate that diagnosis. For example, when treating certain cancer patients, I will commonly modify this formula with Sheng Di Huang and Mu Dan Pi, bringing in the missing elements found in Qing Hao Bie Jia Tang (Artemisia Annua and Soft-Shelled Turtle Decoction), which will also nourish the Heart yin (and Kidney yin), clear Heart fire, and cool and invigorate the blood.

Essential oils and the elemental divergents

As mentioned previously, essential oils have a strong resonance to the yuan level, being the jing-essence of the plant. Additionally, many oils also resonate to the wei/sinew layer as detailed in Chapter 4. Below is a list of essential oils that can resonate to the elemental divergent pairings. Additional oils can, and should, be used to round out the Heart Shock strategies when using the below oils on the confluent points. The previous chapter outlined dozens of oils that can be used for a variety of shen and psycho-emotional issues, and have functions that satisfy the remainder of the strategies. These oils should be mixed into a blend with a carrier oil, generally as a 6–8 percent dilution, and can be applied to the opening confluent points and other points on said channel, as well as other acupoints that resonate with the treatment dynamic.

BL/KI:

>   DSD: celery seed, basil, cypress

>   SDS: jasmine, pine

GB/LR:

>   DSD: angelica seed or vetiver, needle oil (fir, cypress, pine)

>   SDS: chamomile, citrus (orange/tangerine for shen, grapefruit if wind phlegm, bergamot if sensory issues)

ST/SP:

>   DSD: carrot or angelica seed, anise/coriander, cypress

>   SDS: lavender, citrus, coriander, clove or terebinth

SI/HT:

>   DSD: angelica, anise, coriander, caraway, myrrh, needle oil

>   SDS: myrrh, citrus

SJ/PC:

>   DSD: spikenard, cypress, benzoin

>   SDS: frankincense, sandalwood, citrus, peppermint

LI/LU:

>   DSD: cedarwood, cinnamon bark, benzoin

>   SDS: elemi, cistus, peppermint

CHAPTER 8

The 8 Extraordinary Channels

Affecting the Blueprint and Our Sense of Self

8x energetics

In the previous chapters, I have discussed the relationships of the other channel systems to Heart Shock as a representation of the channel systems' specific energetics, e.g., the sinew channels and wei qi, the luo vessels and ying qi, etc. Here, the 8x meridians will be discussed in relation to their domain over the yuan qi and jing-level energetics. But, first, to truly understand the 8x vessels and the jing level, a brief look into the Chinese medical and Daoist cosmology can provide some foundation. As Heart Shock first and foremost affects the spirit, cosmology is instructive in providing its fullest picture.

Prior to an incarnation, it is believed that a spirit in the heavens chooses a particular incarnation.[168] During sexual intercourse, a particular vibration is created which attracts a spirit wishing for a new earthbound life and curriculum. An interested spirit can enter via Du 20 and the original Chong mai (or via a zang fu approach, the Lungs descending the po to the Kidneys), making its way to the uterus and reproductive system, and at the moment a sperm meets and interpenetrates an egg, the spirit becomes encapsulated and, with a new prima material, can become a ling-soul. From here, the alchemical process begins, the spirit-soul sparking and catalyzing the growth and development into embryo, fetus, and person. Each stage within the gestation process is multi-faceted, but it is believed that during the first trimester the soul has a chance to review the conditions of its upcoming life, including its race, ethnicity, gender, genes, parental influences, and curriculum in life. The soul during this time has an opportunity to accept or reject these circumstances, rejection leading to miscarriage. The first trimester is associated with the Earth phase, and one reason why many early symptoms can include rebellious qi, such as nausea and vomiting, prolapses, etc., leading to miscarriage.

During the second trimester, governed by the Fire phase, the soul experiences and acknowledges its curriculum and path in life, and the circumstances around this birth and incarnation become formalized. The third trimester, associated with the Wood phase, formalizes the timing of life experiences, and prepares the fetus for delivery and birth into its new world. The 10th month comes back to water and provides for the actual birth itself.

This very brief cosmological view is profoundly important in providing context to Heart Shock and trauma, as potentially bringing to light a perspective that one's experiences are understood prior to birth and chosen to be experienced towards spiritual growth. This can be a very difficult concept, even one that incites anger and frustration for many. It does not, however, imply any blame on the victim of trauma, nor does it relieve any responsibility to anyone who victimizes another. It does, however, provide some insight into a concept that was discussed earlier in Part I of this text, which is that traumas can be overcome, and one can even grow spiritually from said event(s).

Remembering I Jing Hexagram 51, Wilhelm and Legge both relate that, moving through and past shock, one finds happiness and joy.

> "When the (time of) movement (which it indicates) comes, (its subject) will be found looking out with apprehension:"—that feeling of dread leads to happiness. "And yet smiling and talking cheerfully:"—the issue (of his dread) is that he adopts (proper) laws (for his course).[169]

Much like "playing the hand we were dealt," or applying such Buddhist concepts as "radical acceptance," this Daoist cosmological view can allow one to bypass the process of blame, which can be a significant barrier towards healing. According to Wang Shanren and Liu Yousheng, blame damages the Earth phase and Spleen and Stomach organs, and that which they dominate (digestive system as a whole).[170] In previous chapters it has been demonstrated how vital the Spleen and Stomach are in treating Heart Shock, their health and integrity being one of the treatment strategies that must be addressed. They are also instrumental in dictating one's narrative. Thus, blame not only injures the Spleen and Stomach, but also causes one to reflect on their circumstances as being the victim, blaming the outside world for problems, injuries, illnesses, and difficult circumstances.[171] The earth is influenced by wood, and it is quite common for blame to also include anger towards one's circumstances. Impacting the wood and Liver/Gall Bladder, the manifestations of anger are far reaching, including impacting the nervous system and creating tension, the diaphragm impacting blood circulation, as well as how one magnifies and/or suppresses one's emotions, etc. Of course, the cycle does not end here, but creates the myriad of energetic imbalances that must be addressed within the context of Heart Shock.

Domain of the 8x

As the deepest set of channel systems, the energetics of the 8x vessels use yuan qi and jing as their resource. As such, the 8x is best used for constitutional, long-term, chronic, and deeper-level issues. Jeffrey has mentioned those who use the 8x vessels to treat many surface-level problems, such as external pathogens. From the perspective of this chapter, such treatments would be akin to debiting one's 401k or the cash value of a life insurance policy to pay for grocery bills. While effective in the short term, it weakens one's resources (yuan qi and jing) and takes years off the back end, negatively impacting one's longevity. Applications of the 8x vessels include, but are not limited to:

- congenital issues, constitution, and birth and early life disorders

- issues surrounding growth and development, aging, and longevity

- problems with the Kidneys and Triple Burner mechanism,[172] including bone and structural disorders, and obstetric/gynecological and reproductive conditions

- pediatric conditions

- geriatric disorders

- separation of yin and yang

- genetic disorders and diseases/conditions that run in the family

- issues of temperament and nature (consider also divergent meridians)

- issues of self-exploration and knowing oneself.

The 8x vessels represent in many respects one's genetic and evolutionary foundation, providing the roadmap of one's physiology and the deepest aspect of constitution (combination of genetics/jing and astrology/shen). They have a strong connection to the curious organs (bone, marrow, blood vessels, uterus, brain, Gall Bladder) and assist with adaptations over time. As alluded to above, the 8x vessels impact issues of fate and destiny, potentially giving one the ability to make changes. Through cultivation, they enable one to more fully explore and embody her true self and come to understand her purpose in life.

As roadmaps representing the unfolding of the constitution towards one's destiny, the 8x vessels influence one's ability to adapt and survive. This includes mediating yuan qi's influence over structure (morphology), procreation and sexual energy, mutations and evolution (curious bowels), and the overall drive to maintain survival and avoid death. Critical junctions include the cycles of 7 and 8 (Su Wen), or 10 (Ling Shu), which depict historically important rites of passage,[173] the disjunctive ones often defining our personalities.

In terms of pathology, the 8x vessels are reservoirs and ditches which can hold onto and store toxicity deep within the yuan layer, buying time in some circumstances, or weakening the structure and foundation in others (depending on resources). The 8x vessels, like the divergent meridians, can maintain latency using the heavier yuan and jing-level resources, slowing down pathology. Signs and symptoms associated with each of the 8x vessels appear as the ditches fill up and reach a critical mass.

Additionally, the 8x vessels may need to siphon and convert jing to support post-natal qi in times of great deprivation (or chronic poor lifestyle), or manifest excessive holding in its ditches to accommodate pathogens.

Ancestries

The 8x vessels are commonly grouped within three ancestries. This notion of ancestry also suggests a hierarchy and/or continuum in terms of how the channels develop and, hence, their level of importance to one's physiology. The first ancestry includes the Chong mai, Ren mai, and Du mai. It represents our deepest foundation, blueprint for our existence, and raw materials, including such concepts as genetics. Chong is the blueprint, Ren provides the raw materials, and Du forms the structure. The second includes the Yin Wei mai and the Yang Wei mai, dealing with relationships and experiences, especially the most formative ones. It is the playing out through experiences of the energetics and curriculum set forth in the first ancestry. The third ancestry is made up of the Yin Qiao mai and the Yang Qiao mai, representing the present (how one feels about oneself and one's life), as well as the Dai mai (our unresolved issues). These channels impact our relationship to the world, how we stand up for ourselves and to others, and how we accommodate difficulties in life (our inability to let go).

8x treatments

Needling technique

Generally, as the 8x vessels are reflections of yuan qi and jing, the densest energetic, vibrating, and shaking technique is most appropriate. The needle should be vibrated slowly for tonification, and rapidly to release pathology and to drain. Lifting and thrusting may also be performed, especially if one is attempting to move the 8x vessel energetics to the primary channels. In that case, once qi is obtained, the needle should be lifted to the moderate level. For the Chong mai, the direction of needling is determined by whether or not one is tonifying Chong (or putting something into latency), or to support post-natal qi (or release something from latency). In the former instance, one needles towards the midline. In the latter, needling is directed towards the Stomach channel.

As yuan qi and jing are slower to react, their treatments require a longer duration generally. One often retains the needles for 30–45 minutes. Treatment is typically done one time per week, so as not to disturb the yuan qi repeatedly, potentially draining it. Overall treatment on the 8x vessels is a minimum of three months' duration, re-evaluating after that time. A simple protocol, including sequencing of needles, is given below.

Basic protocol

1. Needle opening point (left for men, right for women; rapid vibrating for sedating, slow for tonification).

2. Treat points along the channel being opened using the vibration technique as above (moxa can be used for deficient points).

3. If needling a paired meridian, needle appropriate points along the trajectory.

4. Needle the confluent point of the paired meridian.

5. If warranted, add points that resonate with yuan qi, such as he-sea points, yuan-source points, mu and shu points, divergent confluent points, etc.

8x vessel ancestries

In this section, I will briefly examine each 8x vessel in terms of its basic energetic, channel pathways, common uses, and representative acupuncture points. It is not my intention to provide as lengthy a discussion of the 8x vessels as has been done for the other complementary channels, as I believe there exists much more information on the 8x vessels currently in print and available. Therefore, the discussion below is to provide simply an orientation to a particular perspective on these vessels. Later in the chapter, I will present more on their uses specifically for Heart Shock.

First ancestry

Chong mai

The Chong mai is the blueprint of the life being lived, storing the curriculum, the foundation, and the unfolding of yin and yang in service of one's destiny. It helps bring jing-essence to the post-natal environment, as evidenced by its other roles as the Sea of Blood and the Sea of the 12 Channels. It provides a strong influence over the abdomen, SP/ST, and post-natal qi, as well as assisting with communication of the Heart and Kidneys. Its deep connections with blood and the Heart provide us with resources, spirit, and the ability to mobilize one's shen and reveal one's nature. Its impact on the chest also provides access to one's ancestral qi. Its opening point, SP 4, "grandfather-grandson," further evidences this relationship. The Chong mai has roots in the lower abdomen and Kidneys (pre-heaven), is influenced by the Spleen and Stomach via its opening point, SP 4, and ST 30, and its channel trajectory through the abdomen (post-heaven), and manifests via the chest and Heart in service of fulfilling its destiny. A full treatment of the Chong mai (and the other 8x vessels) is beyond the scope of this text, which will mostly focus on its uses in Heart Shock, but, briefly, some of the most common usages of the Chong include treating issues of the lower jiao (obstetric/gynecological and reproductive disorders), strengthening post-natal qi, nourishing and invigorating blood and treating its myriad manifestations, communicating Heart and Kidneys, treating running piglet qi, etc.

CHANNEL TRAJECTORY

The Chong mai can be seen as two distinct channel systems, one more pre-natal, the other more post-natal. The pre-natal or original Chong is considered the central channel and traverses the middle of our bodies, from Du 20 down to Ren 1. It is used mostly with qigong and meditative practices, via significant cultivation. The post-natal Chong mai begins in the lower abdomen, travels to the genitalia (said to meet the Liver luo and divergent), and emerges at KI 11. It travels up the Kidney channel to KI 21, diffusing into the chest (connecting to the Heart).

It has five trajectories, as follows:

1. From the lower jiao, the channel contacts the Liver luo (and also divergent as they represent the same trajectory) and branches to KI 11, ST 30, and SP 12. It ascends to the abdomen and middle jiao.

2. A trajectory begins in the chest, ascends to the throat, mouth, and nose, encircling the lips, and ending at the eyes.

3. From the lower abdomen a branch goes to the lower back and Du mai, influencing the spine. This branch is assisted via the communication with Dai mai, which helps it encircle the body.

4. Moving towards the lower body from the lower abdomen at KI 11, it descends through the knees to the medial malleolus (birthing Qiao mai), the heel, and sole (Du mai connection to structure and upright posture).

5. From ST 30 a branch moves to the dorsum of the foot (ST 42), supporting the ascension of body fluids (pure yang of the Stomach) and Spleen qi, as well as LR 1 and SP 1, assisting digestion.

Points along the trajectory: A broad reading of the Chong mai trajectory and areas of its influence include Ren 4, Ren 1, SP 12, ST 30, Ren 7, KI 11–27, Ren 23, BL 40, KI 10, SP 6, SP 1, LR 3, and LR 1

Opening point: SP 4

Sea of Blood points: BL 11, ST 37, ST 39

Associated/connected organs: Kidneys, uterus, Heart, Stomach, Lungs, throat, spine

Ren mai

The Ren mai reflects the raw materials, yin, required to construct the Chong's blueprint. As the Sea of Yin, it is about materialization, as well as bonding and the creation of boundaries. Much like we discussed for the Lung luo previously, the Ren mai is the embodiment of the bonding between mother and newborn, hence LU 7 being the opening point of Ren mai, as well as a reflection of its psycho-social development. The mother cradles her newborn to her chest, and the child suckles the breast and receives nourishment (yin, and raw material of its own), to be further transformed in its own body, eventually creating the distinction of self and other. The Ren mai is responsible for aligning with the energetics of mom, in terms of breathing dynamics and overall contentment. This sets the vibration for which is later recognized as love and safety. Some of the Ren mai's most common uses include reproductive issues, digestive problems, yin deficiency, yin stasis, damp, cold, shan-hernias, respiratory and cardiac issues, disorders of the face and sensory organs, etc.

CHANNEL TRAJECTORY

The Ren channel has two main trajectories. The first begins below Ren 3, travels to the genitals, and traverses the anterior midline of the abdomen and chest to the throat. It continues up to the bottom of the mouth and encircles it, then to the eyes (ST 1 and/or BL 1).

The second trajectory travels from the lower abdomen to the perineum and follows the Du mai up the spine to the nape of the neck.

Points along the trajectory: Ren 1–24, Du 28, ST 1

Opening point: LU 7

Luo point: Ren 15

Associated/connected organs: lower abdomen, umbilicus, upper abdomen, chest, throat, mouth, lips, eyes, Lungs, uterus, genitalia, anus, coccyx, spine, Kidneys, Spleen, Stomach, intestines, Heart

Du mai

The Du mai creates the structure, utilizing the raw materials (Ren) and following the blueprint (Chong) to create the home of the physical body. As the Sea of Yang, it has a strong connection to Kidney yang, willpower, and ming men energetics. Where the Ren mai assists with bonding and boundaries, the Du mai assists with individuation in the process of becoming. Strong similarities exist between this concept from Classical medicine with that of Dr. Hammer's conception of the Metal phase individuation. In Classical terms, Du mai assists with bringing Kidney yang to its paired Bladder channel and taiyang (as discussed earlier), as well as the Triple Burner's dissemination. As such it deals with yang qi supporting wei qi. Separation from the maternal matrix allows for growth and development, taking the raw materials and acting on the blueprint to live one's curriculum. This process of becoming also relies heavily on the Heart, which Du mai's yang supports. Its impact over the brain helps mediate sensory and motor skills as well as impacting the sensory portals overall. General uses for the Du mai include structural issues, Kidney yang deficient symptoms including growth, development, reproduction and aging concerns, wind-stroke, ascending yang symptoms, etc. It warms the body, influences the sensory orifices and brain, as well as the nervous system and shen, strengthens the structure and constitution, and boosts immunity.

CHANNEL TRAJECTORY

The Du mai has multiple trajectories. The first begins in the lower abdomen below Ren 2 (some say Ren 1) and travels to the perineum and up the coccyx and along the spine to Du 16, then into the head and brain. From there the main channel continues to Du 20, the forehead, and nose, terminating at the frenulum of the upper lip. The second emerges from the lower abdomen, and follows the Ren mai trajectory to the navel, abdomen, chest, and throat, encircling the mouth and ending at the eyes. The third is said to begin at BL 1, goes to Du 20 where it enters the brain, and then splits into two trajectories, exiting the head at the nape of the neck and descending along the sides of the spine to the Kidney area. The fourth trajectory starts in the lower abdomen, goes to the genitalia and into the perineum, meeting up with Ren mai, then to the coccyx and Du 1, where it continues to ascend to the gluteus, meets with the Bladder and Kidney channels, goes to the sacrum, and travels up to the lumbar region before entering the Kidneys.

Points along the trajectory: Du 1–8, Ren 1–24, inner Bladder line

Opening point: SI 3

Luo point: Du 1

Associated/connected organs: lower abdomen, perineum and genitalia, anus, coccyx, spine, head and brain, navel, chest, throat, face, eyes, Kidneys, Bladder, lumbar region, forehead, nose, uterus, sacrum, Heart

Second ancestry
Yin Wei mai

As a reflection of one's experiences and aging, the Wei mais reveal the unfolding of the curriculum in the service of life having been lived. It is what contributes to the formation of one's identity, and includes all the formative moments of one's life, the disjunctive ones revealing a lot about one's personality. As the cycles of 7 and 8 unfold, the Yin Wei mai measures the impact of life on one's physical structure. As the yin linking vessel, Yin Wei mai is the patch quilt that weaves together the historical changes to one's physicality over time. The Yin Wei mai channel helps govern the interior domain and the qi of the yin organs. As evidenced by its luo point, PC 6, it can invigorate blood and also regulate the emotions and shen. Common uses for the Yin Wei mai include pathologies in the Stomach, diaphragm, chest, and Heart.

CHANNEL TRAJECTORY

Beginning at KI 9, the channel ascends the Kidney channel to the lower abdomen where it meets up with the Spleen channel, particularly SP 12–16 (some do not include SP 12 or SP 14), then to the hypochondriac region, meeting up with the Liver at LR 14. From here it passes through the diaphragm and chest and ascends to the throat, communicating with Ren 22 and terminating at Ren 23.

The imagery of these points is that the Yin Wei mai provides a glimpse at oneself (self-reflection) and the life being lived (KI 9), as well as societal influences (Spleen). It provides access to how one's jing-essence has been converted to blood, revealing one's shen in terms of experiences and memory/recollection, as well as the ability to let go (LR 14 as the last point on the last channel). The eventuality is a new cycle, returning to the WOS domain on the throat (providing access to the heavens), or a recycling and return to the source of Yin Wei mai, the Ren channel.

Points along the trajectory: KI 9, SP 12–16, LR 14, Ren 22–23; some include SP 6

Opening point: PC 6

Xi-cleft point: KI 9

Associated/connected organs: medial aspect of lower extremities, lateral aspect of lower abdomen, hypochondriac region, chest, throat, tongue, Heart

Yang Wei mai

Similar to the Yin Wei mai above, Yang Wei mai reflects the impact of the cycles of 7 and 8 on one's activities and experiences. Where Yin Wei mai deals with body structure, Yang Wei mai deals with body functioning/coordination/movement. Yang Wei mai governs the exterior, especially the taiyang and shaoyang channels, as they bring wei qi to the surface. It helps circulate jing-essence and balances yang qi as well as the emotions, including manic-depression and obsessive-compulsive disorders. An image of Yang Wei mai is that of a net cast into the world bringing back its experiences to Du mai and the brain. These experiences, and the movements it engenders, allow one to make choices, such as choosing partners to be intimate with, making commitments based on what is important to us, which responsibilities to take on, and overall how to move in the world in a way that allows us to live out our curriculum.

CHANNEL TRAJECTORY

The Yang Wei mai also has conflicting or alternate pathways. It begins at BL 63, then follows the GB primary channel to GB 35, up to GB 29, and then the hypochondriac region, through to the lateral shoulder at LI 14, SI 10, and SJ 15, up to the neck at GB 21, to the retroauricular area, and up to the forehead at ST 8. From there it moves to the back of the head from GB 13–20, ending at the nape and meeting with the Du mai at Du 15–16.

The imagery of the latter part of the trajectory is about depositing one's experiences into the Du mai and brain. Another view, which eliminates the trajectory from GB 14–20 and the Du mai points, is that one is able to be decisive and resolve any conflicts and issues in the moment. In that case, SJ 13 and SJ 14 are added (SJ 15 removed) to the trajectory and it ends at GB 13.

Points along the trajectory: BL 63, GB 35, SI 10, SJ 15, GB 21, ST 8, GB 13–20, Du 15–16

Opening point: SJ 5

Xi-cleft point: GB 35

Associated/connected organs: lateral side of lower extremities, hip, hypochondriac region, lateral shoulder, neck, ear, forehead, lateral head, nape of neck, cheek, outer canthus, brain

Third ancestry

Yin Qiao mai

The Yin Qiao mai represents one's current situation/consciousness and assists with the process of self-reflection and the ability to accept one's circumstances. Having its roots in the Kidney channel below, it provides for self-respect, and trust and faith in ourselves and our curriculum. Yin Qiao mai assists with structure and muscular balance, especially for the medial muscle groups, and also helps regulate the opening and closing of the eyes (Yin Qiao excess showing somnolence) and the throat (vocal cords), as well as certain functions of the brain and nervous system (Yin Qiao excess showing listlessness, apathy, and overall hypoactivity).

CHANNEL TRAJECTORY

The channel starts at the medial ankle and ascends from KI 6 to KI 8, up the medial thigh into the pelvis, passing through the genitalia, up the abdomen and chest to ST 12, and passing through the throat at ST 9, into the face, ending at BL 1, where it meets Yang Qiao mai. From there it is said that both channels travel together to GB 20 and enter the brain at Du 16. KI 2 is often included within Yin Qiao mai's trajectory. It is often thought to be an extension of the KI channel.

The imagery behind the Yin Qiao mai is that one is able to look at oneself (Kidney-water), and see and own who one really is. The Yin Qiao mai operates in present time and is about acceptance.

Points along the trajectory: KI 2, KI 6, KI 8, ST 12, ST 9, BL 1

Opening point: KI 6

Xi-cleft point: KI 8

Associated/connected organs: medial ankle and lower extremity, genitalia, abdomen, chest, throat, face, lateral head, eyes, brain

Yang Qiao mai

The Yang Qiao mai represents one's stance in the world and how one stands up to others. It reflects how engaged we are with the outside world, how active or passive we are, and the kinds of conflicts engendered (e.g., being a martyr, a rebel or activist, a hermit, etc.). It assists with structure and muscular balance, especially for the lateral muscle groups, and also helps regulate the opening and closing of the eyes (Yang Qiao excess showing insomnia and/or red irritated eyes), as well as certain functions of the brain and nervous system (Yang Qiao excess showing hyperactivity, restlessness and irritability, convulsions, etc.). It is often thought to be an extension of the BL channel.

CHANNEL TRAJECTORY

The channel starts at the lateral ankle at BL 62 and moves to BL 61, ascending the lateral leg to BL 59, up the thigh to the hip at GB 29, passing through the lateral abdomen and hypochondriac region, and traveling to the lateral aspect of the scapula and shoulder, where it meets SI 10, LI 16, and LI 15. It follows the lateral side of the neck to the corner of the mouth at ST 4, and continues to ST 3 and ST 1, then to the inner canthus at BL 1, where it meets with Yin Qiao mai. From there it is said that both channels travel together to GB 20 and enter the brain at Du 16.

Points along the trajectory: BL 62, BL 61, BL 59, GB 29, SI 10, LI 16, LI 15, ST 4, ST 3, ST 1, BL 1, GB 20, Du 16

Opening point: BL 62

Xi-cleft point: BL 59

Associated/connected organs: lateral ankle and lower extremity, hip, hypochondriac region, lateral scapula and shoulder, lateral aspect of head, eyes, brain

Dai mai

The Dai mai assists with draining stagnation and long-term holdings, including damp (heat and cold), regulates the GB channel, lower back, and lower abdomen, including the reproductive organs and organs of elimination, and regulates qi and circulation to the lower body. It is a channel of latency that often accumulates and absorbs pathology (mental-emotional and physical) to be stored for a future time when resources can be brought to bear towards it. Inability to move this stagnation weighs one down, limits and restricts the ability to move, impacts decision-making, and prevents the ability to contain suppressed issues. It is often used for reproductive and obstetric/gynecological issues, muscle weakness or pain, abdominal fullness, lower back issues, etc.

CHANNEL TRAJECTORY

The Dai mai also has multiple trajectories. Typically, the Dai mai consists of a continuous loop from Du 4 around to the front of the body and including GB 26–28. This channel is most commonly used to drain pathology from the Dai mai. LR 13 (influential point of the zang and front mu point of the Spleen) was added to this trajectory at a later time and is often included for this purpose.

If one seeks to use the Dai to consolidate, the original Dai mai is more likely to be used. It consists of GB 26, SP 15, ST 25, KI 16, Ren 8, and wrapping all around the body, including BL 23 and Du 4.

The skeletal structure of the body and its upper (head), middle (thorax), and lower (legs) aspects are held together by various muscle structures, i.e., the SCM (connecting the head to the thorax), diaphragm (connecting the chest to the abdomen), and iliopsoas (connecting the lower back and abdomen to the legs), all mediated by the paravertebral muscles. One can view the Dai mai as influencing all these connections: the SCM (upper Dai mai), including GB 20, GB 12, SJ 16, SI 17, SI 16, ST 9, LI 18, ST 10, and ST 11; the diaphragm, which is consistent with the Da Bao or great wrap (in earlier chapters, I have demonstrated how the Da Bao, Bao mai, and Dai mai are often combined into a single treatment); and the area of the psoas (the Dai mai most spoken of). With this conception, the Dai is almost like a spiral that encircles the body at these three critical junctures.

Some believe that the Dai mai is created as part of the KI DM, originating from Du 4, providing another strong connection to the Kidneys.

Points along the trajectory: LR 13, GB 26–28, SP 15, ST 25, KI 16, Du 4, BL 23, BL 52

Opening point: GB 41

Associated/connected organs: Kidneys, uterus, lower back and lumbar vertebrae, hypochondriac region, navel, inguinal area, lower abdomen

8x pulses

Pulses reflecting the 8x vessels are pulses that must resonate to the yuan and jing levels. These are energies that do not necessarily reveal themselves without some prodding, and they are also more resistant and harder to influence simply with one's intention. As a reflection of the deepest energetics of an individual, the most precise reading requires some time, attention, and cultivation. In terms of mapping, the yuan level is represented in the deeper aspects of the vessel. As one presses from superficial to deep, pressure should be exerted also medially toward the tendon moving down towards the bone. Moving medially ensures one is accessing the interior aspects of physiology. Lateral aspects typically reflect more superficial energetics, as is observed, for example, when accessing the sinew meridians at the 3 and 6 beans of pressure. The yuan-level pulses require vibration, as evidenced also by its needling techniques. To access this deep reservoir, one should slide their hands back and forth along the bone at the deep level represented by the 15 beans of pressure. The bone level images a stone or rock, and the way to uproot it is to shake it or vibrate it. As the stone is rocked and vibrated, it begins to reveal its pulses. Additionally, to assess the yuan level and the 8x vessels, the placement of the arm should be with the palm facing upwards.

Some pulse images for the 8x channels can be found in the Mai Jing, scroll 2, Chapter 4, but Wang Shu-he was not very definitive about them and many contradictions can be found, especially between the Chong mai (which he calls the "sea of yin" and notes it starting at Ren 4, traveling up the abdomen to the chest and throat) and the Ren mai. Later versions of the Mai Jing teach the Chong starting at ST 30.[174]

First ancestry pulses

Pulses of the first ancestry are considered Long pulses. A Long pulse is one that is not confined to one position, but extends into others, suggesting the boundaries have been breached and limits have been exceeded. Ditches begin to be created and become filled up. Long pulses are taxing on the constitutional yuan level.

Du mai pulse

This is Long from cun to chi on the floating level. This pulse can be Full or Wiry (Tight-Tense in Shen-Hammer). It may also be Vibrating, suggesting a more active pathology (i.e., can ask if there is stiffness along the spine).

Chong mai pulse

This pulse is Long from cun to chi on the moderate[175] level, often Wiry (Tense-Tight in Shen-Hammer). This pulse may also be Firm (pressing from moderate to deep may feel Leathery).

If Chong mai is found on the right wrist only, that would relate more to its role as the Sea of Blood.

If Chong mai is found on the left wrist only, that would relate more to its role as the Sea of the 12 Primary Meridians and the zang fu. Points chosen to treat should relate more to qi and one can add moxa to the treatment.

Ren mai pulse

This is Long from cun to chi on the deep level, often Wiry (Tense-Tight in Shen-Hammer).

Second ancestry pulses

The Wei mai pulses reflect relationships, hence where things meet and exchange. They, too, are Long pulses, but extend to only two positions, not three like the first ancestry.

Yang Wei mai pulse

This is Deep and Long at cun and guan. A second configuration for this channel is a pulse that moves laterally from the chi position to the cun position, starting off medially at the chi and moving towards the Lung channel at the cun.

Yin Wei mai pulse

This is Deep and Long at guan and chi. A second configuration for this channel is a pulse that moves medially from the chi position to the cun position, starting off radially at the chi and moving towards the Pericardium channel at the cun.

Third ancestry pulses

Vessels of excess are the Yang and Yin Qiao and Dai. Ditches are created. There is the pressure of something trying to siphon inwards but cannot. It is like a finger on a vacuum cleaner when the vacuum is trying to suck your finger in and you are trying to resist.

Yang Qiao mai pulse

This pulse is Deep at cun and Vibrating, and often Short. It is a sign of yang excess.

Yin Qiao mai pulse

Deep at chi and Vibrating, and often Short, this pulse is a sign of yin excess/yin stasis, though some consider it to be a reflection of yin deficiency.

The Qiao mai's pulses can also be reflected by a weakness on the deep levels, demonstrating no inner reserves or capacity to self-reflect. Here pulses are Floating and Weak. With a poor self-image, a Wiry pulse may also present on the surface, showing that the person does not feel comfortable with himself.

Dai mai pulse

Deep at guan and Vibrating, and often Short, this pulse reflects yin and yang excess and damp-heat. The Dai mai pulse may also show itself in the moderate level. In that scenario, the pulse will feel as if it is coming from under the tendon at an angle into one's finger.

Methodology for assessing second and third ancestry pulses and distinguishing from DM

8x and DM pulses are both assessed by first checking the 15 beans of pressure. As one releases to 14 beans and presses back down towards the bone, the DM pulses will disappear, reflecting the capacity to hide and the process of latency. When pressing back down to the bone, if the pulses are still present, there is 8x vessel activity, namely the Yin and Yang Qiao, or Dai mai (Short pulses), or the Yin and Yang Wei mai (Long pulses). 8x vessel pulses are also characterized by a Vibrating quality when there is active pathology. Additionally, at the 14 beans of pressure, should one find a Long pulse from the cun to the chi, a Ren mai pulse is present. Then one may lift to the moderate level, checking for a Chong mai pulse, and on to the wei level to check for a Du mai pulse.

Distinguishing between Wei mai pulses and occurrence of Qiao mai and Dai mai pulses

- If guan and chi have different qualities, can be Yin Qiao and Dai mai.
- If cun and guan have different qualities, can be Yang Qiao and Dai mai.

Pulses that indicate discrepancies between yin and yang can also signify 8x vessel activity. For example, if the pulse reflects exuberance of yang above and below, it suggests that yang has gone to where it should be relatively quiet, e.g., Floating and Full/Big/Long and at same time Deep and Full/Big/Long. Similarly, if there are no pulses on the floating and deep levels or if they are very weak, it means the yin quality has gone to the yang.

Full above and below: Du mai and Ren mai pulse images. Often seen in the elderly, especially in those with Alzheimer's. The pulse is of feeble-mindedness, and if not treated it is believed the person will develop multiple personalities (e.g., schizophrenia or personality disorders), with constant fluctuation of yin becoming yang and yang becoming yin. If yin becomes yang, memories stored in blood become lost.

Weak above and below: Faint/Thready/Very Thin/Short pulses above and below suggest a person is possessed by an evil entity/ghost. It is believed that this pulse threatens the 8x vessels and constitution.

Pulses dictating side of treatment

When the 8x vessel pulse is found only on the left wrist, use points on the left side of the body. When it is found on the right side, use trajectory points on the right side of the body. For the Ren and Du, the left wrist is considered yin (pre-natal) and the right is yang (pre-natal). If the Ren mai pulse is found on the right side reflecting yang, because the Ren has a trajectory that gives birth to the Du, Ren points that reflect more of a qi-yang dynamic should be needled (and moxa may be used). If the Du mai pulse is found on the left wrist reflecting yin, as it also has a trajectory that gives birth to the Ren, Du mai points that can engender yin and fluids may be needled.

chi   guan   cun

Ren mai

15 beans

Du mai

15 beans

Chong mai

15 beans

Yin Wei mai 1

_____ 15 beans

Yin Wei mai 2 (depicting medial lateral, not depth)

_____ medial

Yang Wei mai 1

_____ 15 beans

Yin Wei mai 2 (depicting medial lateral, not depth)

_____ medial

Dai mai

_____ 15 beans

Yin Qiao mai

_____15 beans

Yang Qiao mai

_____15 beans

8x channel uses in Heart Shock

Chong mai

Chong mai is instrumental in the treatment of Heart Shock. It represents the original blueprint and sets the stage for who we are, what our path is, and our overall curriculum. Heart Shock and trauma hit one at his core and to some degree represents the antithesis of what the Chong mai stands for. Trauma diverts us from our particular paths and can alter one's personality, preventing the realization of what the Chong has mapped out. Using Chong mai, one seeks to reset the blueprint, re-enliven the spirit and one's nature, and align it back with one's curriculum. It seeks to re-establish communication between the Heart and Kidneys and bring us back in touch with intuition, trust, faith, and an overall sense of comfort.

In terms of comfort, Chong mai also regulates the Spleen and Stomach, stabilizing the center and providing us with a stronger root. As we become more stabilized and the foundation strengthens, we are able to derive more nutrients from food and drink. The vectors of the qi dynamic are more optimized, the Stomach descends its turbidity, and the Spleen ascends its ying qi, red substance, and fluids in the creation of more blood and qi, and hence greater vitality, immunity, and longevity. As the Chong mai assists with the ascension of Spleen qi, one is able to overcome dampness and turbidity, which often manifests psychologically as depression, apathy, lethargy, etc.

Another important aspect of the Chong mai's assistance with raising the Spleen qi is that this ascension also helps the Spleen bring the red substance it creates up to the chest and Heart to become finalized into blood. This substance is primarily fluid-based and serves as a counterbalance to the heat/fire produced in the Heart, in the form of desires, etc. Thus, the Spleen's ascension cools off desires and the resultant heat that is generated in the Heart, creating symptoms such as palpitations, insomnia, irritability, etc. (Gui Pi Tang is instructive in this regard as a representative Chong mai formula.)

Additionally, as the pure yang of the Stomach ascends, we see greater health in the sensory portals, and hence greater clarity of perceptions, including the production of wei qi and its influence over one's mood. The pure yang of the Stomach is instrumental in nourishing the sensory portals, the root of which resides in the fluids of the Stomach. And Chong mai includes a trajectory that brings its resources to the eyes themselves, further enhancing and building on the nourishment received from the pure yang of the Stomach. Another benefit of the ascension of the pure yang of the Stomach and the red substance rising to the chest and Heart for final blood production is that it allows for an increased animation of spirit. Nourished by blood and healthier sensory portals providing clearer perceptions of the external and internal environments, one is able to allow the spirit to accord with one's true nature, blueprint, and the heavenly qi.

With the nourishment of the eyes and portals, and impact on the Spleen-Stomach systems, the Chong mai can help one to process, digest, and assimilate information, experiences, and perceptions in a healthier manner. This becomes a crucial component in the resolution of trauma's impact on the senses, as well as the capacity to take in nourishment (both from our experiences and what we put into our mouths, both having a role in one's health and well-being). Without such capacity, one tends towards rebellious qi, not being willing or able to take and utilize the best of what has been offered.

The trajectories of the Chong mai also provide information as to its usefulness in the realm of Heart Shock treatments. First, it originates in the lower abdomen and communicates with the Liver luo and DM, providing usages consistent with those channels (see Chapters 5 and 7), including a major influence on the lower abdomen, and potentially traumas thereto (e.g., rapes, incest, physical traumas to the lower abdomen, genitalia, and reproductive organs).

The Chong mai also descends from the lower abdomen, making communication at BL 40 and KI 10 and providing some access to the BL/KI DM. The BL/KI DM births the Dai mai as well, providing a whole complex network of channel systems to tap into. Treatments combining the Chong mai, BL/KI DM, and Dai mai are extremely effective for a host of disorders related to trauma, one being infertility. In such cases, right SP 4 can be combined with BL 40, BL 10, and KI 10, plus right GB 41, to open all these channels. Points on these channels can be needled as appropriate, including the use of LR 13 (which will also assist in Chong's influence over the Spleen), GB 26–28 if trying to rid stagnation, or SP 15, ST 25, and KI 16 if one is seeking to consolidate, plus ST 30, and Kidney channel points on the lower abdomen. I often add KI 19 to strengthen the influence over the Spleen and Stomach where appropriate, and the upper Kidney shu points provide access to the Heart dynamics. Where appropriate, the great luo of the Spleen can be included, as can Bao mai, to provide a very powerful treatment, anchoring the Heart and Kidneys, invigorating blood in the diaphragm, abdomen, and uterus, etc.

Chong mai's lower trajectories also include the passing of SP 6, ST 42, LR 3, SP 1, and LR 1. This trajectory can be very useful with the above treatment, but without Dai mai and the BL/KI DM, it can be used to strengthen blood production and invigorate blood. SP 6 and LR 3 also have the benefit of regulating the emotions, relieving pain, calming the shen, and treating insomnia and palpitations, as well as relaxing the nervous system overall. Its connection to ST 42 further solidifies its use to nourish yin and support the ascension of the pure yang of the Stomach and the production of post-natal qi in general. Additionally, the lower trajectory moves to the heel and arch, providing connection to the Yin Qiao mai and all that it treats, especially in terms of providing a strong structure and support.

The Chong's upper trajectory creates a strong influence over the chest and Heart and includes the Kidney front shu points. These points have been detailed in Chapter 6, but briefly, they have a profound impact over the shen and emotions, and create a strong communication between the Heart and Kidneys. When needled outwards laterally, they can also promote circulation and rid yin stasis in the associated shu points' organ system. These points can be very successful in regulating rate and rhythm issues as well. This trajectory into the chest also communicates the Chong mai to the ancestral qi, a function further strengthened by its opening point, SP 4, "grandfather-grandson." The upper trajectory of Chong mai has multi-faceted uses within the realm of Heart Shock, as each of the Kidney front shu points relate to one of the Five Phase organ systems. As such, each of these organ systems can be tapped into depending on the unique presentation of the patient. Where there is anxiety, panic, insomnia, etc., KI 25 is most commonly used; with allergies, shortness of breath, grief, and an inability to let go, KI 26 can be used; where there is nervous system tension, anger, armoring, etc., KI 24 can be needled; with obsessive-compulsive behavior, clouded thinking, and clinginess, KI 23 is useful; and with phobias and deep-seated fears, KI 22 is most helpful. Where one is unsure which shu point to needle, KI 27 can be used as the master point. When the upper trajectory is used, one should close the treatment with PC 6 (the often-used coupled point belonging to Yin Wei mai) to solidify the impact on the chest. Otherwise, PC 6 need not be used; SP 4 does not need to be "closed" with any coupled point. Likewise, if Chong mai is paired with another 8x vessel besides Yin Wei mai, that channel's opening point would be used in conjunction with the treatment.

The trajectory of the Chong mai also shares part of the Kidney luo vessel trajectory, running from the lower abdomen to KI 21. Thus, it shares many of the same uses, including the treatment of panic attacks and running piglet qi, phobias, paranoia, depression, etc. The Chong mai and the Kidney luo can be combined together in the same treatment as well for these concerns.

The Chong mai, as the original blueprint, and part of the first ancestry, is extremely influential during gestation and the first few years of life. Anything that intervenes in the proper formation of all the myriad stages of development from the meeting of sperm and egg to gestation, birth and delivery, early life nurturing, bonding, and boundary formation has profound impact. These are some of the most influential of traumas and are best treated by Chong mai.

Many of the cases of Heart Shock that I treat may have their initiating traumas decades prior to my meeting with the patient. Often these traumas have their roots in birthing or gestational issues, such as cord being wrapped around neck, breech presentation and stuck in birth canal, placenta previa, trauma to mother during pregnancy, etc. Many include traumas from the first few years of life, including death of a caregiver or parent, traumatic injuries, etc. As discussed in Part I, the earlier a trauma happens in the developmental process, the more potential problems it can create. These types of traumas are well suited for Chong mai.

As the Chong tends to mature in the first seven-to-eight-year cycle, early life support and nourishment are critical to it providing a solid foundation. And with its role post-natally and relationship to the Spleen and Stomach (Mother Earth), early and substantive mothering/caregiving is essential to its health. Where early bonding, nourishment, and boundary formation is lacking, disorders can range from minor issues such as digestive problems, learning delays, colic, etc. to significant disorders such as schizophrenia. For traumas that occur within this time frame, Chong mai becomes a first-choice option in its treatment. I find often in patients with traumas rooted in early life nurturing that the digestive system also bears a significant brunt, with a host of possible GI problems. The Chong mai is well suited to treat these disorders, and points on the lower and middle abdomen (especially KI 19) are important in its treatment.

Oftentimes, traumas impact one's ability to find purpose in life. An alteration of the blueprint, or one's inability to merge back onto the major highway of life (rather than a collateral), Chong mai can be used to help a patient find her purpose in life. In these scenarios, I often make sure to utilize the upper Kidney shu points to revitalize and reanimate the shen. Ge Hong's 9 Flower treatments (discussed in the previous chapter) can also be combined into the Chong mai treatment in that regard. In that case one can needle SP 4 (left for male, right for female), followed by Ge Hong's points of KI 21, KI 19, ST 19, KI 23, and Ren 17, and then followed by opposite-side PC 6.

Where a lot of blood stasis presents, one can also combine the great luo of the Spleen into a Chong mai treatment. Adding in SP 21 further enhances the impact of the earth, as well as providing an additional motivation/catalyst to invigorating the blood and releasing trapped circulation in the chest and diaphragm. Where the lower part of the Chong mai is impacted, using Bao mai and Dai mai can serve as additional treatment points.

With blood stasis, I often also utilize the relationship of the Chong to the Yin Wei mai, using points along Yin Wei mai's trajectory as well. This can further the impact of treatment where a patient experiences significant anxiety, panic, insomnia, etc., especially when there is Liver involvement. SP 21 or GB 22 (the original great luo of the Spleen) can be added to this treatment as well when there is significant stagnation in the diaphragm. (Wang Shu-he's blood-invigorating formulas can be instructive in this regard as a herbal approximation.) As traumas tend to be some of the disjunctive and formative periods in one's life, the Yin Wei mai combination with Chong mai can be quite powerful.

As the Chong shares all its acupuncture points from other channels, as do all the other 8x vessels except the Ren and Du, its acupuncture point functions for its trajectory points can be found in the preceding chapters.

Ren mai

Ren mai plays a major role in growth and development within the first year of life as mom cradles baby against her chest, feeding and nurturing her, and creating the first post-natal bond. The child's existence is completely dependent on this primary caregiver, and it is this bond that sets the stage for the ultimate boundary and distinction of who she is as a separate individual. The quality of the bonding, however, impacts the quality of the baby's ability to be content, receive and assimilate nourishment, and eventually individuate (Du mai reliant on Ren mai). Additionally, the mother's energy at this time of bonding becomes imprinted on the baby, creating the sense of what love, safety, and nurturing feels like. Thus, if mom is very anxious or suffers emotional instability, the baby often will seek that energy later in life in relationships as it is most familiar, representing love and security, despite how dysfunctional it may be, and the suffering it may cause.

This instrumental time in the baby's life becomes a determining factor in how safe a person feels throughout life, how dependent she is on others, her strength of identity and ability to take control and responsibility, and her ability to feel content and nourished with what she has. Traumas during this critical formative time (including lack of nourishment, shelter, caregiving, bonding, etc.) can create a host of personality disorders (see also the Earth phase imbalances from the DRRBF perspective) and feelings of victimization. Common scenarios where these traumas create impact later in life are with babies born prematurely or those born with health issues requiring time in the NICU without significant early contact and bonding with mom. Not uncommonly, premature births prevent the Lungs from maturing, again creating an overlap between the use of LU 7 as the opening point of Ren mai, and the host of energetics ascribed to the Metal phase, including safety and vulnerability. The Heart Shock patient can often experience difficulty bonding or holding onto relationships, and feeling incomplete when unable to do so. This lack of completeness and inability to hold onto relationships often results in grief, so is well treated by LU 7 and the upper Ren mai points, especially Ren 22 (WOS point to diffuse the Lungs) and Ren 17.

With traumas affecting the development of Ren mai early in life, or later life traumas shaking one's capacity to feel secure (e.g., traumatic injuries such as car accidents), or betrayals (e.g., infidelity), an individual may lose the capacity to connect with others and trust. Symptoms expressing lack of nourishment (yin-deficient signs and symptoms), or distorted responses to it (yin stasis, dampness and turbidity), may prevail. Treating Ren mai to re-establish the feelings of safety and bonding is warranted in these circumstances. A Heart Shock patient from lack of early life bonding with her mom came to see me for issues of anxiety and palpitations. Extremely sensitive to the energies of others, she would often somatically and emotionally feel the negative emotions and energies of others with whom were nearby. Even reading words written by such individuals would cause her to experience anxiety as the underlying emotions were transmitted to her. Initially, I worked on settling the spirit, strengthening Heart yin and blood, and calming the nervous system. Much improvement was gained, but it was not until I worked on Ren mai that the largest shift occurred.

The use of Ren mai in treating Heart Shock helps to stabilize a patient's resources, in particular the yin, especially when points such as Ren 23, Ren 17, and Ren 15 are included in the treatment. Ren 23 is the termination point for shaoyin, and also affects the tongue, allowing one to speak, giving words to release the trauma stuck in the chest. Ren 17 provides access to the Pericardium, Lungs, and Heart, affecting rate and rhythm, clearing heat, and stabilizing the shen. Ren mai's access to yin can cool off Heart/Pericardium fire from harassing the spirit. Ren 15 is the luo point and strongly nourishes yin.

Ren mai also helps to communicate the Heart and Kidneys, its trajectory including the termination point for shaoyin, as well as traversing the chest, making a direct connection to the Heart, and the lower abdomen and burner, providing access to Kidney dynamics. As with the chest points listed in the preceding paragraph, the lower points include Ren 8 through Ren 1, each of them having a significant impact on Kidney yin, yang, or qi, each of which can root and anchor its associated resource back to the lower burner and Kidneys. With traumas, as the adrenals become hyperactive, qi and yang are constantly being leaked, creating heat, anxiety, and shen disturbances. These points help with its consolidation back to its source. Their point functions are addressed below. It's not uncommon to see people who have experienced traumas to Ren mai suffer from anxiety and tachycardia. Oftentimes those who have been abandoned early in life will carry these wounds with them, and when they experience the threat of abandonment in the future (e.g., loss of friendship, potential break-up of an intimate relationship, etc.), signs and symptoms of trauma can become heightened, including anxiety, rapid heart rate, arrhythmias, insomnia, etc. Using Ren mai and re-establishing the connection between the Heart and Kidneys, as well as managing the energetics of the Lungs (loss, worry, and grief), become important aspects of patient management.

Ren mai's connection to the Lungs provides access to the Po, which can become scattered during and after the experience of a trauma. A scattered Po prevents one from feeling grounded, especially in its residence of the chest, and also creates an inability to be present in the moment. As discussed in other parts of this text, trauma often causes one to live in the past, re-experiencing traumas and projecting that into the future. Wen Dan Tang was noted earlier for treating this dynamic and can serve as a prototype that can be modified to treat this aspect of a Ren mai imbalance.

Ren mai can consolidate the qi of the digestive system as it traverses the abdomen. This provides further connection to its use in bonding and boundary formation (see the Earth phase section of DRRBF from Chapter 6) and provides stability and comfort. Points such as Ren 13, Ren 12, and Ren 10 are major points for regulating qi in the abdomen, helping to assimilate nourishment, strengthen the Lungs, etc. They help with the patients who require support with feeling nourished/nurtured, bonded, and loved. Too much desired connection creates an inability to let go and can create turbidity, as well as constant seeking of nourishment (including addictions). Focusing on the abdominal trajectory, one can treat this lack of connectedness, and the inability to find comfort.

Ren mai's upper trajectory helps to bring fluids up to the sensory portals, especially the eyes and mouth. Part of the breastfeeding dynamics includes bonding via the stimulation of the baby's orbicular muscles in the suckling of the breast, as well as via making eye contact with mom. This connection, when lost or deprived, can create distortions in seeking nourishment and bonding and include a host of addictive behaviors (e.g., food addiction, smoking, alcohol, visual addictions such as pornography, etc.). As with the overall energetics of the 8x vessels, it is the lack of control which allows for pathology to extend past its borders, creating the ditches and long pulses reflected of 8x vessel pathology.

In addition to the muscles of the eyes and mouth, the Ren mai channel influences the ring muscles of the digestive tract as well as the perineum. Patients who become uptight and anal post trauma trying to control their environment and circumstances often experience tightness in these areas. The result can be inability to move the bowels easily (constipation), or those who react to foods with hypersensitivities and allergies, as well as difficulty relaxing, enjoying sexual intercourse, and experiencing orgasm. The latter is especially the case when traumas have been of a sexual origin or where there has been a betrayal of intimacy.

Bringing the pure yang of the Stomach's energetics to the mouth and eyes assists with the health and integrity of the portals, allowing for proper assimilation of nutrients and visual stimuli to nourish not only the physical body, but also the mind and spirit. Those who have felt victimized, uncared for, or betrayed often see the world through a negative lens, and Ren mai can be useful in providing a different view as it taps into a deeper reservoir of nourishment for these patients.

Ren mai provides the yin for the entire body, including its structure, moisture of internal organs and glands, fluid for the joints, spinal canal, hormones, etc. When lacking, the myriad dryness pathologies can present themselves (yin-fluid deficiencies), some manifesting in the form of feeling unsatisfied, unprotected, and overall insufficient or unable to accomplish one's curriculum as set forth by Chong mai. Additionally, dryness leads to distorted compensation in the form of yin stasis and the accumulation of damp, phlegm, and turbidity. Patients become lethargic, depressed, overweight, bored, needy, and dependent. Ren mai can be used to promote self-discovery, security, trust, and contentment in those in search of these qualities.

Ren mai points most applicable to Heart Shock

Ren 1: The "meeting of yin," Ren 1 is the origin of the Ren, Chong, and Du mai. It regulates the Ren and Chong, nourishes yin, benefits essence, and promotes resuscitation. It is an important point for grounding, treating the separation of yin and yang, and anchoring qi, yin, and yang to the lower abdomen. It can play an important role in the treatment of sexual traumas, as well as birthing traumas, but caution, discretion, professionalism, and tact are required for needling such a vulnerable area. It can be used with Du 20 as a central channel Chong mai treatment, and together with Du 20 allows for heavenly qi interaction while keeping man grounded on earth.

Ren 2: The meeting of the Ren and Liver (including its luo vessel), it is also the confluent of the GB/LR DM and can be used in conjunction with these channels to support blood and essence, and invigorate blood in the pelvis. It warms yang, strengthens the Kidneys, and also regulates reproductive functioning.

Ren 3: The front mu of the Bladder, Ren 3 is also the meeting point for SP/LR/KI with Ren mai. It regulates the blood chamber, warms the womb, and releases stagnant fluid from the Bladder.

Ren 4: The front mu of the Small Intestine, and meeting point of the SP/LR/KI with Ren mai. It banks the Kidney yang, strengthens the root, supplements qi, regulates the blood chamber, dispels cold and damp, separates the pure and turbid, regulates original qi, nourishes blood, strengthens yang, and roots the Hun. Ren 4 is one of my most commonly used points for treating trauma for its ability to root yang qi in the abdomen. It is a very grounding point, and its connection to the Small Intestine, the paired Fire phase channel with the Heart, provides an added incentive to use it. The Small Intestine is also taiyang, and is paired with the Bladder channel, its internally–externally paired channel being the Kidneys. Thus Ren 4 with its connection to the Small Intestine, Bladder, Heart, and Kidneys makes it a powerful point for anchoring the entire taiyang–shaoyin axis, with a marked ability to nourish and anchor yang qi.

Ren 5: The front mu of the Triple Burner, Ren 5 warms the Kidneys, invigorates yang, regulates menstruation, strengthens original qi, and regulates the waterways. I tend to favor Ren 5 when focusing on the Triple Burner's dissemination or harnessing yang qi in the context of a Triple Burner focused treatment.

Ren 6: The lower source of qi, Ren 6 regulates qi and strengthens yang, anchors the Kidneys and supplements qi, harmonizes ying qi, warms the lower burner, rids damp and turbidity, and tonifies qi and yang. Another very commonly used point, Ren 6 has a more active nature than the points below it, also harmonizing and strengthening the Spleen and Stomach as well as moving qi.

Ren 7: The yin intersection, Ren 7 is a meeting point of Ren and Chong. It's an important point in alchemical acupuncture for providing yin resources to stabilize and contain yang to allow for its transformation.

Ren 8: This point, while not needled, can be treated with moxa to warm and free yang qi, open the portals, restore consciousness, move GI qi, transform cold and damp accumulations/stagnations, and strengthen the Spleen and original qi. The energetics of Ren 8 provide deep access into the pre-natal environment, holding the energetic signatures of nourishment and safety in utero. The cutting of this cord can be seen as one of the first traumas, cutting one off from pre-heaven energetics and the safety of the womb. Once cut, the baby must breathe on her own, and this sparks the movement of Kidneys grasping Lung qi, pulling down the oxygen to stoke the fire of ming men, to be distributed by the Triple Burner. Symbolically, the cutting of the cord can represent letting go of attachments and moving on. It can be used to anchor Lung and ancestral qi, stimulate the Kidneys and anchor yang qi, and regulate metabolism. It can be used to provide a connection to original qi and the safety of the womb and/or motherly embrace. And it can be used to provide the nourishment and bonding necessary to learn to individuate and "breathe on one's own."

Ren 9: In the context of trauma, I mostly use Ren 9 to assist with moving damp and stagnation and regulating the Spleen's water transformative functions.

Ren 10: A meeting point of the Ren and Spleen, Ren 10 moves and transforms Stomach and intestinal qi, promotes descension of the Stomach, and tonifies the Spleen. I use it mostly symptomatically in the context of the larger Heart Shock dynamic.

Ren 12: The front mu of the Stomach, Ren 12 moves Spleen qi, rectifies qi in the middle burner, harmonizes the Stomach, and promotes the rotting and ripening of digestate to assist with processing and assimilation. It can treat insomnia secondary to food stagnation and Stomach heat. As a major point for strengthening and stabilizing the earth, it also nourishes the Lung qi and allows for the formation of bonds and boundaries necessary to feel safe and individuate.

Ren 13: Having a function of rectifying the Spleen and Stomach, Ren 13 also transforms turbidity and phlegm. Additionally, Ren 13 can stabilize the spirit and mood.

Ren 14: The front mu of the Heart, Ren 14 disperses phlegm in the chest and diaphragm, transforms damp in the middle burner, clears the Heart and stabilizes the spirit, benefits the diaphragm, and descends rebellious Stomach qi. As Ren 14 taps right into the Emperor, caution should be used. Typically, one would not approach the Heart directly, but via the Pericardium (Ren 17 is a much more commonly used point). As such, it is often better to develop a relationship and rapport with a patient prior to releasing what is stored in the Heart.

Ren 15: The luo point of the Ren mai, Ren 15 has been discussed in the luo vessels chapter.

Ren 17: The front mu of the Pericardium, and the influential point of qi, Ren 17 downbears counterflow qi, clears the Lungs and transforms phlegm, tonfies qi, loosens the chest, and regulates the diaphragm. It can also be used to help synchronize the Lungs' relationship to the Heart and Pericardium and wei qi's influence over smooth muscle contractions (i.e., heartbeat, rate, and rhythm). It's a first-choice point for anxiety, insomnia, irritability, qi deficiency, depression, etc. as it creates a general impact over the entire chest, Lungs, Pericardium, and Heart.

Ren 18–21: These points can loosen and relax the chest and rectify the qi dynamic.

Ren 22: A Ren/Yin Wei mai meeting point, Ren 22 diffuses the Lung qi, transforms phlegm, and restores the voice. A WOS point, Ren 22, the celestial chimney, provides access to heaven's influence and the sensory portals. Needled down and behind the sternum, it can descend qi.

Ren 23: A Ren/Yin Wei mai meeting and termination point for shaoyin, Ren 23 nourishes yin, and impacts the throat and voice, allowing one to release traumas via speech and connection to others.

Ren 24: A Ren/Du/ST/LI meeting point, Ren 24 dispels wind, and diffuses fluids to the face and sensory portals.

Du mai

The Du mai utilizes the raw materials from Ren mai and the blueprint of Chong to create a solid structure/home with a strong foundation. With this stability in place and healthy bonds and boundaries, Du mai can seek to explore the external environment and world. This process allows for the process of individuation in service of growth, development, and the pursuit of one's destiny. Relying on Ren mai, and also sharing its trajectory in part, Du mai provides the safe structure of home in which to return, bringing back its experiences and relationships and further discovering oneself.

The experience of trauma often impacts the individual's ability and desire to explore the outside world, once considered safe, now considered dangerous. Curiosity and the need to form new experiences become damaged. The Du mai's interest in seeking newness and the drive to conquer the world becomes replaced with a defensive attitude, fearing the outside and finding it threatening. Simultaneously, a person also cannot find the same familiar comfort she once experienced prior to the trauma, making her feel unsafe and have a constant need for vigilance. Thus, Du mai encompasses both an ability to move outwards towards the external world or inwards to avoid excessive stimuli. Traumas can cause either of these directions to become predominant, often excessively moving in one direction at the expense of the other. A very common example is the child who is overstimulated from birth, often with bright lights, mobiles, loud music, and constant interactions, developing ADD or ADHD, or the common hypersensitivities and allergic responses. Insufficient stimulation creates the opposite dynamic with lack of motivation to the yang and a surplus of yin which can become stagnant.

Du mai's relationship with wei qi as a subset of yang qi, and its mediation of the Kidney yang and shaoyin connection to the Bladder taiyang, can create a hyperactivity of yang as a protective defensive measure. Hyperactivity often manifests with rebelliousness and the ascension of yang qi, creating such symptoms as dizziness, headaches and migraines, stiffness in the back from constant readiness for action, neck and occipital tension, and even wind and seizures at its extreme. Treating Du mai can help settle the hyperactive floating yang and anchor it to the Kidneys/ming men and lower back, utilizing yang's capacity for consolidating and preventing leakage.

Similarly, this tension in the nervous system creates an inability to relax within one's own body, causing tightness along the back, neck, sacrum, and even lower orifices where the Du mai traverses. Such tension here creates the proverbial anal personality type who is over-controlling, cannot relax or "let go" emotionally, and who often suffers constipation from this inability to let go physically. The drain on yang qi can often create a coldness in personality or an aloofness, and physically can create frigidity and/or impotence with attempted relationships. Needling the Du mai to release this tension and free up yang qi can ease one back into his body, relaxing the nervous system and mind.

Some individuals respond to broken boundaries, experiencing damage to their yang qi, often manifesting as lack of will, depression, and an inability to move forward in life. Here, the Triple Burner mechanism has become impacted, unable to properly disseminate. Frozen yang qi weakens the adrenals and one loses her animation and zest for life. The Triple Burner is tasked with disseminating yuan qi to the various back shu points of each of the zang fu. The quantity and quality of this dissemination determines the element/phase and personality type for a given individual. Trauma impacts this dissemination, and the normal (for the individual) amount of yuan qi to the organs is often displaced. A once fire constitution with confidence and a gregarious personality may become fearful, phobic, and withdrawn. Using Du mai, yang qi can be freed up to allow for one's constitutional displacement of yuan qi to be restored.

While some retreat inwards post trauma and assert strong boundaries, others exert a constant dissemination of wei qi by releasing any seeming care to his health and well-being. Such individuals become risk takers, seeking adrenaline rushes and partaking in dangerous activities, often ones that can be life-threatening. This can take the form of partying and substance abuse, constant sexual activity and encounters, extreme sports, and any such activity and behavior that causes a chronic loss/expenditure of yang qi. Here, the Triple Burner mechanism is working at full tilt, driving its yang qi to the extreme and depleting resources via constant adrenaline secretions.

As the source of yang qi, Du mai can either bring up and out (dissemination of yang and/or transformation of yang qi to wei qi), or descend and anchor yang qi in the Kidneys and ming men. Utilizing Du mai for either of these possibilities relies on different strategies. For the excessively vigilant patient, Du mai can be needled downwards, helping to anchor rebellious and floating yang qi into the lower back, ming men, and the Kidneys. For the patient with loss of animation, depression, lethargy, and lack of will, Du must be tonified to stoke the fire, often accomplished with the use of moxibustion as part of the treatment. In either of these scenarios, there may be the need to utilize the Bladder channel, often the sinew channel and its domain of the wei qi. As Du mai shares a trajectory, descending along the inner Bladder line, this can enhance the descension of yang back to its home. Alternatively, the Bladder sinew channel can be needled to release nervous system tension, muscle armoring, and any stagnation preventing yang qi from circulating to the exterior.

Combinations with Du mai for these purposes are many. One such option is to use the BL/KI DM in conjunction, using SDS needling when looking to release trapped yang qi or latency, and using DSD needling when seeking to anchor to the Kidneys or put the patient into a state of latency. With the BL/KI DM, or without, Dai mai can also be included, especially as it originates from the BL/KI DM, and traverses through Du 4, providing an additional Kidney energetic to a given treatment. Dai mai is often added when further releasing latency, or when one seeks to use it to store latency for a future time, as it is one of the most common places to do so.

With Ren mai, of course, the Du channel treatments go full circle, encompassing the nurturance of yin, security, bonding, etc. with either the ability to move out into the world and explore, or delve into the comforts offered by internalizing its yang into the yin. With Yang Wei mai, the two channels can be used to reconcile the painful and traumatic past experiences of life, bringing forth the yang needed to move forward. In this instance, as Yang Wei mai has a strong connection to the shaoyang and Du mai via its curvature, and axes allow for choices to be made via directional movement, these channels can be used together to harness one's ability to make decisions in service of seeing the blueprint fulfilled. As mentioned above, the Du mai is about independence, requiring the ability to stand upright; thus its use with the Yang Qiao mai is often to affect the integrity of the structure, providing a strong foundation with groundedness and stability. Yang Qiao assists with our ability to stand up to the world with confidence, and this requires a solid structural foundation. With both Yang Qiao mai and Yang Wei mai, Du mai promotes structural movement, a prerequisite for exploring the world and living with independence. Anyone can attest to the correlation with mood and particular postures; those who are depressed are often slumped over and the chest hollowed. Traumas and injuries to the back, especially near Du 4 and Du 14, can impact this integrity, and the reflexes required to control and use one's legs to move forward, and to initiate the head movement necessary to move towards that which one sees and desires. Using these two points as part of a Du mai treatment can assist with providing this much-needed motivation and desire.

Impact to the Du mai can also impact the yang of the Heart, creating either a rapid heartbeat (where stagnation and rebelliousness create hyperactivity and heat) or a slowing down (as yang qi becomes depressed). Its connection to the Heart's paired channel and the Fire phase yang channel, the Small Intestine, via its opening point SI 3 is instructive here. This provides an additional influence from Du mai's yang (and also that from the shaoyin Kidneys and their relationship to the Small Intestine's paired taiyang partner, the Bladder). How the Heart responds depends in part on how the patient experiences and/or attempts to reconcile one's traumas. For example, should the Kidneys be already in a weakened state, the capacity of yang qi may either be already impaired (showing for example a Deep pulse in the proximal positions), or unanchored (showing an Empty pulse in the proximals). With the first scenario a slow heartbeat is more common as Kidney yang is unable to support Heart yang; with the latter, a more rapid one, as yang qi floats away uncontrolled by yin. An additional connection based on Du mai's trajectory (especially Du 15), and the relationship to the Heart, is the influence over the throat and speech. Promoting the capacity for speech allows one to give voice and articulate one's pain in service of expressing and releasing it. Often traumas include the victim's inability to speak about it, or very commonly during a traumatic experience, one loses the capacity to speak, or yell, as they become frozen.

Du mai's trajectory, especially its upper one, strongly impacts the head, brain, and sensory portals. Its ability to bring yang qi up and/or down can modulate how yang qi functions. Common Du mai symptoms from excess yang qi in the head include red swollen eyes, headaches, and seizures. The nourishment of the portals themselves can help impact a patient's perspective and ability to see her life (and her past trauma(s)) in a new light, providing the initiating catalyst towards healing. These trajectories also traverse the lower brain (important for survival instincts and the will to live), the middle brain (the ability and desire to create relationships), and the upper brain (that which controls differentiation, likes, dislikes, etc.). Thus, utilizing points on any of these zones (or combination thereof) can influence these functions. Its trajectory along the spine, or course, also influences the sensory-motor tracts and assists one with promoting movement and allowing a patient to pursue one's goals and dreams. Senses and motor expressions are intimately linked; the more one senses and desires, the more inclination to move towards realizing those desires. Post trauma, there is often an imbalance in this expression, e.g., hypersensitivity or dulled senses and expressions. Du mai can be activated to mediate this relationship.

Du mai points most applicable to Heart Shock

Du 1: The luo point, and meeting point of KI/LR/GB, Du 1 harmonizes yin and yang, courses qi, regulates the intestines, relieves pain, regulates the Ren and Du, and calms the mind. Not needled as often as can be helpful due to its location, Du 1 can provide a strong release of yang qi, one that initiates a more positive mood, and call to action, unfreezing yang left immobilized from traumas.

Du 2–3: Used less often than Du 4, and mostly when it doubles as a local ashi point, Du 2 and 3 both strengthen the lower back, regulate the blood chamber and palace of essence, and tonify yang.

Du 4: One of the most influential of Du mai points, ming men is an instrumental point in strengthening the Kidney qi and yang, regulating the Triple Burner dissemination, securing essence, warming and nourishing one's vitality, benefitting essence, providing willpower and drive, and expelling cold (fright and paralysis). It can strengthen the shen by providing yang qi to support Heart yang, and also calms the mind and relaxes the nervous system.

Du 5–8: While used less often than some of the other Du mai points, these points can strengthen the Spleen and Stomach, address dampness, supplement the Kidneys, and calm the spirit. Where digestive issues present, these points can be a nice addition to a Heart Shock treatment focused on Du mai.

Du 9: At the level of the diaphragm shu, Du 9 rectifies qi and loosens the chest and diaphragm, and also regulates the activity of the Liver and Gall Bladder. Du 9 is a junction point and often used to help assist with either the upward movement of yang qi or its descension depending on the angle of needling.

Du 10: At the level of BL 16, Du 10 has an excellent use of being able to diffuse the Lung qi.

Du 11: At the same level as BL 15, Du 11 quiets and clears heat from the Heart and spirit, relaxes the nervous system, calms wind, relieves pain, and calms the mind.

Du 12–13: These points can calm the spirit, clear heat from the Heart and blood, nourish the Lungs, and regulate the shaoyang.

Du 14: Along with Du 4, Du 14 is probably the most influential point on the Du mai. It is a meeting point of all the yang channels; it clears heat, strengthens yang qi, clears the Heart and calms the spirit, regulates qi, clears the mind and brain (opens the portals), frees circulation of yang qi throughout the body, and brings yang qi up to the head.

Du 15: The first point on the head, Du 15 relaxes the joints, frees the portals, clears the spirit disposition, stimulates speech, clears the senses, and restores consciousness. It can be used for mental disorders, spirit problems, wind symptoms, paralysis, etc.

Du 16: A meeting point of Du/Yang Wei/BL, Du 16 rids wind and cold, relaxes the joints, clears the spirit, and benefits the brain. One of the four sea points for the marrow, it relaxes the nervous system.

Du 17: The "brain door," Du 17 dispels wind, settles tetany, rouses the brain, and opens the portals.

Du 18–19: These points calm the Liver, extinguish wind, soothe the sinews and channels, and quiet the Heart and spirit. Good for restlessness, agitation, confusion, obsessiveness, insomnia, etc.

Du 20: With Du 4 and Du 14, Du 20 is probably the most commonly used point on the Du mai. It extinguishes Liver wind and subdues Liver yang, clears the spirit disposition, returns inversion, lifts fallen yang qi, discharges heat in the yang channels (especially with Du 14), clears the senses and calms the spirit, tonifies yang, strengthens the ascending function of the Spleen, and brings the clear yang to the head and brain to promote clarity (of vision and perceptions/understanding). Du 20 allows one to communicate with heaven and accord with one's curriculum. It also lifts the mood, and helps with concentration and memory.

Du 21–23: These points strengthen the mind, calm the Liver, open the portals, and treat insomnia, anxiety, etc. Du 22 is noted for settling fright. Du 23 is used for freeing the portals, especially the nose and eyes.

Du 24: A meeting of Du and Bladder, Du 24 calms the Liver, extinguishes wind, quiets the Heart and spirit, clears the mind, and opens the portals (especially clearing the nose, and even treating polyps). ST 8 has a trajectory to Du 24, enabling it to deposit one's perceptions into the brain. Using these points together can help to create a fresh start, wiping clean old ways of viewing the world.

Du 25: Du 25 opens the portals, returns yang and stems counterflow, clears the senses, and raises yang qi, especially for restoring consciousness.

Du 26: A meeting of Du/ST/LI, Du 26 returns inversion, clears the spirit, resuscitates, benefits the lower back and lumbar spine, resonates with Du 4, and clears the senses. It can be used for mental disorders, epilepsy, hysteria, etc.

Du 27–28: These points nourish yin, quiet the spirit, diffuse the Lungs, and free the portals, especially the eyes. They can also relieve itching (all itchy painful sores that impact the Heart).

Yin Wei mai

As we move into the second ancestry, the Yin Wei mai is tasked with linking all the yin of the body together, ultimately returning back to Ren mai at the throat, and internalizing its resources to maintain proper nourishment and stability. Yin Wei mai reflects the playing out of Ren's resources in the cycles of 7 and 8 and how those resources have been used over time.

Not everyone ages at the same rate, and most people will probably agree that those who have experienced hardships and traumas tend to age more quickly and seem older than they are physically. This is a reflection of the toll on Yin Wei mai from Heart Shock. The first point on the trajectory of Yin Wei mai is KI 9, which represents the astringing of the yin-essence lost, and consolidating that into the lower abdomen as it moves upwards.

One of the most important functions of Yin Wei mai in the service of treating Heart Shock is its ability to bring yin to the Heart. As one of the primary treatment strategies in treating trauma, Yin Wei mai becomes a very important treatment option. As it brings yin to the Heart, it helps to stabilize runaway yang, slow down an elevated heartbeat, calm the shen, and provide comfort and calm. It also brings yin to that which the Heart regulates, the tongue. As it goes to Ren 23, Yin Wei mai brings nourishment to the throat and tongue to allow one to speak and release traumas through connection with others.

Part of this connection to others is further rooted in the bonding and security of the Earth phase, and the lower abdominal trajectory of Yin Wei mai. This establishes Yin Wei mai's role in socialization and connection with others, specifically from the Spleen points on the abdomen. This includes traumas associated with socialization, bullying, peer pressure, being humiliated, etc. As was discussed earlier in this chapter, the Spleen also becomes damaged with blame, a common scenario post trauma as the victim seeks to understand and rationalize his suffering. Stagnation and turbidity in the Spleen and abdomen can also manifest with obsessiveness and overthinking, a feeling of being stuck in the possibilities of what could have been, and a lack of acceptance of one's past, or a longing to relive the past prior to being damaged by trauma.

Yin Wei mai is tasked with bringing its essence up to the lower abdomen and the earth, to provide the context and narrative that Spleen mediates, then up to the Liver and wood to invigorate the blood (and the shen carried within it), and into the chest and throat, eventually back into the Ren mai as a new foundation/narrative/ perspective. This trajectory (of Ren mai) then moves to the eyes so that one sees life differently going forward. This communication back into the Ren mai is also a return of nourishment and contentment and a pacifying of spirit.

Yin Wei mai can be used to treat the nine Heart pains. These include the issues of life and parts of one's curriculum that have not been able to be completed. This can create the result, of course, of traumas and life events preventing this realization. As part of this failure to achieve a desired end, patients often present with frustration, irritability, anger, poor self-esteem, and feelings of inadequacy. Heat from stagnation can develop, as can yin deficiency as the heat burns off yin over time. Oppressive heat can result in compensation, causing dampness as a response. Another chronic manifestation is blood stagnation. Common symptoms that can attend to the heat, damp-heat, blood stasis, or yin deficiency can include angina, palpitations, shortness of breath or heaviness in the chest, anxiety, etc.

Yin Wei mai influences how an individual evaluates themselves and their life, where it has been and projecting where it is going. Often the disjunctive aspects play a major role in this analysis, and traumas are some of the most disjunctive and influential events. In addition to the specifics of a traumatic event, Yin Wei mai also influences how a person views her curriculum, including how she feels about her genetics, how that influences her socialization (embracing or rebelling against it), and the potential stagnation of blood (and the shen within) as a result. Yin Wei mai links together the essence/genetics (Kidney) with socialization (Spleen), and how that is invigorated to the chest (Liver and diaphragm) for animation and return to Ren mai. Where rebellion exists, symptoms such as running piglet qi can present, and Yin Wei mai is often combined with Chong mai for this purpose. Some individuals suffer trauma and significant fear from the potential playing out of genetic diseases, unable to relax and think of much else except succumbing to a disease that runs in the family. Yin Wei mai with Chong mai can be treated to quell these fears. It can also potentially enable someone to utilize their essence and will (Kidneys) to alter the way one sees things (Spleen narrative), and change the way they perceive these fears, utilizing an epigenetic approach to alter the future expression of disease.

A part of one's internal evaluation of self, Yin Wei mai is looking to the past and how one used to be as the barometer for how one should still be. Traumas of course can dramatically alter one's life and path, including relationships that may no longer exist, as well as physical structures and capabilities that are no longer there. Part of Yin Wei mai's imbalance is holding onto the past, reliving old memories, and being unable to be in the present. Its trajectory on the diaphragm/Liver and throat is about invigorating the blood and shen to release these holdings, as well as diffusing the Lungs (Ren 22) to be in the moment, and connect back to the heavenly qi (WOS point). Thus, one can let go of an old, and unserving, sense of self.

Yin Wei mai plays a role in invigorating blood, as it can utilize the Liver's energetics to release blood stagnation in the diaphragm and chest, where many traumas are held. When seeking this as a primary strategy, I will often combine Yin Wei mai with either Chong mai and/or the great luo of the Spleen. Using SP 21 and/or GB 22, and tapping into the Da Bao/Great Wrap, and LR 14 from Yin Wei mai, one can further enhance the blood-invigorating aspect of Yin Wei mai and promote significant movement in the diaphragm and chest to release trauma. Utilizing the lower portion of the trajectory (the Spleen points), one also creates a resonance to the SP 21 (great luo) and Chong mai (SP 4 and ST 30), creating a multi-faceted approach with many potential uses. It also opens the possibility to further the impact on the chest with Chong mai's upper trajectory connecting to the Kidney shu points. If looking to consolidate, these Kidney shu points can be needled towards the midline and Ren channel, and Yin Wei mai's KI 22 and KI 23 can be incorporated.

The Yin Wei mai also has a domain over the humors as a channel that links all aspects of yin together. That includes the yin-essence, jin-ye, and blood. In terms of this role, and coupled with how it regulates and adjusts to the cycles of 7 and 8, including the recording of one's experience, Yin Wei mai impacts the memory. Memory, of course, is often selective and can be quite fluid. What one remembers and how one remembers it can be influenced by many factors, trauma being one major factor that can distort it significantly. As mentioned above, Yin Wei mai can be used to tap into one's narrative and the entire contextual framework it resides in. Moving the blood and yin in this part of the trajectory can alter that framework, bringing it to the Liver (blood storage) to be recorded for later recall/retrieval. For this context, Yin Wei mai can be coupled with the Chong mai, or Dai mai, to move the yin-blood stasis in the abdomen.

Yang Wei mai

The Yang Wei mai links us with our past and represents changes to our ability to move and function over the cycles of 7 and 8. Like Yin Wei mai, it helps us to reconcile and process some of the most significant traumas and events of our lives and rites of passage.

An inability to link together yang of the body, often created by trauma, can create a leakage of yang qi. Yang qi that cannot be consolidated can result in symptoms such as wei qi deficiency/insufficiency, loss of will and motivation (and depression), and lack of self-control. The Yang Wei mai, as an 8x vessel, is created via the process of an overflow of one's boundaries, resulting in a ditch being created. The Long pulse of Yang Wei mai is one such energetic sign that the individual cannot maintain control of her yang qi.

Additional Classical signs of a Yang Wei mai imbalance include alternating chills and fever, indecisiveness, and dizziness (especially visual). All three of these symptoms have an association with the Gall Bladder and the ability to make decisions based upon a deep intuitive sense of what is right for oneself. This dynamic and ability relies heavily on the communication of the Heart and Kidneys, the fire–water axis that everything else revolves around. On the five element sheng cycle, wood lies between water and fire, and the yang aspect of wood, the Gall Bladder, acts as an intermediary. This role provides an ability to decide, based upon one's knowledge of self (Kidneys), and bringing that forth to the Heart in service of the curriculum. Alternation of chills (cold) and fever (heat) demonstrates a lack of regulation in this role. Visual dizziness also suggests an inability to see which direction to move in, and can result in a feeling of being scattered and out of control. Here, the Gall Bladder is forced to consider and evaluate the myriad options and contingency plans, stressing the Liver, obsessing about the future, yet creating an inability to move forward.

Lack of regulation of yang qi also creates vulnerability, instability, and insecurity. Wei qi's domain over the exterior becomes compromised, and its circulation to the head weakened, furthering the dizziness and alternating temperatures. This insecurity of the borders/boundaries is destabilizing physically as well as mentally. Susceptibility to colds and EPFs is common, as is a general sense of caution and fear of the outside and external world. A person becomes unable to manifest her curriculum or exert her five element constitution, feeling as if she cannot reach her potential. Stagnation of both the physical structure, as well as mental-emotional faculties, develops. The patient becomes trapped in the past and depressed, and potentially anxious and afraid of the future (or creating the tendency to daydream, or a longing for some future fantasy). Another option, similar to one experienced via Du mai, is that the lack of wei qi and defensive boundary creates a constant moving up and out, not stopping to link back to Du mai, but rather to keep one's yang directed towards the external. Here, decision-making does not serve the constitution, or the directed efforts of yang in service of the curriculum, but rather is a constant drain on yang qi via behaviors that are risky and depleting. These can include frequent and/or risky sexual encounters, addictive behaviors including drug use, over-exercising to the point of depleting reserves and damaging the body structure, etc. This lack of consolidation and return creates ongoing leakage and depletion.

Yang Wei mai's traversing of the head and brain influences the portals. Utilizing its trajectory allows one to reinforce the proper movement of yang qi to nourish the brain, and deposit one's experiences thereto. Influencing this dynamic, one can assist with allowing a change of perceptions post trauma, one consistent with the communication between the Heart and Kidneys. Bringing yang qi back to the source can influence the marrow and a patient's overall memory of their experiences. Insufficient yang qi circulating to the head can also create brain fog and damp obstructing the orifices.

As actions and movement are heavily dictated by one's experiences, trauma can have a profound impact on how a person behaves or views their reality. Often, the impact is to become anxious about the future, unhappy or unsatisfied with the present, including one's responsibilities and tasks/commitments. Constant comparisons are made based on previous experiences and abilities. Yang Wei mai helps with coming to terms with how things have changed over time. This includes bodily movement and coordination, so often dictated by one's comfort (both physically and emotionally) doing the movements, as well as determining how graceful one can be (which is in large part determined by how readily one can accommodate change).

Yin Qiao mai

As part of the third ancestry, the Yin Qiao mai is about self-reflection in the present. As such, it mobilizes its resources towards current consciousness and gazes deeply into the self, learning to trust oneself and regain faith.

Trauma shakes one to his core and often alters one's life moving forward. It can be difficult to accept the changes to oneself, one's environment and surroundings, relationships, etc. The myriad of emotions can present themselves, all rooted in a lack of acceptance, and oftentimes blame (here, usually to oneself). For the person who believes their trauma was a result of their own action, Yin Qiao mai can assist with providing a new perspective of acceptance, for oneself and for what one has experienced. A focus on KI 8 can assist with this dynamic.

The Yin Qiao mai person is one whose trauma has created an introvert, frustrated at his circumstances, and now feels the need to blame. Unable to stand up for himself, he becomes stagnant internally, outwardly often seeming apathetic and impotent. Internally, he becomes tight and restricted (medial muscle groups hypertonic), and his fight/flight/freeze muscles flaccid and weakened. His eyes become heavy, he has little motivation, and he seeks to sleep away his days. Adding KI 2 into this trajectory can help re-ignite one's fire and provide a boost to the will and yang.

The Qiao vessels meeting at BL 1 demonstrate their influence over wei qi arousal/stimulation and/or sedation/internalization. Yin Qiao mai also affects how one sees herself and includes aspects of self-esteem and self-worth, of course influenced by traumatic experiences and the sense of responsibility (guilt/blame) or acceptance one feels about it. As such, it plays a role in one's internal narrative (trajectory in the abdomen and Earth phase) and how one stands up to oneself in the wake of such experiences and perceptions. Its trajectory to ST 12 also influences the integrity of the canopy of the Lungs and how one fully inhales and receives inspiration. Guilt and blame often result in low self-esteem and depression and a sinking of the earth and integrity of the canopy. Lung and Heart qi become weakened, dampness and phlegm obstruct or mist the orifices, and one's capacity to animate and have confidence is impaired. Feelings of vulnerability are heightened and self-worth declines. Wei qi internalizes; one retreats inwards and feels depressed and sleepy.

In others it may create a need to compensate, creating an angry and boisterous quality the more insecure one feels. The need to prove oneself and gather accomplishments to offset feelings of worthlessness may result in aggressiveness.

This stimulation of wei qi can create hypervigilance and sensitivity as well as a rapid heart rate, and blood sugar, thyroid, and blood pressure issues. ST 9 can be influential in treating these.

Its meeting at BL 1 also suggests its influence over the hormonal system. This provides connection and synergy with the divergent channels as well. One popular treatment that can assist with the impact on the hormonal system is the combination with the SI/HT DM, as both utilize BL 1 as a major point. Similarly, the ST/SP DM can have useful combinations with the Qiao vessels, sharing BL 1 as well as ST 12 and ST 9, as well as regulating the impact of hypervigilance on depleting the fluids, resulting in chronic dehydration from constant financing of the wei qi (rooted in Stomach fluids). ST 9 and its proximity to the thyroid creates constant adjustments to the stimulation of wei qi (the thyroid sharing many wei qi functions). Symptoms of imbalance include those of an underactive thyroid (e.g., fatigue, hair loss, constipation, etc.).

Yang Qiao mai

Like the Yin Qiao mai above, the Yang Qiao mai reflects how one stands up to the world. Often, the compensatory aggressive personality trying to achieve to boost self-worth is reflective of Yang Qiao mai. But mostly, where Yin Qiao mai blames herself, Yang Qiao mai blames the world and seeks to change it. With wei qi at the exterior, BL 1 is always activated, looking to engage with the world. Classical symptoms of this constant engagement include insomnia, headaches, tremors, etc.

Exuberance of yang and the desire to change the world often result in the experience of conflict. This conflict with the outside world, and constantly seeing it as threatening, creates the ongoing response and sensitivity to it. Here, hypervigilance creates hypersensitivity to all external stimulants, including EPFs, another metaphor for what's wrong with the external environment reinforcing a need to fight.

The Yang Qiao mai person often becomes the rebel. With constant rebellious qi, however, come stagnation and the resultant heat. When excessive, this may engender wind and unpredictability. Should one come to the conclusion that his efforts are in vain, that his is unable to change the world, suicidal ideations and tendencies are a possible concern.

Yang Qiao mai assists Du mai with maintaining structure and mobilizing the muscle articulations to go out into the world. Often the obsession with moving yang outwards creates tension and stagnation from overuse, and an eventual depletion of yang qi and the structure. The yang muscle groups become hypertonic, while the yin ones become weak and flaccid, as wei qi's internal circulation is compromised to finance the constant hypervigilance. One may see changes to the posture and gait.

Via this connection to the skeletal system, one can also combine the Qiao vessels with the divergent channels in treatments. This can include the BL/KI DM providing a strong connection to the jing-essence and skeletal system, and can also tap into all the Bladder shu points and/or the wei qi and yuan qi aspects of the BL/KI dynamic.

One can also easily tap the SI/HT DM which provides access to the hypervigilance resulting in allergic responses to the external world and hypersensitivities and shares SI 10 as a trajectory point. It also strengthens the impact of yang qi on the chest. Combining with the GB/LR DM helps to tap into Liver blood and its control over the sinews, and adds a further connection to the eyes at GB 1, and to the reproductive and pelvic organs at Ren 2 which the Qiao and Ren mai regulate.

The Qiao vessels together have a strong connection to the hormonal system. Yang Qiao mai's trajectories traverse the thymus, breast, and thyroid glands and via their connection to BL 1, influence the pituitary and entire hormonal system, including the adrenals (connection to ming men and the Kidneys) and one's muscle tone. Via the adrenals and muscle tone, one is also mediating the release of adrenaline in terms of the fight/flight/freeze muscles, and hence activation of the nervous system.

Yang Qiao also traverses the portals, BL 1 as mentioned already, but also the mouth, nose, and eyes via ST 4, 3, and 1. It influences the way one assimilates sensory information and looks out into the world. Constant activation of the portals from hypervigilance and wei qi activity can create irritation to the eyes (red irritated eyes), nasal mucosa (allergies, polyps, sinusitis), and mouth (apthous ulcers, bleeding gums, digestive sensitivities) as so often seen in patients who have experienced trauma.

BL 1, as a major point reflecting wei qi, has far-reaching significance. The amount of light our eyes pick up plays a major role in how our organ systems function. As noted above, with its connection to wei qi and the thyroid, Yang Qiao excess often manifests in hyperthyroid symptoms (e.g., insomnia, high blood pressure, bulging eyes, etc.), as well as symptoms of Heart fire which are common post trauma.

Dai mai

One of the main functions of Dai mai is to absorb excesses that cannot be processed and move them into a state of latency. One of the major causes of these excesses is emotional (and physical) traumas.

With the capacity to accumulate that which we cannot let go of (including guilt and our inadequacies, loss and grief, etc.), Dai mai becomes the rug that pain, discomforts, and unresolved issues get swept under. As it fills up, it can exert pressure on the lower abdomen, cinching the waist (and diaphragm) and causing other systems to dysfunction. It can create pain in the lower back and/or abdomen, pressure or heaviness or a sinking feeling in the abdomen, and poor digestion and assimilation preventing the ascension of pure yang and the descension of the turbid. When filled to capacity, leakage can occur, as with vaginal discharges below, and outbursts of anger and/or crying above.

A recent patient experienced the death of his young child a few years ago, but continues to work tirelessly in a high-powered job, requiring constant travel and a relentless work schedule. He presented with Diaphragm, Dai mai, and Yin Wei mai pulses and acknowledged his inability to let go of the loss. The restrictions in the diaphragm (ancestral sinew) and Dai mai have created digestive and assimilation problems, along with guilt, and the inability to be in the moment with his other child; he is constantly focused on how life would be different if his son were still alive. At capacity with his suppression, he leaks tears easily, as well as experiencing anxiety. Using Dai mai, with Da Bao/great luo of the Spleen and Yin Wei mai, helped to move the stagnation, release the suppression, purge the diaphragm, and process this part of his life to help him move on.

Dai mai can be used in the context of trauma to rid and purge toxicity and long-term physical and emotional holdings. It can release the burden on the digestive system and help assist with assimilation (via food and nutrition and thoughts and ideas). In the context of releasing stagnant holdings, Dai mai can be used in relationship to the Gall Bladder to move and release stagnation and toxicity therein. As such it can also influence the hun (and po as reflected in the discussion on Wen Dan Tang in Chapter 6), which plays a major role in the recording of experiences to one's memory.

Dai mai can be used to free up space to allow for yang to descend and anchor into the lower abdomen. Often rebellious qi cannot be anchored if Dai mai is closed and full, preventing a clear communication to the lower burner. In these cases, we see symptoms of ascendant yang and a harassing of the shen in the chest with heat from stagnation causing anxiety, panic, insomnia, palpitations, tachycardia, etc. Pent-up emotions causing Liver and Gall Bladder qi stagnation and resultant tightness and restriction in the diaphragm can further the heat from stagnation and impact the chest. Releasing the Dai mai and the diaphragm with needling, gua sha, or herbs can remove the restrictions and provide space for yang qi to return home.

Dai mai can also be used to free up space to allow for additional areas of latency to be stored as necessary. It is often used with the GB/LR DM for this purpose, transferring latent pathogens to and from the divergent meridian system. When adding to Dai mai, the GB/LR DM is released via SDS and the pathogen is brought to Dai mai with a slow vibration technique to tonify. When releasing Dai mai, the pathogen can be removed with a rapid vibration technique and the GB/LR DM can be needled with SDS and a jing-well to release it externally, or via DSD to store it in the divergent for a later time.

As mentioned earlier, the Dai mai actually consists of three channel branches, the waist and pelvis, the diaphragm, and the SCM area. When the Dai mai becomes restricted, movement between the three burners becomes impaired. These three regions of Dai mai relate to the communication of the jing and qi (lower abdomen to chest), and the qi to the shen (chest to the head/brain and big shen). This communication is instrumental in alchemical and longevity practices, but also for mediating the relationship between our deepest self (jing), our relationships (qi), and our spirit (shen). The Triple Burner mechanism works to maintain the smooth transition and flow between these regions.

When too slack, the Dai mai can be consolidated and yang qi anchored to the abdomen. Here, the SJ/PC DM can be used in conjunction with the Dai mai treatment, needling it with DSD into the abdomen (Ren 12, lower confluent point), and also adding Ren 5 (Triple Burner mu point).

The Dai mai when full creates burden and turbidity. The weighing down of the functions of the Spleen and Stomach impact the effect of dampness, and can create a lack of clarity in one's thinking, congesting the portals. With Dai mai's influence over the Gall Bladder and Liver, this dampening of the portals can also impair creativity (which involves the ability to look/see into the future), clouding perceptions and how one moves towards what one sees. What maintains the latency in Dai mai is also jing-essence, which becomes stagnant and impairs circulation to the reproductive organs (one interpretation of the ancestral sinew impacted by Dai mai). Lethargy, indecisiveness, depression, and infertility can follow as one becomes stagnant and blocked. Releasing Dai mai and purging the turbidity can ease this process for those unable to move forward in life.

8x herbs and herbal formulas

Herbs that resonate with the 8x vessels

While not discussed in Bensky and Gamble's *Materia Medica*, others have taught on the various correlations of herbs to the 8x vessels. The list below is a compilation of teachings from Jeffrey Yuen as well as a couple other sources, including Bob Flaws' article summarizing the Ye Tian Shi Zhen Zhi Da Quan (*A Great Collection of Ye Tian-shi's Diagnoses and Treatments*), as well as Maciocia,[176] a compilation of readings, and my own experience.

In some cases, the lists of herbs said to resonate with the 8x vessels can be lengthy, especially when consolidating multiple sources. While this may seem to make some of these connections potentially less reliable, my perspective is to look at the herbs from the potential functions and usages of the 8x vessel in question, and see how the herbal functions may be used to strengthen that certain aspect of an 8x channel. For instance, Chong mai can be accessed via its blood nourishment functions with Shu Di Huang, Bai Shao, Dang Gui, Shan Zhu Yu, etc. But for its relationship to the Spleen and Kidneys, Bai Zhu, Bu Gu Zhi, Yi Zhi Ren, and Ren Shen are more appropriate. In many cases, herbs are said to resonate with multiple 8x vessels, also creating confusion and potential uncertainty as to their use. The key to understanding the herbs and their relationships is based on the combinations with other herbs. For example, while Shu Di Huang can resonate with the Chong, Ren, and Du, it will move to the Chong when combined with Mai Men Dong, the Du when combined with Gan Jiang, and it will be more focused to the Ren mai when coupled with Xuan Shen.

While the lists below are provided to the reader to begin the process of understanding the particular affinities of the herbs to the 8x channels, it is beyond the scope of this text to analyze each of the herbs and its relationships. It is trusted to the reader's understanding of herbal medicine to further delineate the connections of the herbal functions to the particular energetics of the 8x vessels as described above. The lists are simply a starting point in that process. The lists below are basic classifications, and many of the herbs can be included in multiple categories. They are provided as is for ease of reference only.

Chong mai

Herbs that regulate the SP/ST, nourish or strengthen blood, invigorate blood, astringe the Spleen and, Kidneys, strengthen the Heart and Kidneys, and affect the chest.

SP/ST	Tonify blood	Move qi/blood	SP/KI	HT/KI
Bai Zhu	Shan Zhu Yu	Bie Jia	Ba Ji Tian	Ren Shen
Ban Xia	Bai Shao	Chuan Lian Zi	Qian Shi	Fu Zi
Cang Zhu	Shu Di Huang	Chuan Xiong	Bu Gu Zhi	Rou Gui
Ren Shen	Gou Qi Zi	Shan Zha	Yi Zhi Ren	Wu Wei Zi
Wu Zhu Yu	Dang Gui	Lai Fu Zi	Shan Yao	
Mai Men Dong	Bai Zi Ren	Mu Dan Pi	Huang Jing	**LR/KI**
Xiao Hui Xiang		Xiang Fu	Rou Cong Rong	Shan Zhu Yu
Dai Zhe Shi			Huang Bai	Hu Tao Ren
Ge Gen			Fu Ling	Sha Yuan Zi
				LU/KI
				Ge Jie

Ren mai

Herbs that nourish yin and/or move yin stasis, strengthen the Lungs and impact the chest, and nourish the Spleen/Stomach and Liver/Kidneys.

Nourish yin	Yin stasis	Lungs/Chest	SP/ST	LR/KI
Gui Ban	Bie Jia	E Jiao	Bai Zhu	Ba Ji Tian
Shu Di Huang	Cang Zhu	Gan Jiang	Cang Zhu	Fu Pen Zi
Sheng Di Huang	Chen Pi	Dan Shen	Ding Xiang	Zi He Che
Mai Men Dong	Huang Bai	Chuan Xiong	Mu Xiang	Chuan Lian Zi
Xuan Shen			Xiao Hui Xiang	
			Wu Zhu Yu	
			Hou Po	
			Zhi Shi	
			Chen Pi	

Du mai

Herbs that strengthen yang, impact the spine, portals, and brain, and regulate bones.

Yang	Spine/Muscles	Portals	Brain	Bones/Essence
Lu Rong	Qiang Huo	Cang Er Zi	Gou Qi Zi	Gou Qi Zi
Zi He Che	Du Huo	Chuan Jiao	Chuan Xiong	Du Zhong
Lu Jiao (Jiao)	Gao Ben		Gao Ben	Xu Duan
Lu Jiao Shuang	Ge Gen		Tian Ma	Gou Ji
Rou Gui				Shu Di Huang
Fu Zi				
Yin Yang Huo				
Suo Yang				
Gui Zhi				
Yang Gou				
Yang Waishen				

Yang	Spine/Muscles	Portals	Brain	Bones/Essence
Huang Qi				
Rou Cong Rong				
Gan Jiang				

Yin Wei mai

Herbs that nourish the Heart, regulate KI/SP/LR, invigorate blood, nourish yin, clear heat from the Heart and spirit, and open the portals.

Heart	KI/SP/LR	Blood	Yin	Heat/Portals
Gui Zhi	Yi Zhi Ren	Bai Shao	Bai Shao	Lian Zi (Xin)
Huang Qi	Xiao Hui Xiang	Dang Gui	Nu Zhen Zi	Dan Shen
Long Yan Rou	Fu Ling	Chuan Xiong	Sha Yuan Zi	Chi Shao
Bai Zi Ren	Nu Zhen Zi	Dan Shen		Yu Jin
Lu Jiao Shuang	Sha Yuan Zi	Chi Shao		Dan Nan Xing
		Mu Dan Pi		Shi Chang Pu
		Long Yan Rou		Mu Dan Pi

Yang Wei mai

Herbs that affect yang, the Triple Burner, things that are astringent/internalizing, hyperactive wei qi, and Heart pains.

Yang	Triple Burner	Astringe/ Internalize	Wei qi	HT pain
Gui Zhi	Xiang Fu	Bai Shao	Jue Ming Zi	Ku Shen
Huang Qi	Chuan Xiong	Suan Zao Ren	Di Gu Pi	Bai Zi Ren
		Dai Zhe Shi		Suan Zao Ren
		Mu Li		

Yin Qiao mai

Herbs that nourish yin, move yin stasis, affect the head, portals, and throat/chest, and treats prolapse and heat from stagnation of yin.

Yin	Yin stasis	Head/Portals/Eyes	Clear heat	Throat/Chest
Bie Jia	Bie Jia	Tian Ma	Mu Dan Pi	Wang Bu Liu Xing
Shi Jue Ming	Zhu Ling	Yuan Zhi	Sheng Ma	Kun Bu
Bai Shao	Qu Mai	Zhu Ling	Gan Cao	Hai Zao
Shu Di Huang	Ze Xie			
Gui Ban	Huang Bai			**Lift qi/Hernia**
Shan Zhu Yu	Fu Ling			Sheng Ma
Wu Wei Zi	Kun Bu			Chuan Lian Zi
Da Zao	Hai Zao			
	Bu Gu Zhi[177]			

Yang Qiao mai

Herbs that anchor and descend, or lift qi-yang, impact the eyes, and affect fluids and movement/sinews/bones (including essence which nourishes).

Descend	Lift	Eyes	Fluids	Movement
Di Fu Zi	Jiang Huang	Che Qian Zi	Wu Wei Zi	Ren Dong Tang
Che Qian Zi	Bai Zhi	Bai Zhi	Fu Ling	Qin Jiao
Fu Ling		Ren Dong Tang	Huang Bai	Gui Ban
Gui Ban			Mu Tong/Tong Cao	Shu Di Huang

Dai mai

Herbs to drain, impact the Gall Bladder and Triple Burner, astringe, nourish SP/ST/ KI qi, protect yin, and move stagnation (food, blood, etc.).

Drain	Astringe	GB/SJ	KI qi	SP/ST qi
Yin Chen Hao	Wu Wei Zi	Chai Hu	Huang Jing	Bai Zhu
Long Dan Cao	Qian Shi	Qin Jiao	Fu Pen Zi	Sheng Ma
Tao Ren	Lian Zi	Shan Yao	Xu Duan	
	Jin Ying Zi	Ai Ye		
	Wu Mei	Wu Zhu Yu	**Stagnation**	**Protect yin**
	Sang Piao Xiao	Sha Yuan Zi	E Zhu	Zhi Mu
	Long Gu		Tao Ren	Bai Shao
	Mu Li		Dang Gui	Shi Hu
	Fu Pen Zi			
	Sha Yuan Zi			

8x vessel formulas

There are a number of formulas that have been noted to impact the 8x vessels, most notably the Chong, Ren, and Dai mai. In addition to those, below I correlate a number of other formulas to the 8x channels based on their properties and the formula constituents, focusing on the ones more relevant to Heart Shock. While one can link many formulas to the 8x channels based on the information in this chapter, I will simply list a few representative formulas, leaving the reader to further explore the 8x energetics and herbs.

Chong mai and Ren mai

Wen Jing Tang (Warm the Menses Decoction)

Wu Zhu Yu	9g
Gui Zhi	6g
Dang Gui	9g
Chuan Xiong	6g
Bai Shao	6g
E Jiao	6g
Mai Men Dong	9g

Mu Dan Pi	6g
Ren Shen	6g
Ban Xia	6g
Gan Cao	6g

Classically used for deficiency and cold in the Chong and Ren from blood stasis, Wen Jing Tang warms the uterus and dispels cold, nourishes blood, and moves blood stasis. As a Heart Shock formula, it also strengthens the Heart qi (Ren Shen and Gui Zhi, and indirectly via Liver blood with Dang Gui, Bai Shao, and E Jiao) and Heart yin and blood (Mai Men Dong and E Jiao). It strengthens the Kidneys and anchors yang (Ren Shen, Wu Zhu Yu), calms the nervous system (Bai Shao, Mu Dan Pi), and supplements and unburdens the earth (Ren Shen, Wu Zhu Yu, Ban Xia, Gan Cao). Ban Xia and Wu Zhu Yu also have an impact on the portals by treating phlegm-damp and accessing the brain.

Gui Pi Tang (Restore the Spleen Decoction)

Ren Shen	15g
Huang Qi	30g
Bai Zhu	30g
Zhi Gan Cao	7.5g
Long Yan Rou	30g
Dang Gui	30g
Suan Zao Ren	30g
Fu Ling/Fu Shen	30g
Zhi Yuan Zhi	30g
Mu Xiang	15g
Sheng Jiang	5pcs
Da Zao	1pc

Gui Pi Tang is a classic formula for Spleen qi and Heart blood deficiency with symptoms such as palpitations, forgetfulness, anxiety, poor appetite, insomnia, etc. As a Chong mai formula, it can be used where the middle trajectory of Chong mai fails to ascend to the chest and Heart, creating the above symptoms. As a Heart Shock formula, it has been analyzed in the previous chapter.

Chong mai and Yin Wei mai

Together the Chong and Ren strongly influence the circulation of blood, thus resonating with Wang Qin-ren's blood-moving formulas. They have already been discussed in Chapter 5.

Xue Fu Zhu Yu Tang (see Chapter 5)

Ge Xia Zhu Yu Tang (see Chapter 5)

Shao Fu Zhu Yu Tang (see Chapter 5)

Shen Tong Zhu Yu Tang (see Chapter 5)

Ren mai

Da Bu Yin Wan (Great Tonify the Yin Pill)

Shu Di Huang	180g
Su Jiu Gui Ban	180g
Chao Huang Bai	120g
Jiu Chao Zhi Mu	120g
Marrow from pig's vertebrae	

Da Bu Yin Wan contains a few of the Ren mai herbs, including Shu Di Huang, Gui Ban, and Huang Bai. This formula strongly nourishes the yin of the Liver and Kidneys, while clearing and descending heat. Gui Ban will also nourish yin and tonify the Heart. A simple formula, additional herbs can be added to round out the Heart Shock strategies.

Liu Wei Di Huang Wan (Six Ingredient Pill with Rehmannia)

Shu Di Huang	240g
Shan Zhu Yu	120g
Shan Yao	120g
Ze Xie	90g
Mu Dan Pi	90g
Fu Ling	90g

This is a classic formula for Liver and Kidney yin deficiency with a weak marrow. Slightly different than Da Bu Yin Wan above, this formula contains astringents to help preserve the yin (Shan Zhu Yu), as well as blood invigoration (Mu Dan Pi), and herbs to strengthen the earth (Shan Yao, Fu Ling).

Mai Wei Di Huang Wan (Ophiopogonis Schisadra and Rehmmania Decoction)

Adding Mai Men Dong and Wu Wei Zi, this formula includes some of the SMS energetics, adding to our treatment strategies for Heart Shock, with the exception of opening the portals.

Du mai

Du Huo Ji Sheng Tang (Angelica Pubescens and Sangisheng Decoction)

Du Huo	9g
Xi Xin	6g
Fang Feng	6g
Qin Jiao	6g
Sang Ji Sheng	6g
Du Zhong	6g
Niu Xi	6g
Rou Gui	6g
Dang Gui	6g
Chuan Xiong	6g
Sheng Di Huang	6g
Bai Shao	6g
Ren Shen	6g
Fu Ling	6g
Zhi Gan Cao	6g

Du Huo Ji Sheng Tang is often used for damp-cold bi-obstruction syndrome with Liver and Kidney deficiency presenting with heavy and painful back and limbs, weakness, palpitations, etc. It opens the Du mai with its characteristic herbs Du Huo and Qiang Huo. Du Huo opens the lower spine and Qiang Huo the upper; both help move yang upwards along the spine. Rou Gui stimulates ming men (one can also utilize Fu Zi for this purpose); Fang Feng is used to settle any wind and to protect the exterior. Xi Xin and Qin Jiao assist with scattering cold and wind-damp in the sinews and release to the exterior. Si Wu Tang (Dang Gui, Bai Shao, Sheng Di Huang, Chuan Xiong) and Si Jun Zi Tang (Ren Shen, Fu Ling, Zhi Gan Cao) are included to nourish and move qi and blood with dosages adjusted to prioritizing movement over nourishment. As a Heart Shock formula it assists with strengthening Kidney yang (Rou Gui, Du Huo, Qiang Huo, Du Zhong), promoting individuation and movement into the world, and strengthening the structure so that one can stand on his own. It opens the orifices (Xi Xin), strengthens Heart yin and qi (Sheng Di Huang, Bai Shao, Ren Shen, Zhi Gan Cao), invigorates blood (Dang Gui, Chuan Xiong), protects the earth (Fu Ling, Rou Gui, Zhi Gan Cao), and calms the nervous system (Bai Shao, Qiang Huo, Du Huo, Qin Jiao).

Juan Bi Tang (Remove Painful Obstruction Decoction)

Qiang Huo	3g
Du Huo	3g
Qin Jiao	3g
Sang Zhi	9g
Hai Feng Tang	9g
Chuan Xiong	2.1g
Dang Gui	6g
Ru Xiang	2.5g
Mu Xiang	2.4g
Rou Gui/Gui Zhi	1.5g
Zhi Gan Cao	1.5g

While Du Huo Ji Sheng Tang above manages low back and extremity pain, Juan Bi Tang focuses more on the joints and upper limbs, both opening Du mai with Qiang Huo and Du Huo. In accordance with the Heart Shock principles, Kidney yang is further strengthened by Rou Gui/Gui Zhi, blood invigorated with Dang Gui, Chuan Xiong, and Ru Xiang, earth managed by Mu Xiang and Zhi Gan Cao, and the nervous system and sinews with Qiang Huo, Du Huo, Qin Jiao, Hai Feng Tang, Chuan Xiong, Sang Zhi, and Ru Xiang. Ideally, an herb for Heart yin can be incorporated here, Shu Di Huang being a good addition which will also warm and strengthen. Ru Xiang is also a fragrant herb which can open the orifices, and as a resin is instrumental in healing wounds.

Dai mai

Jiao Ai Tang (Ass-Hide Gelatin and Mugwort Decoction): Dai/Chong/Ren

E Jiao	6g
Ai Ye	9g
Sheng Di Huang	18g
Dang Gui	9g
Chuan Xiong	6g
Bai Shao	12g
Gan Cao	6g
Rice Wine	3 parts

Jiao Ai Tang treats abdominal pain with uterine bleeding, post-partum bleeding, and weakness in the lower back. Its sister formula, Ding Xiang Jiao Ai Tang, treats more uterine bleeding with an ice-cold sensation in the lower abdomen from a combination of blood deficiency and cold. Both formulas contain Si Wu Tang

(Jiao Ai Tang using Sheng Di instead of Shu Di), thus can nourish and tonify the blood while also invigorating. Sheng Di Huang in Jiao Ai Tang also nourishes the Heart yin and clears heat from the Heart, blood, and spirit. E Jiao further strengthens the blood and helps impact, and helps to stop bleeding (in Heart Shock this can be metaphorical wherein the patient is unable to soothe herself). The rice wine assists with keeping the blood moving and warming the circulation and creates an impact on the spirit. Ai Ye warms the Kidneys and unfreezes yang.

Ding Xiang Jiao Ai Tang (Clove Ass-Hide Gelatin and Mugwort)

Shu Di Huang	6–9g
Bai Shao	6–9g
Chuan Xiong	3–9g
Ding Xiang	3–6g
Ai Ye	6g
Dang Gui	6–9g
E Jiao	3–9g

Yin Qiao mai

Qing Gu San (Cool the Bones Powder)

Yin Chai Hu	1.5g
Zhi Mu	1g
Hu Huang Lian	1g
Di Gu Pi	1g
Qing Hao	1g
Qin Jiao	1g
Zhi Bie Jia	1g
Gan Cao	0.5g

Qing Gu San is the classic formula for steaming bone syndrome from Liver and Kidney yin deficiency, with such symptoms as tidal fevers, heat sensation in the bones, irritability, insomnia, night sweats, etc. It was also discussed in the divergent meridians chapter as it contains two DM signature herbs, Di Gu Pi and Bie Jia. Bie Jia also resonates with the Yin Qiao mai due to its ability to nourish yin and anchor yang, and also move yin stasis. This formula strongly clears heat from deficiency and nourishes yin. Its resonance to Yin Qiao mai helps to see oneself more clearly by comforting (yin nourishment) and clearing the vexing heat burning the structure. This formula is useful for those with poor self-image who are constantly beating themselves up and internalizing their emotions in a destructive way. This often leads to autoimmune diseases and cancers of the blood and lymph, which I often use this formula to treat. Modifications, of course, can be made to accord with the other Heart Shock strategies as needed, but this formula can be used for more acute presentations and a secondary formula added alternately. As is, the formula calms the nervous system, assists the Spleen, nourishes yin, anchors yang, and invigorates the blood.

Qing Hao Bie Jia Tang (Artemesia Annua and Soft-Shelled Turtle Decoction)

Bie Jia	5g
Qing Hao	2g
Sheng Di Huang	4g
Zhi Mu	2g
Mu Dan Pi	3g

Similar to Qing Gu San above, Qing Hao Bie Jia Tang clears heat from deficiency smoldering in the yin aspects of the body with night fevers and morning coolness, absence of sweat, emaciation, loss of appetite, etc. This formula nourishes yin, including the Heart (Sheng Di Huang, Bie Jia, Zhi Mu), clears heat from the Heart and from deficiency (Sheng Di Huang, Zhi Mu, Qing Hao, Mu Dan Pi), calms the nervous system (Mu Dan Pi, Sheng Di Huang), and invigorates blood (Mu Dan Pi, Bie Jia). Like Qing Gu San, it can be used alternately with a second formula to accommodate the missing Heart Shock strategies as needed.

Yang Wei mai

Xiao Chai Hu Tang (Minor Bupleurum Decoction)

Chai Hu	24g
Huang Qin	9g
Ban Xia	24g
Sheng Jiang	9g
Ren Shen	9g
Zhi Gan Cao	9g
Da Zao	12pcs

Xiao Chai Hu Tang is the classic formula for shaoyang syndrome with alternating fever and chills, bitter taste, hypochondriac pain, irritability, nausea, vomiting, and visual dizziness. In the context of Yang Wei mai and Heart Shock, it treats the bitterness one feels towards life post trauma, and the ultimate confusion regarding which direction to move in. Dampness and heat linger, creating irritability, with an inability to resolve one's symptoms and situation. This formula helps to remove obstructions in the healing process. It can be combined or alternated with a formula to satisfy the remainder of the Heart Shock strategies.

Yin Wei and Yang Wei mai

Dang Gui Gui Zhi Tang (Dang Gui and Cinnamon Twig Decoction)

Dang Gui	9g
Gui Zhi	1g
Bai Shao	3g
Ban Xia	6g
Zhi Gan Cao	0.6g
Pao Jiang	2pcs
Da Zao	3pcs
+	
Lu Jiao Shuang	
Sha Yuan Zi	
Gou Qi Zi	
Xiao Hui Xiang	
Bai Zi Ren	
Fu Ling	

Dang Gui Gui Zhi Tang, with the additions noted as per Ye Tian Shi,[178] resonates to the Wei mais. It nourishes Heart yin and blood (Bai Zi Ren), Heart qi (directly via Gui Zhi and Zhi Gan Cao, and indirectly with Dang Gui, Bai Shao, and Gou Qi Zi), strengthens, anchors, and consolidates the Kidneys (Lu Jiao Shuang, Sha Yuan Zi, Xiao Hui Xiang), benefits the earth (Ban Xia, Pao Jiang, Da Zao, Zhi Gan Cao, Fu Ling, Xiao Hui Xiang), affects the portals (Gou Qi Zi), and astringes to stop bleeding (Pao Jiang, Lu Jiao Shuang) and thus the nine Heart pains.

Yin Wei mai

Yi Guan Jian (Linking Decoction)

Sheng Di Huang	18g
Gou Qi Zi	9g
Sha Shen	9g
Mai Men Dong	9g
Dang Gui	9g
Chuan Lian Zi	4.5g

Yi Guan Jian serves as a Heart Shock formula consistent with Yin Wei mai's functions of securing essence, and linking the Kidneys, Spleen, and Liver. Used often for yin deficiency with heat symptoms from stagnation, including hypochondriac pain, epigastric pain or distension, dry mouth and throat, acid reflux, etc., Yi Guan Jian demonstrates its influence over the major aspects of Yin Wei mai's trajectory. It strongly nourishes Heart yin (Sheng Di Huang, Mai Men Dong, Sha Shen), nourishes and invigorates blood (Dang Gui, Gou Qi Zi), stabilizes the earth (Sha Shen, Mai Men Dong), calms the nervous system (Sheng Di Huang, Dang Gui, Chuan Lian Zi), and impacts the brain and eye portals (Gou Qi Zi). An additional herb can be added to protect Kidney yang if necessary.

Dang Gui Si Ni Tang (Tangkuei Decoction for Frigid Extremities)[179]

Dang Gui	9g
Gui Zhi	9g
Bai Shao	9g
Xi Xin	3g
Zhi Gan Cao	6g
Da Zao	25pcs
Mu Tong/ Tong Cao	6g

Dang Gui Si Ni Tang is used for blood deficiency and cold in the channels with cold hands and feet from poor circulation, as well as joint pain, menstrual irregularities, etc. It can be used in the context of Heart Shock where long-term stagnation from traumatic injuries damages the circulation. Additional nourishment to Heart yin can be warranted, as can further Kidney yang tonification as needed (Xi Xin warms the yang). The chest is opened with Gui Zhi and Mu Tong, blood nourished by Dang Gui, Bai Shao, and Da Zao, and invigorated by Dang Gui, Gui Zhi, and Mu Tong, the Spleen and Stomach addressed with Zhi Gan Cao and Da Zao, portals opened by Xi Xin, and the nervous system calmed by Bai Shao.

8x essential oils

Utilizing the essential oils with the 8x vessels creates a strong resonance to yuan qi and jing, as that is what essential oils represent as part of the plant they are derived from. Like always, we are creating essential oil blends which are then diluted and applied to the opening points and channel points associated with the respective 8x channel being entered. One drop of the diluted blend should be applied to each point, opening point first, with a vibration technique for approximately one minute.

Chong mai

Angelica: strengthens blood, communicates HT/KI, invigorates
blood, impacts the chest, nourishes the SP/ST

Patchouli: unburdens the SP/ST, impacts the chest and shen

Savory: strengthens the SP/ST, transforms damp, rids worms

Fennel: communicates HT/KI, strengthens the SP/ST/LR/KI, regulates fluids

Ren mai

Neroli/Orange Blossom: strengthens LU/SP, clears HT fire, calms shen

Ginger: warming, moves yin stasis and neediness,
harmonizes SP/ST, invigorates blood

Oakmoss: nourishes yin and moves yin stasis, breaks phlegm from LU

Du mai

Cedarwood: descends and clears heat toxins and inflammation from bone

Cinnamon Leaf: strengthens ming men, warms middle
and lower burner, invigorates blood

Rosemary: lifts yang qi, promotes yang qi and wei qi to the surface, opens the
diaphragm, stimulates LR/GB; chemotype camphor strengthens Heart yang

Yin Wei mai

Rose: communicates HT/KI, clears HT/LR fire

Melissa: clears heat in HT/LR and blood, relaxes chest

Clary Sage: communicates HT/KI, nourishes yin,
clears heat in blood, calms LR wind

Vetiver: nourishes and invigorates the blood, clears heat in blood,
calms shen, regulates LR qi and tones the sinews

Frankincense: invigorates blood, heals wounds, relaxes the diaphragm,
clears heat in and promotes circulation of LU, calms the shen

Vanilla: nourishes LR and hun, and KI and willpower, calms shen and comforts

Yang Wei mai

Rosemary: lifts yang qi, promotes yang qi and wei qi to the surface, opens the diaphragm, stimulates LR/GB; chemotype camphor strengthens Heart yang

Citronella: clears heat in wei level, resolves hot bi-obstruction syndrome

Rosalina: clears wind-heat and allergic responses, calms ST fire

Yin Qiao mai

Narcissus: communicates HT/KI, calms shen, promotes self-love

Jasmine: nourishes KI yin, communicates HT/KI, promotes comfort with self, clears LR fire

Juniper: nourishes and warms LR blood, promotes circulation and menstruation, moves wind-damp-cold bi-obstruction and drains damp-cold

Yang Qiao mai

Basil: strengthens KI yang and wei qi, resolves wind-cold, descends ST qi

Cinnamon Leaf: strengthens ming men, warms middle and lower burner, invigorates blood

Dai mai

Mugwort: warms uterus, promotes menstruation, expels cold in abdomen and Dai mai

Sandalwood: clears damp-heat in lower burner, opens the diaphragm, calms shen

Niaouli: clears damp-heat in lower burner, tonifies LU/KI qi

Patchouli: clears damp-heat and fermentation

Savory: strengthens SP/ST and transforms damp

Cypress: consolidates/astringes

CHAPTER 9

Gui and Gu

Trauma as a Ghost/Parasite

Gui/ghosts and gu/parasites

As discussed earlier in this text, one can conceive of trauma as a pathogen that has entered into the interior aspects of the body and gained residence. As such, it interferes with and impacts physiology and psychology on a very profound level. The concepts of "gu"/parasites and "gui"/ghosts are two possible manifestations of this pathogen concept. In the discussion below, I will first present the concept of gui and discuss acupuncture, herbal, and essential oil therapies followed by the same with regard to gu. Both gu and gui can provoke substantial mental-emotional and psychological reactions. The discussion of gui below demonstrates some of the extreme symptoms that it can create.

The nature of the relationship to Heart Shock is a bit different with each of these concepts. Often, with gui, an experience of Heart Shock makes one vulnerable to the influence of a gui. It is not uncommon for Heart Shock to create a scenario wherein the individual becomes depressed, introverted, and extremely vulnerable. It can also create issues of altered or lack of consciousness, as well as dissociation, which leaves one vulnerable to the gui entering. Additionally, surgeries and other medical procedures that alter consciousness (e.g., anesthesia) pose a heightened threat to gui.

Gu, on the other hand, is more often the catalyst in the creation of Heart Shock. Being exposed to the varied hosts that can enter and colonize within one's body can be extremely disheartening and challenging on a mental-emotional level. Where there is vulnerability preexisting, even a relatively minor infestation of gu (parasites, worms, etc.) can provoke a significant response. And of course, many infestations of gu can be extremely recalcitrant and difficult to treat. Living for extended (or even short) periods of time where the internal landscape has been shifted to accommodate gu can create physical symptoms, too, that can be quite dispiriting and traumatic. And many of these gu-type infestations can provoke profound symptoms (e.g., Lyme's disease with joint pains, fatigue, brain fog and difficulty thinking/concentrating, debilitating headaches, central and peripheral nervous system dysfunctions, etc.).

It is important to acknowledge that the wear and tear of such symptoms can be the cause of a Heart Shock diagnosis.

Gu and gui share many similarities as well as a number of treatment strategies with Heart Shock, as delineated in Part I. But, due to the unusual nature of these issues, they also require some additional information in order to strategize their successful treatments with the Heart Shock context. Below is a discussion of each concept with its unique strategies for successful integration into the Heart Shock framework.

Gui

Gui are referred to as ghosts or demons (which contains the character for gui with an additional radical signifying an infestation with increased severity). Gu and chong are referring to worms or insects. Daoist literature describes what these different kinds of worms look like, but they can also act as metaphors for the temptations in our lives. Hexagram 18 of the I Jing (Gu, Wind, and Mountain trigrams) relates to gu which becomes a receptive host to parasitic infestations and blocks the possibility of change just as a mountain blocks the wind. Gu is generally something that can be contracted from food/drink, especially things high in sugar (i.e., dampness). It is associated with decay and could also be contracted from areas where a lot of people are sick and dying, and even traditionally from brothels. Venomous animals (including scorpions) and horns were also used to detect and treat the presence of gu, especially when used in black magic or as poisons. Gu has the capacity to damage the jing-essence and required strong treatments historically. Gui were often contracted in areas of the sick and dying as well, but also in places generally considered cold and damp (yin influences) or in people with an internal yin condition, e.g., dampness, phlegm, cold, sadness, fear, obsession, etc. Gui are said to loiter in areas such as bars, brothels, and places where people are depressed, drinking alcohol, and altering their consciousness. Another common time people contract gui is when they themselves are sick and weak or during medical procedures under anesthesia, etc. They are often contracted via the sensory orifices. There are three types of gui:

- Wandering ghosts: someone who died while traveling, or any spirit that feels he did not complete his journey or mission in life and felt incomplete at the time of passing

- Hungry ghosts: someone who dies unsatisfied, having failed to learn to control or relinquish one's desires and appetites

- Sexual ghosts: someone who is clinging to sexual and/or romantic feelings and cannot leave that person behind.

What gui and gu both have in common is that they tend to create mental and emotional imbalances and disturb the spirit (shen), creating a lack of control over one's life. They also can disturb the soul (ling) and create growth and developmental issues. Earlier we discussed a little bit about the hun and the po; both characters contain the radical for gui (hun has "cloud" next to it; po has "white" next to it). Hun depicts the image of clouds. Rain ascends from earth and creates clouds which are considered the intermediaries to heaven. Hun is collective consciousness, accumulating a "cloud" of personal experience. At death it leaves the body to a dimension between heaven and earth and serves as a database or central reservoir that collects your memories and experiences during your lifetime. Shamans and psychics tap into this to gain information. The Liver ascends, and shamanic dances tend to use twirling and spiraling to ascend their spirits and astro-project. This can be done with internal techniques to allow one's qi to go upward towards the upper realms. Needling techniques (see below) for gui mimic this action.

Po are more yin, and are said to linger around the earth for 49 days after death. This is why families of lost loved ones should refrain from demonstrating grief or sadness towards the end of this period, as doing so could encourage the po to linger and miss its ascension into the next realm. Po are earthbound entities/spirits and can become suspended in this realm because of attachments. Once this happens, they seek out others to use to take them to the next dimension. They are said to look for people that are very yin, sad, depressed, isolated, lonely, etc. Entities come in via the orifices, particularly during times of vulnerability (i.e., illness), and encourage their hosts to engage in behaviors that are likely to accelerate death and entry into the next realm. A person might then demonstrate reduced appetite or even anorexia or starvation and withdraw from the world. They may also engage in activities that would quickly deplete jing-essence (e.g., masturbation, increased sexual intercourse, drug and alcohol abuse), weaken the immune system, and create scenarios in which they will catch diseases, as well as partake in activities that are risky and life threatening. Eventually, latent issues will manifest, notably cancers and other significant illnesses, as the po attempts to piggyback on the departing soul.

Diagnosis

Diagnosis of gui is made based on the psycho-emotional profiles as delineated below. However, there are a couple other factors to consider, including pulse and diagnosis of the eyes.

Pulse

In general, heaven is associated with the shen and myriad spirits (as well as gui/ghosts). Heaven animates us; its influence comes through our breath (Lungs and wei qi), and we animate this influence through the vessel as Lung/wei qi moves the blood. Yang from heaven moves to the moderate level, pulsates our blood, and gives us our animation of life, then further descends to the bone level (Kidneys) to light the darkness in order to reveal one's destiny. So, a strong influence of heaven is present when the yuan level of the pulse is substantial. If there is no pulse in the interior (i.e., only on the floating/wei level), this is a sign that there might be a ghost/possession/infestation. Note that this configuration is what the Shen-Hammer lineage calls the Empty pulse (see Figure 3.1 in Chapter 3). It is a sign of extreme dysfunction, instability, and chaos.

Another pulse configuration is one in which the pulse is weak above as well as below, being Faint/Thready/Very Thin or Short. This indicates a person who lives in a house that has an evil entity/ghost or where someone recently died. As their house is possessed, they are in danger; this pulse is a sign that the person's 8x vessels and constitution are threatened.

A third configuration is that if one's pulse is Superficial/Floating in the cun and chi with nothing underneath (Empty) and Deep in the guan (only felt at the deep level), a ghost invasion is possible.

I have also encountered a fourth scenario in which the borders of the pulse are palpable, but the pulse has no texture or substance inside. Different from the Empty pulse described above, where as one presses the pulse disappears, with this Ghost pulse, the borders of the pulse (diameter) are present on the different depths, but there is no substance or anything palpable in between the borders. I have mostly found this pulse quality in the right distal position and thus far in my experience it has been confined to the experience of significant grief where one cannot let go of a deceased loved one, and once where a woman could not forgive herself for having an abortion decades earlier. The Ghost pulse I describe here has a similar shape, but much like the archetypical image for a ghost under a white blanket, the pulse retains the shape, but has nothing inside.

Eyes

As the shen is often manifested in the eyes, the "ghost eye" (gui yan) reflects a new distorted way that the individual is seeing and perceiving one's world and that one's shen has been altered. The eyes begin to look glassy or lose their shine/sparkle/glitter.

Gui treatments[180]

Acupuncture

Treatments for gui have centered around a group of acupuncture points discussed by Sun Si-miao (590–682 CE, Shui to Tang dynasty), called the 13 Ghost points. Often these points were used with moxa, or utilizing the fire needle with shallow insertions (3–5 fen) to entice the entities out. The insertion technique is the "flying needle" technique, also referred to as the "flying corpse" technique, which uses a constant flicking motion with the hand positioned like a wing to create a spiraling tornado effect to draw the entity upwards. Part of the ritual of this treatment is that the practitioner wears white (color of the po and the Lungs) to demonstrate to the person an image of safety and that no harm will come to them. After the treatment, the needles are to be quickly removed and either buried in the earth or thrown onto the floor and stomped on. Historically, there were three needles, one buried, one burned, and the last thrown into a river (representing heaven, earth, and water, the three humanities). If done indoors, a window or door to the outside should be left open to allow for the spirit to exit and return to its proper dimension. For women one is to start on the right side; for men the left. The fire needle was often used, especially on BL 62 (yang activity on yin water), Du 16, and LI 11, where the point was often cauterized several times (three to seven times in one treatment), utilizing heat to bring fire back to the eyes and expel the yin factor (which remember often enters from the sensory orifices).

The Daoist belief is that inside our bodies we have worms as well as internal gods/ entities which maintain our health and can come to our rescue (an internal resource of spirits/angelic presences that manifest through us). We can have access to these deities as well as our own inner and outer light to help expel these ghosts/devils/ demons.

The Ghost point treatment usually consists of retaining these needles for 30 minutes as we are needling the wei level and wei qi completes its cycle within approximately 23 minutes. Because of the shallowness of insertion, needles can and often do fall out, which is also an indication that the wind/entity is coming out. After the treatment has concluded, one is to wait three days, and on the fourth day (the fourth day represents death) treat again. This is repeated nine times, and a course of treatment will last roughly a month.

Typically, the 13 Ghost points, when used for an exorcism, are needled in a series of three points reflecting and tapping into the depth the entity is considered to be residing at. Each trinity represents a stage of progression, and the three points needled are dependent on which trinity addresses the particular stage. The first trinity should be needled in the initial treatment, despite which trinity one believes the ghost to reside in, as this will provide a window out (alternatively, one can include a WOS point).

The 13 Ghost points contain four trinities. The first is comprised of Du 26, SP 1, and LU 11; the second, PC 7, BL 62, and Du 16; the third, ST 6, Ren 24, and PC 8; the fourth, Du 23, Ren 1, LI 11, and Haiquan (later changed to Yintang). What these trinities show us is that first there is an impact on the sensory organs. This eventually impacts the throat and the WOS energetics that also control speech, and the articulation of thoughts/ideas, and results in a change of voice, often one of negativity and "ghost talk." Next the ghost progresses to take control over the chest, which controls the blood, the Heart, and one's interaction with the world. As the blood/shen moves in a different direction according to the will of the ghost, we see a change in one's will and, hence, destiny. Ultimately, the ghost makes its way to the lower jiao and corrupts the jing.

FIRST TRINITY

Du 26—gui gong/gui ke ting: This point reflects that the ghost has invaded the living space of the person's body and begins to disrupt and stunt his development. It's called the palace of the ghost. Ghosts enter through the orifices (e.g., mouth, nose, etc.), and Du 26, also named Ren Zhong (center of humanity), lies between where we breathe (nose) and eat (mouth/earth). Ghosts disrupt our way of maintaining post-natal qi, and this relationship also brings us to yangming which is commonly seen with shen disturbances (e.g., dian kuang syndrome). Du 26 is typically needled towards the nose and can induce trembling in the lips, reflecting the entity starting to come out. Nasal discharge is an additional sign.

LU 11—gui xin/trust or faith in ghost: At this point the ghost is now talking to the person and she cannot distinguish it as separate from herself. She begins hearing voices and seeing things but doesn't recognize them as hallucinations. The ghost begins to gain her trust and access to becoming her. Here it is very common to see a change in a person's voice as well as a change in disposition. Ghosts tend to "deaden" the responses of their hosts who then show indifference to their environment and a lack of reaction/reactivity in their orifices. The orifices are controlled by the throat and the WOS points and we may begin seeing a choking sensation/throat bi obstruction or plum pit qi. If so, we can add a WOS point into the treatment to open up the window (bring in some fresh air) and create more reactivity.

SP 1—gui lei/fortress, hidden white (po, entity hiding): By this point the ghost has positioned the person to create distance from the world. The Spleen is about boundaries and assimilation, and SP 1 has been referred to as ghost eye (gui yan). The ghost has changed the way he assimilates the world. The eyes begin to look glassy or lose their shine/sparkle/glitter (shen as manifested in the eyes). They are leaking qi, dreaming excessively about things that involve the deceased or other yin influences. Occasionally, this leakage may manifest with yang being released in explosive episodes where the po comes out and enters the level of blood (the Spleen as the manager of the blood). Hemorrhoids can also develop in the gastrointestinal tract as ghosts reside in burial grounds and areas of decay (e.g., stool). Women may experience increased menstrual bleeding with the inability of the Spleen to manage the blood. There arises a strong need to support the digestive functions and to tonify post-natal qi. This support is supposed to come from the Lungs partly, which have also been impacted from the preceding point energetic.

All the foregoing points are distal, as we want to keep things external and push out this inward progressive energetic dynamic. One of the first elements that we see here is a clouding of the portals due to an excess of phlegm from the taiyin. Du 26 attempts to open the chest region and resuscitate yang to expectorate the phlegm contamination of the gui. As the po reflects our immediate consciousness, it has a strong relationship to the present moment, the Lungs, and the breath. As it is also earthbound, it has a relationship to the Spleen as well. These taiyin jing-well points, as a reflection of the most distal aspects of the taiyin, attempt to thrust out these yin influences.

This first trinity reflects the initial infestation where a person changes overnight with an acute change in emotional demeanor. This initial disturbance of the shen can manifest with laughing/crying for no reason, irritability, restlessness, talking to oneself, and introversion. We see a person hiding something and beginning to create a fortress around themselves. The ghost alters one's inner voice as the sensory orifices become affected. The excessive yin influence also begins to challenge yang qi at Du mai and we often see a stiffness in the spine, low back pain, knee pain, and an overall disruption of the Triple Burner's mechanism.

Treatment at this trinity attempts to clear the pathogenic factor, resuscitate and ground one's consciousness, and open the portals and senses. In addition to the flying needle technique, at this trinity one can also bleed the tips of each finger. Du 20 can also be combined and used to awaken the senses and address the sensory motor internalization. If the focus is more on the Lung component, one can add in WOS points. And if the focus is more on the Spleen and post-natal impact, one can add in ST 42, SP 6, and SP 10.

SECOND TRINITY

PC 7 (some commentators say it should be LU 9)—gui xin/heart of the ghost: Here the gui enters the blood level and the Heart. The prior trinity dealt with how the person perceives the external world, but now the gui impacts her internal world. The eyes show dimming of spirit and photosensitivity, and she experiences chest stuffiness, labored breathing, and potentially a sensation as if something is sitting on top of the chest when laying down. The individual has difficulty controlling (shen deals with control) her emotions and experiences labile laughter, crying, anger, and fear. In the first trinity the individual was withdrawing; here she is actually fearful of others. As the gui impacts the blood level we may even see uncontrolled mania (dian kuang syndrome). The yin aspect of the gui can overcome the yang qi of the person, resulting in depression, darkness, turbidity, phlegm, internalization, etc.

BL 62 (some commentators say PC 5)—gui lou road/path of ghost: At this stage a gui-infested person begins to visit places the ghost frequented while alive. BL 62 utilizes the energy of taiyang to arouse and break through the obstructions. BL 62 also reflects the beginning of Yang Qiao mai which, as discussed previously, addresses the ability to stand up for ourselves and more importantly to extend our selves to stand up to the world. Moxa can be applied on this point to add more yang/fire to bring light into that darkness of the ghostly world and burn up the yin/phlegmatic quality one is moving into.

Du 16—gui jin/ghost pillow: The metaphor here is that the ghost lies down with you. It is also called feng fu/warehouse of wind. We see an increase in unpredictable behavior, and the impact of wind on the person's body (e.g., shaking, anger, seizures, etc.). Du 16 is also the meeting point for Yang Wei mai and we begin to see the loss of yang's ability to link yang impacting one's coordination/gait, and creating a lack of synchronization of one's body (e.g., dizziness, dropping things, inability to regulate wind, indecisiveness, cloudiness, migraines, nervousness, tongue thrusting, incessant speech, etc.). The person's rationale and reasoning become impacted and we may even see suicidal tendencies creeping in and the idea of death wind (the best way to change is by dying). They also experience memory loss and increasingly fear and fright. Additional points to add in this level would be GB 20 and GB 13 (points of Yang Wei mai) treated with moxa or fire needle to exorcise the ghost. In the second trinity we start to see change in the person's eyes as they become hollow and bloodshot (like they haven't slept for a long time), headaches, going to places they never did before, doing things with a degree of hostility, wind stirring up, etc. If the patient's eyes are hollow, the webs of the hands and feet can be bled with the points of the second trinity. BL 62 as a Yang Qiao mai point manifests in the eyes, but we can also see upper jiao symptoms as pathology further enters Du mai, and even changes in facial features and expressions. We may see very yang-exuberant behavior with unpredictability (wind), talking to oneself, further sensory changes, and even schizophrenia. Here the gui has penetrated the level of blood and the individual becomes more protective of self/gui. External contact is avoided and the inner dialogue becomes more corrupted. In this trinity we are trying to arouse yang to break through obstruction in this blood level (BL 62). But as the qi and blood become stagnated, blood heat is produced, causing episodes of mania, violence, and aggression. As the blood heat stirs wind we see seizures, epilepsy, and even loss of consciousness. We may see broken blood vessels around the cheeks and eyes (BL 1) and the BL 62 area. Emphasis is also placed on invigorating blood (and to some degree production of blood via proper digestive capacity) as the blood stagnation traps the shen, causing less and less engagement in life, and violence when it is engaged.

It is important to note that one need not progress from the first trinity to second to third, etc. The second trinity of symptoms can occur without having experienced the first, especially where a person feels betrayed and/or heart-broken or when there is insufficient yang qi, requiring internalization of pathology. Also, moxa can be done at the points within the first two trinities, but not the third. It can be done on the fourth trinity, but one will also have to concurrently nourish yin.

THIRD TRINITY

ST 6—gui chuang/ghost bed: Here the ghost and pathology are moving into yangming. The ghost has gained residence and is in every aspect of the body, consuming flesh and blood/yin, and causing wasting. We see a dark complexion, dark rings around the eyes, pale complexion, dryness, shifty eyes, and movements of the nose and mouth reflecting the entity trying to express itself. The person has difficulty chewing, doesn't eat much due to loss of appetite, becomes emaciated while retaining turbidity in the abdomen (malnutrition disorder, swollen abdomen, parasites flourishing, and fermentation taking place), and there is foaming of the mouth from an inability to separate the pure from turbid, discomfort in the abdomen which feels like something moving when pressed, borborygmus, drum distension, focal distension, retention of phlegm, changes in consciousness, etc. Here we need to help the body separate the pure from turbid. Additional points that can be added in are Stomach and Small Intestine points, e.g., SI 18 for consciousness/phlegm in mouth, sinew meridian points to arouse yang to separate the pure from turbid, SI 20 to separate the pure from turbid, and ST 42 to allow the pure yang of the Stomach to ascend.

Ren 24—gui xi/shi/market of ghost, source pan/receptacle: At this stage the ghost is now searching for others who are also possessed. The Ren channel is now affected and body fluids are being dried up. The individual becomes attracted to yin things like dirty, stale, contaminated foods and other individuals like them. We see a numbing of yang qi and craving for things that are antidepressive, numbing the Liver which brings yang qi up and out. Addictions come into play and, as satisfied, create more yin stagnation and turbidity in the middle. Blood pressure can become elevated (yin-fluids being retained) and there is increased risk of stroke. The ghost increasingly gains control.

PC 8—gui ku/ghost cave, lao gong: Here we see the individual become catatonic, a complete withdrawal from the world, with no desire to eat or engage. The Pericardium suggests blood involvement. Lao suggests consumption/exhaustion as the person is fatigued and tends to lie in bed all curled up (ghost cave) retreating inward. He has become very yin, cold, and numb (emotionally and physically). Digestion is impaired and the person has undigested food in the stool or may even vomit what is eaten. They experience nausea and vomiting, increased pressure in the diaphragm with shortness of breath, asthma, palpitations, etc. An attempt can be made to warm them at this stage, but not with moxa, as it will consume yin that is already extremely deficient. BL 48 can be added with moxa (yang guang/yang shield) to arouse the yang. One may also use LI 11 (fourth trinity point) with moxa to utilize the fourth trinity to assist with the third. But otherwise there is heat consumption of yin, causing yang deficiency signs as yin and yang begin to separate.

In this trinity, we find our patient in bed (cave), gravitating to things that are parasitic. They are introverted, catatonic, paranoid, phobic, attracted to darkness, and avoiding all yang, with dark rings around their eyes and purplish nails (occluded blood blocking access of the jing-wells to the exterior), tossing and turning as if fighting with themselves. We are using Ren mai to support the patient's resources as Du mai (burning up the gui) wasn't sufficient in the prior trinities. We are also tapping into yangming to support post-natal qi and, with the Pericardium, ridding the internal heat from the blood which is disturbing the soul.

FOURTH TRINITY

Du 23—gui tang/hallway of ghost: In the fourth trinity, the ghost has now claimed the entire chest (LU 5, also called hallway of ghost) and has become the sovereign ruler. The ghost has control not only of the soul, but also the shen (here referring to the brain, not the Heart), where Du mai and yang qi meet up with Ren mai and yin. Here we see fluctuations between manic and depressive states with the shen being severely disturbed. Multiple personality disorders can occur as the individual becomes a different person, the entity. The portals have been blocked for some time and the person can no longer perceive their old life. Sensory orifices become numb, with declined vision and hearing, including memory (amnesia, dementia, Alzheimer's, etc.). Points that can be added here would be the first trinity points and others to affect the portals and the four limbs, e.g., WOS points, master points to control the extremities (e.g., LI 15 for arms, GB 31 for lower limbs, etc.), and other Du mai points like Du 17 (doorway to the brain) and GB 20 (relationship to yang wei/qiao and to the eyes).

Ren 1—gui zang/ghost burial/hiding: Some commentaries say Ren 1 for men and the clitoris (jade spring) for women. Here the ghost is ready to bury your body and piggyback on your spirit ascending to the next realm. One becomes very suicidal, engaging in risky behaviors; inviting death. Ren 1 is the meeting of the Ren, Chong, and Du (the first ancestry) and one feels a need to destroy one's ancestry. Ren 1 historically was used to resuscitate (from drowning, comatose state, etc.). In terms of point energetics, Du 23 above seeks to disengage from life, whereas Ren 1 engages one's thought processes towards suicide.

LI 11—gui tui/leg of the ghost: Here we see restless leg syndrome and internal heat manifesting. One has become demonized. The yang meridians start with the legs. As the ghost moves one towards this introverted yin state, the legs begin to lose sensation and one can experience neuropathy, swellings, edema/leg qi, etc. LI 11 was indicated by Sun Si-miao for such leg symptoms. It is also associated with yangming and can treat the intermittent fevers that can develop. At this late stage, there is a high likelihood that the person will contract additional pestilent qi due to the body fermenting/decaying, which attracts parasitic entities. So, here, an alternative to dying by suicide is death by infection. This infection can appear to be exogenous (wind-heat) like meningitis and encephalitis (swellings now move away from the abdomen and go to the head). LI 11 is often cauterized to clear heat as well as invigorate the yang.

Hai Quan—gui feng/ghost seal: This is an extra point located under the tongue, sometimes described as the tip of the tongue. This point signifies that the ghost has stamped its seal; one is now a certified ghost. The Daoists replaced Hai Quan with Yin Tang. The person returns back to a mindset of suicide, attempting to harm himself without being rescued (not taking risks like above, but doing it directly).

The ghost has sealed his fate and his spirit has been stolen by the ghost. The ghost is in total control with an intent to kill its host.

In the fourth trinity, the root of yang and yin have both been compromised and we see a separation of yin and yang, with a longing for death. Yin and yang aspects of the personality fluctuate and the person is unable to recognize people/things/places that were once familiar. They themselves become unrecognizable (physically and/or emotionally). In the third trinity the person might try to commit suicide, but knows someone will come and save them. Here, they make sure no one will stop them or find them until they are dead. In terms of adding additional points to arouse the memory, if the person's issue is forgetting the space/earth they are in, add Spleen points. If forgetting time, add Liver points. If they forget people and their family members, add Kidney points.

As always, acupuncture involves the cultivation of the practitioner and one's ability to impose our shen towards the individual being treated. In the scenarios described above, many practitioners can become frightened and concerned and one must look beyond the fear in order to be successful with the treatment. You must see and treat the patient as you see and would treat yourself, envisioning the success of your treatment. Just like in the practice of taiji, when we push or strike someone, we imagine striking/pushing through them, and that intention is paramount to the success of the technique. The same is true for the treatment of gui and gu. We envision the light of yang and the thunder of yin to strike deep and exorcise the demons and parasitic influences. Sun Si-miao believed that we could also utilize the ghost points as an invitation to angelic deities for guidance, inviting an authority that you can relate to within yourself or an external deity of some religious faith that has the ability to cleanse you and illuminate your inner light to eradicate the yin factors that gui can cause—inviting a degree of healing that you haven't had access to. Give the patient a way of affirming their own inner healing rather than their disease!

What I hope is clear from the foregoing explication of the 13 Ghost points and their energetic trinities is the similarity that much of the profiles have in common with those suffering from extreme traumas. And while most practitioners will not have the opportunity to witness patients in the third and fourth trinities as by this time these patients are hospitalized or not seeking treatments, the treatment strategies are nevertheless consistent with much that I have laid out in Part I of this book. Treatments for gui focus on bringing the individual back to the present moment, opening the portals of consciousness, invigorating blood and clearing heat, nourishing the yin and focusing on the shen-spirit and ling-soul, nourishing yang qi, and supporting the proper dissemination of the Triple Burner mechanism. Often guilt can be a significant factor obstructing the po and preventing one from moving on from one's trauma. Addressing the hun and po become important.

Herbal treatments for gui

Besides the acupuncture perspective on the 13 Ghost points, there are also herbal accompaniments to the four trinities. Each formula and the individual herbal modifications are designed to establish the same connection to the treatment strategies and energetics to the corresponding trinities.

FIRST TRINITY

The focus of this trinity is to impact and open the orifices. Herbal representatives include:

- *Yuan Zhi*: Radix Polygalae Tenuifoliae. It's bitter, acrid, slightly warm, and slightly toxic. It homes to the Lungs and Heart. It calms the spirit and quiets the Heart, expels phlegm and clears the orifices, expels phlegm from the Lungs, reduces abscesses, and dissipates swellings.

- *Shi Chang Pu*: Rhizoma Acori Graminei. It's acrid, slightly warm, and aromatic. It homes to the Spleen and Heart. It opens the orifices and vaporizes phlegm and quiets the spirit, harmonizes the middle jiao and transforms turbid damp, and treats shen disturbances like depression, mania, paranoia, and unclear and foggy thinking.

- *Yu Jin*: Radix (Tuber) Curcuma. It's bitter, arid, and cool and homes to the Lungs, Liver, and Heart. It invigorates the blood and breaks up blood stagnation, promotes the movement of qi, clears the Heart and cools the blood, benefits the Gall Bladder, and reduces jaundice.

- *Dan Nan Xing*: Pulvis Arisaemae cum Felle Bovis. It's bitter and cool and homes to the Liver and Gall Bladder. It clears heat and resolves phlegm, dispels wind, and relieves convulsions.

- *Tian Zhu Huang*: Bamboo secretions. It's sweet and cold and homes to the Liver, Gall Bladder, and Heart. It clears and transforms phlegm, clears the Heart, and relaxes spasms.

The herbal formula associated with this trinity is Ding Zhi Wan (Settle the Emotions Pill).

Ding Zhi Wan (Settle the Emotions Pill)

Ren Shen	90g
Fu Ling	90g
Shi Chang Pu	60g
Yuan Zhi	60g

Ding Zhi Wan assists in building the qi of the Lungs and Spleen as well as the body's upright qi (Ren Shen and Fu Ling). It also focuses on opening the portals/orifices, remedying confusion (Shi Chang Pu and Yuan Zhi), strengthening the Kidneys and the will, and communicating the Heart and Kidneys (Ren Shen and Yuan Zhi). Thus, it contains a number of our treatment strategies for Heart Shock as well. Ding Zhi Wan can be modified to add Dan Nan Xing and Tian Zhu Huang to penetrate the orifices and expel wind phlegm, and if there is any mania. If the person is more depressed we can add Tian Nan Xing and Bai Fu Zi to treat cold phlegm. According to Jeffrey Yuen, many of these herbs were used to treat gui/gu, and in the Song dynasty the Imperial Academy took out all references to religious spiritual aspects as Confucianism took hold. With blood stagnation in the picture, Yu Jin should be added to address that while simultaneously addressing the phlegm misting the orifices.

SECOND TRINITY

The second trinity dynamics demonstrate the gui moving into the chest (PC 7) and impacting how one conducts and prioritizes one's life with control shifting to the entity. As the entity has gained access to the Heart, we want to start moving blood and qi back out to the exterior. Opening the exterior is typically our first charge, hence treating the first trinity prior to this one. The primary treatment strategy here is to tonify qi, move blood, and open the exterior. The representative herbal formula is Du Huo Ji Sheng Tang.

Du Huo Ji Sheng Tang (Angelica Pubescens and Sangjisheng Decoction)

Du Juo	9g
Xi Xin	6g
Fang Feng	6g
Qin Jiao	6g
Sang Ji Sheng	6g (15–30g)
Du Zhong	6g
Nui Xi	6g
Rou Gui	6g
Dang Gui	6g
Chuan Xiong	6g
Sheng Di Huang	6g
Bai Shao	6g
Ren Shen	6g
Fu Ling	6g
Zhi Gan Cao	6g

Du Huo opens the lower spine (Du mai) and Qiang Huo the upper; both help move yang upwards along the spine. Rou Gui stimulates ming men (one can also utilize Fu Zi); Fang Feng is used to settle any wind and to protect the exterior while you try to release. Xi Xin and Qin Jiao assist with scattering cold and wind-damp in the sinews and release to the exterior. Si Wu Tang (Dang Gui, Bai Shao, Sheng Di Huang, Chuan Xiong) and Si Jun Zi Tang (Ren Shen, Fu Ling, Zhi Gan Cao) are included to nourish and move qi and blood, with dosages adjusted to prioritizing movement over nourishment. Other herbs can be added to assist movement out to the four limbs such as Yi Yi Ren, which will also further strengthen the Spleen energetic and manage dampness from the first trinity. This formula can nourish qi and address bi-obstruction in the bones/spine with underlying exhaustion of blood and qi, as well as addressing the four limbs and sensory orifices.

THIRD TRINITY

At this trinity the Ren mai becomes implicated as the gui enters the yangming and then into the yin level, and the level of essential qi. At this point we need to nourish fluids and direct to the exterior (Ren 24 symptoms include dry skin, withering, aging, decreased humors, leakage of qi; Ren 1 in the fourth trinity reflects the internal humors being affected), as well as address the turbid damp. ST 6 reflects the jaw, a major region where toxins get trapped and become latent (e.g., gums, teeth, parasites: Chao Yan Fang's treatise in 610 CE on etiology of diseases spoke about worms you can't see with the naked eye that hide in the area of gums), with symptoms such as teeth grinding, TMJ, and latent heat from yin consumption deteriorating the marrow, bones, and source qi. This can create wei atrophy syndrome and wasting disease (PC 8, lao gong and consumption). So, we need to nourish yin, deal with turbidity, move the pathology back out to the exterior, and at the same time clear heat in the blood that has gone latent. A representative formula is Wei Rui Tang.

Wei Rui Tang (Solomon's Seal Decoction)

Wei Rui/Yu Zhu	6g
Bai Wei	6g
Ma Huang	6g
Cong Bai	0.6g
Du Huo	6g
Xing Ren	6g
Chuan Xiong	6g
Gan Cao	6g
Mu Xiang	6g
Shi Gao	9g

Yu Zhu nourishes the Heart/Lung/Stomach yin; Ma Huang moves the yin to the exterior for release; Xing Ren accesses and opens the chest to allow for the diffusion of Lung/wei qi; Chuan Xiong invigorates blood and expels wind out to the exterior; Du Huo opens the spine; Bai Wei clears the intermittent residual heat from latency (i.e., irritability, restlessness, shortness of breath, occasional explosive belching, throat clearing, shouting, weeping, emotional lability, etc.); Mu Xiang moves qi from the chest to the abdomen (jing is rooted in the lower burner, reflected in Ren 1 in the next trinity and is precautionary); and Shi Gao and Gan Cao clear heat and harmonize. Herbs to address damp and turbidity include Ban Xia (damp, cold, phlegm), Zhi Shi (for descension, focal distension), Ju Pi (citrus peel of mandarin orange to regulate qi), and also Ren Shen for tonification of qi and blood as all this takes place against a backdrop of deficiency.

As Jeffrey Yuen has taught, the "Wei" from Wei Zhu Tang means to overcome, accomplish, and achieve, and the "Zhu" means to expel (e.g., expel blood stasis, water, evil), and represents in Classical terms getting rid of something impacting/violating one's life.

FOURTH TRINITY

In the fourth trinity we have yin and yang separating as we have consumed exterior/upper yin and now the Kidney and Liver yin of the lower burner. One sees floating yang with such symptoms as seizures, high blood pressure, epilepsy, etc., representing yang overwhelming the Heart with severe shen disturbance, etc. The representative formula is Xi Jiao Di Huang Tang.

Xi Jiao Di Huang Tang (Rhinoceros Horn and Rehmannia Decoction)

Xi Jiao (or Shui Niu Jiao)	1q/30–120g
Sheng Di Huang	8q
Chi Shao	3q
Mu Dan Pi	2q

The treatment strategies here are to nourish Liver and Kidney yin, cool heat and move the blood, and extinguish wind. (One may also need to clear damp heat.)

Sheng Di Huang nourishes yin and weighs down the yang. Xi Jiao expels gu and evil and used to be powdered and put into liquids and foods that were suspected to be poisoned. If it foamed it would reveal the presence of poison. It would also be used to test the Emperor's food. Xi Jiao cools heat in the blood and stops bleeding and clears wind (horns and thorns clear wind). Sheng Di Huang also cools heat in blood and stops bleeding (including someone who wants to hemorrhage, e.g., cut themselves, etc.). Mu Dan Pi and Chi Shao invigorate and clear heat in the blood and are included as part of the intention is to keep things moving during the exorcism to prevent against an excess of yin causing depression. Huang Lian or Huang Qin and Da Huang may be added if mania is present.

Dietary recommendations for gui

Along with the internal herbal formulations, there are also dietary recommendations which should accompany any treatment of gu or gui. They mostly include avoiding the following:

- sugar and damp-producing food and drink (includes a number of fruits, especially tropical fruits)

- Da Zao/dates

- meat (except for pork which tonifies yin, and yang animal of water/KI; pigs develop a bond with humans unlike cattle—pigs seen as more human) or lamb (invigorates yang and warms, not like beef—see below)

- fish, as it produces phlegm

- chicken, as it is also phlegm producing (turkey is similar to pheasant and would be ok)

- beef, as it produces too much heat in the blood

- duck, as it is too damp and heat producing

- grains, because they are hard to digest. If one eats grains it must be combined with herbs to deal with food stagnation as well as sprouts. Only small portions would be appropriate as grains can create dampness.

Essential oil treatments for gui

Essential oils are a huge topic and anything more than a short introduction would be outside the scope of this book. But it should be noted that essential oils are excellent treatments for gui and gu as many are anti-parasitic, e.g., Thuja, Camphor, and Mugwort (which also happens to have some toxicity as it is high in ketones). More information about essential oils can be found in the preceding chapters.

Typically, essential oils are used in blends. When approaching the treatment of gui, one often will include essential oils that treat toxins, such as Mugwort, Thuja, Camphor, and Helichrysum (also known as Everlast or Immortelle). The process is that one will utilize the essential oils most relevant to the particular trinity one is seeking to treat (see below), with the addition of these toxin/gui oils added to the blend. The blends are created initially with a 4 percent dilution (40 drops per one ounce of carrier oil), then increasing to a 10 percent dilution (100 drops per one ounce of carrier oil) in later stages. Resins such as Myrrh and Frankincense can also be used as they assist in the treatment of recalcitrant and knotty problems, including non-healing wounds. They can act like the invitation of a divine presence to assist with the treatment. For this reason, Angelica Archangel can also be added to a blend. Lavender absolute is another option to add as it treats fire toxins and wound healing, and is a very calming oil which can also invigorate the blood.

FIRST TRINITY

Essential oils that resonate with the first trinity work on our main strategy of opening the portals of consciousness and communication. They include the following.

- Camphor: a top note which opens the portals and treats fire toxins. Camphor wood has been used for making coffins to prevent bugs from getting in and prevents decay. It is antiparasitic, antifungal, and an insecticide

- Rosalina: a middle note which opens the portals

Here we also want to use a mucolytic carrier oil such as castor oil.

SECOND TRINITY

Essential oils that resonate with the second trinity work on our main strategies of opening the chest and affecting the blood level, nourishing qi and blood, and moving the pathogen back to the exterior. One can also choose oils to open the spine.

- Pine
- Thyme Linalool
- Angelica Archangel for impacting the blood level as it invigorates as well as nourishes, and it invites divine angelic spirits
- Carrot Seed to invigorate/nourish blood only
- Bay Laurel: moves blood and phlegm

Here we want to use a carrier oil to invigorate the blood, so we would choose safflower oil.

THIRD TRINITY

Essential oils that resonate with the third trinity work on our main strategies of clearing heat and empty heat, nourishing yin, and calming the shen.

- Geranium
- Rose
- Lemon Balm/Melissa

Here we want to use a carrier oil to clear heat and nourish yin (LU/ST/HT), so we can use sweet almond oil or a thicker oil like hazelnut oil to nourish the barrenness/dryness. Carrot oil is used for blood.

FOURTH TRINITY

Essential oils that resonate with the fourth trinity work on our main strategy of nourishing yin, anchoring yang, and clearing heat.

- Clary Sage: nourishes yin and is also mucolytic (use with caution as this oil is also estrogenic)

- Cypress: astringent as well as anchoring yang

- Cedarwood

Here we want to use a carrier oil that will nourish yin, is heavy enough to anchor yang, and may address complications such as damp heat, so we choose jojoba oil which drains as well as moistens.

To take the pathogen/gui out of latency we can also add Terebinth and Clove into the third and fourth trinities to assist with the expulsion of the gui.

Additional essential oil treatment

A blend that Jeffrey Yuen has recommended and that I have used on many occasions has proven successful for the treatment of gui as well as for nightmares, night terrors, and insomnia due to fear (especially in children). It can be used on the first trinity of gui points and massaged in, or alternatively, and especially with children, mixed with grain alcohol and water in a misting bottle and sprayed in the bedroom and on the pillow (6–8% dilution).

Rosemary

Terebinth

Eucalyptus dives (or ½ polybractea; ½ smithii)

Lavender

Angelica Archangel (I add this to the blend to invite the angelic spirits)

Fumigation

Fumigation, or the burning of herbs, is another strategy used to treat gui, especially if it was contracted from something external like someone's bed or clothing. In this case, one returns back to the original source of infestation to fumigate. For example, if the gui was picked up in a particular home or location, that location as well as the individual should be fumigated.

Gu (and Zhu)

These two terms are often used interchangeably, but are slightly different. Gu is deliberately inflicted (e.g., poisoning). This was often associated with black magic where toxic venomous animals were cultivated and kept in a vessel (e.g., venomous cobras, scorpions, and centipedes kept together and whichever one survived absorbed the toxins/poisons from the other). The surviving animal was killed and drained of its blood, which was dried and formed into a powder to be used to poison people. Zhu is contracted accidentally. As gu is the more popular term being currently used in Chinese medicine, I will refer to both these terms collectively as gu.

Gu can be contracted from a contaminated space (environment) and food (dietary), or from coming in contact with a dead body or a person who is very sick (interaction). Chao Yuan Fang, an Imperial physician, wrote one of the first textbooks to classify diseases (noting 2000 disorders), in which zhu/gu was first classified. The most common cause was from something that ascends/flies out of a corpse (flying corpse syndrome/fei xi; germs). Within the character for zhu is the radical for host and for disease, the implication being that not everyone contracts it as not everyone is a receptive host. A receptive host is one needing to be embraced/soothed/hugged/held, commonly seen in those with depression, sadness, or grief, reflecting needs, external attachments, and vulnerabilities that similarly attract gui. Gu often becomes chronic due to its ability to penetrate and hide in crevices and shield itself from effective treatments. Patients often experience relapses and chronic manifestations.

There are four types of gu/zhu:

- Food gu/zhu

- Qi gu/zhu

- Blood gu/zhu: exchange of blood/sexually transmitted diseases; can be passed on from people to people. This comprised one of the early theories on epidemics

- Hot/cold/water climatic gu/zhu.

Contraction of gu/zhu can create:

- fainting wind, creating fainting fits and loss of consciousness, seizures, epilepsy, etc.

- falling wind/lack of coordination wind, presenting as disorientation, mania, violent outbursts, etc.

- madness wind, wherein a person screams, shouts, curses at everyone, laughs, and talks to themselves, e.g., dian kuang.

One of the initial signs that one has contracted zhu is that they experience a stabbing pain in the chest reflecting that something has taken hold of the axis of qi. Other symptoms consistent with qi stagnation in the chest or dehydration/exhaustion may manifest.

Thus, there are overlapping signs and symptoms for both gui and gu. A key feature is that the person who was relatively healthy gets sick quickly from some external contraction (Sun Si-miao characterized gu as a Lung external disease) in contrast to disorders of the shen/ling which are considered internal factors. Gu is commonly seen contracted when one travels to other regions, as traveling can tax wei qi, making one more vulnerable to external disorders. Gu are actual/tangible substances that invade the body. Sun Si-miao, in his descriptions on treating zhu, says that if you give one of his formulas with realgar and cinnamon the patient will literally spit out tadpole-like substances or mini frog reptilian-looking animals.[181] Some of the organisms that live in the body were classified by size (some 3 fen, others 1 cun), and others were said to look like long tapeworms and other protozoans and parasites.

One of the key symptoms of gu is that when one places one's hand on the patient's chest (above or below) there is a general sense of discomfort and the patient doesn't want your hand there. This is not so with gui. Gu tries first and foremost to have access to the chest (the portals for gui). Bowel symptoms are more prevalent due to the connection of the Lungs and wei qi to the Large Intestine and bowels (bloody mucus, mucus in stools, etc.); the person has labile emotions and prefers darkness, and experiences achiness in limbs, lethargy, lassitude, etc. Other mental-emotional symptoms identified by Sun Si-miao include depression, suicidal thoughts, unpredictable emotions (unlike gui), restlessness, irritability, being most active at nighttime during the dark, etc. (insomnia), angry outbursts, confusion, and auditory and visual hallucinations.

Gui, if not treated, progressively worsens, whereas gu infestations, even if untreated, appear to resolve, but then relapse repeatedly despite treatment as gu multiplies and infests by finding crevices and laying eggs. Gu needs shelter in the body. As gu infestations inhabit the intestines, they encase themselves within the lining to protect themselves. Intestinal abscesses, polyps in the intestines/nasal cavity, and scars can form because they gnaw away at the gut lining, creating ulcers, and eventually scar tissue, as they heal. These polyps tend to manifest in areas governed by yangming (Stomach/Large Intestine organ/meridians). Chronic sinusitis can be viewed as a parasitic condition from this lens. As it goes internally, it goes to the intestines. Parasitic symptoms of the Stomach channel include styes, nodules under the jaw, and goiters. People with thyroid issues (nodules, etc.) can have many of these mental/emotional symptoms associated with gu and gui, including irritability, mania, depression, etc. Lesions can form in the head around ST 8 or in the brain as a result of these infestations.

One of the major treatments for gu utilizes the yangming channel, especially as it also goes to the portals (yangming deals with all sensory organs, but in particular the sinuses). One of the principal herbs for gu infestations is Bai Zhi (white analgesic), which is aromatic, opens the sinuses, has a Stomach affinity, is spicy, and expels/discharges pus and pushes out lingering dampness. Aromatic herbs penetrate turbidity as parasites are attracted to strong flavors and smells. Other herbs are then combined to destroy the gu. (See below for treatment strategies.) Phlegm is produced by dampness and has a relationship to the Spleen. The Stomach, however, is associated with turbidity, which is a different concept. Turbidity (duo) vs. dampness (shi); Gu vs. gui. Gu is associated with yangming, and the focus is on turbidity and the Stomach rather than phlegm/dampness (which we saw more with gui). So treatment-wise we are looking more at aromatics to transform and penetrate turbidity and to move the pathology back out to the exterior.

Diagnosis
Looking/palpation

Diagnosis really comes from looking at the spirit and touching the abdomen, looking for borborygmus and a lot of movement going on. Typically, with gu, there are chronic digestive issues like gas, bloating, assimilation issues, fatigue, heaviness, fogginess, clouded thinking, and weakness of the limbs. There are also pulse configurations associated with gu. Sun Si-miao believed that gu presented with Rough and Choppy pulse configurations. These qualities represent the damage to the tissue (Rough reflecting parenchymal tissue damage; Choppy reflecting blood stasis, a major consequence of gu). In my experience, there are additional qualities that are more suggestive of gu. They include the Slippery pulse quality as well as the Sticky pulse quality. The Slippery pulse has the sensation of sliding past your fingers like an oil slick. It signifies dampness and with gu is a product of the turbidity created in the Stomach. We can also see a strong Slippery quality in the organ depth of the left middle positions with the release of eggs. The Sticky pulse is a quality that I started documenting around 2010. The primary sensation of this pulse is that it feels waterlogged or rubbery or sticky in that the pulsation of the artery seems to linger on your fingertip. It is a quality of the vessel and its texture and is distinguishable from the Leisurely pulse which feels as if its movement is slowed down or exaggerated. One of my colleagues helped describe it as the "Peanut Butter" quality as your finger sticks to it. I consider the Sticky pulse to be a progression and accumulation of phlegm-heat. In the Liver, it can reflect phlegm-heat toxins; in the Stomach and Spleen potentially candida and malabsorption and gluten intolerance (manifestations of gu). It is most often found in the middle positions, but I have found it mostly everywhere by now. I consider this pulse quality a more recent expression of toxicity in general whereby the lymphatic system attempts to trap pathogenic (including gu) influences (as opposed to Choppy which reflects the influence on blood circulation).

Treatments

As with any diagnosis, treatments can be performed with whichever modality one is most comfortable with. Below, I provide options for herbal treatments, acupuncture, essential oils, and diet.

Herbal treatments/acupuncture/essential oils

In terms of herbal medicine, there are three herbs that are most popular for treating gu: Zi Su Ye, Bai Zhi, and Bo He. They deal with cold/heat/dampness. Cold and damp eventually transform to heat (which tends to fluctuate). Heat creates emotional irritability, cold creates emotional depression and indifference, and damp creates emotional cloudiness and indecisiveness requiring one to penetrate the turbidity.

Chao Yuan Fang believed that gu are intelligent. They have an ability to mutate, change form, and hide in the body for a long time. Gu symptoms constantly and stubbornly recur (e.g., candida), and often create lots of digestive, wind-type, and sexual symptoms (i.e., hungry, wandering, and sexual). Because of this, one needs to constantly adjust the herbs and acupuncture treatments to maintain efficacy. Similarly, it is also very important to rotate the diet. Gu are able to reproduce as a consequence of the turbidity of the yangming Stomach, which also controls the yi/mind. As they are intelligent, it is believed that gu can read your mind and affect your consciousness. You have to trick your consciousness/mind, and as turbidity clouds the mind, aromatics must be a consistent component of the treatment.

Gu treatments contain five strategies. And while this five-fold strategy must be consistent, the actual treatments require variety and must be changed often. For the herbal formula, one should use at least five herbs and rotate the herbs as one begins to see change. The strategies and their representative herbs/acupoints/oils are:[182]

1. *Dissipate poisons/toxins*: get rid of poison/toxin/infestation with the use of strong aromatic herbs that penetrate turbidity causing dilation and release to the exterior. These herbs love the sun and can bring light into the darkness.

   Herbs: Qing Hao, Gao Ben, Sheng Ma, Lian Qiao, Zi Su Ye (or Zi Su Zi), Bai Zhi, Bo He, Ju Hua

   Acupuncture points: LI 7, BL 57, GB 36, Du 10

   Essential oils: Rosemary Verbena, Camphor, Peppermint

2. *Rid infestation, destroy parasites, and kill demons*: sha (to kill gui, gu).

   Herbs: Antiparasitic herbs such as She Chuang Zi (seed of snake bed), Da Suan/garlic, Bing Lang, Ding Xiang/clove, Chuan Shan Jia, Ku Shen, Qing Hao, Huai Hua, He Zi, Chuan Shan Jia, Yu Jin, Jin Yin Hua, Shi Chang Pu, Lei Wan, Ku Gua, Gui Jian Yu, Guan Zhong, and Hu Zhang

Acupuncture points: ST 4, LI 7

Essential oils: Clove (as essential oil, clove rids fire toxin and parasites)

3. *Calm shen by nourishing yin/blood*: the shen is always disturbed with gu (remember that one of the cardinal symptoms of the person is not liking the placement of a hand on his chest).

Herbs: especially herbs that nourish the Lungs and Heart (impact on chest), such as Huang Jing (Sun Si-miao believed it had a calming effect on shen, and Hua Tou used it to calm the shen during meditation and prevent one from contracting parasites/entities during that time),[183] Bai He, Sha Shen, Xuan Shen, Sheng Di Huang, Xi Yang Shen, Fu Shen, and Jiang Xiang

Acupuncture points: ST 30, BL 45, SP 10

Essential oils: Carrot Seed, Savory

4. *Tonify qi and blood*: qi and blood are being consumed by accommodating this host, so one needs to tonify.

Herbs: Dang Gui, Bai Shao, He Shou Wu, Huang Qi, Suan Zao Ren, Bai Zi Ren, Gan Cao, Wu Jia Pi (brain gu, body pain)

Acupuncture points: ST 36, LU 9, SP 3, SP 6, ST 42, PC 7

Essential oils: Pine, Thyme Linalool, Tea Tree

5. *Break up barriers (fortress) that parasites have created*: move qi to break up blood stasis and phlegm. As discussed above, the worms cause the shen to become distressed. This causes qi stagnation (chest distress) and one becomes depressed. The stagnation also creates heat and one becomes irritable and anxious. The heat burns off/consumes qi and one cycles back to becoming depressed, creating this cycle of behavior. Thus, the moving of the qi and the breaking up and dissipating of the blood stasis has a two-fold responsibility of assisting with calming the shen while also breaking up the barriers parasites have used for protection (e.g., biofilms).

Herbs: Lai Fu Zi, San Qi/Tian Qi, E Zhu, Si Gua Lou, Chuan Xiong, Chai Hu, Chen Pi, Mu Xiang, Ze Lan

Acupuncture points: SP 8 and SP 10 and extra point Bai Chong Wo

Essential oils: Roman Chamomile, resins (Myrrh, Frankincense, or Myrtle for mucolytic effect, Angelica Archangel or Elemi to exorcise)

Additional acupuncture treatments

There are a few other options available for utilizing acupuncture in the treatment of gu. One is to do garlic moxa on BL 43/gaohuangshu. Garlic moxa can also be used on Ren 15, ST 32, ST 8, ST 25 (yangming connection to the Large Intestine), and LI 20. Sometimes Sichuan pepper was given, which destroys and burns up turbidity. In general, one should use one point at a time and rotate the points. With acupuncture one can also alternate sides in treatment to maintain unpredictability.

Yet another option is the use of points with the name gu/valley or bai/white. Jeffrey Yuen has detailed some of these treatments and they are summarized below.

ACUPUNCTURE POINTS WITH GU IN THE NAME

LI 4 (He Gu) = union valley. Treats damp-heat in the Large Intestine, with constrained Liver insulting the Lungs, preventing descension to the Large Intestine.

ST 43 (Xian Gu) = sunken valley. Wood shu-stream point which powerfully descends gu and treats food stasis, rebellious Stomach qi, reflux, nausea, and vomiting.

SP 7 (Lou Gu) = leaking valley. Treats malabsorption, ascends Spleen yang to treat diarrhea and loss of fluids, assists the Spleen in transforming and transporting, prevents weight loss, and secures leaky gut, spermatorrhea, and Bladder.

SP 8 (Di Hi) = earth pivot. Treats acute abdominal pain, ascends sinking Spleen/Gu qi, puts earth into flight, and treats prolapse, bloating, uterine prolapse, etc.

SI 2 (Qian Gu) = front valley. Water of fire, mobilizes damp in the lower heater and guides heat out of the Gall Bladder (when bled), separates the pure and impure fluids and drains damp-heat via the Bladder, and treats irritable bowel and iliocecal valve problems.

SI 5 (Yang Gu) = yang valley. Ascends yang, treats wei qi deficiency.

BL 66 (Zu Tong Gu) = foot passage valley. Water of water, mobilizes and treats symptoms of damp-heat in the Bladder.

KI 2 (Ran Gu) = blazing valley. Fire of water, stimulates hunger, the will to live, and will power, boosts ming men, and brings yang to the Spleen via a branch to SP 8.

KI 10 (Yin Gu) = yin valley. Treats yin qi deficiency.

KI 20 (Fu Tong Gu) = abdominal passage valley. Treat with moxa for deficient Kidney yang from Spleen yang deficiency and dampness; treats abdominal stagnation and undigested food in the stool accompanied by pain.

GB 8 (Shuai Gu) = leading valley. Directs the Liver to descend, treats damp-heat jaundice and difficulty digesting fat with nausea and headache, and assists decision-making clouded by dampness.

Acupuncture points with Bai in the name

LU 4 (Xia Bai) = *guarding white.* Treats/disperses phlegm in the upper heater.

SP 3 (Tai Bai) = *supreme white.* Source point which transforms/transports damp.

In this treatment, generally ST 43 is needled first, followed by KI 2, SP 7 or 8, and LI 4. The first three points are needled on the exhale and removed on the inhale to tonify. LI 4 is sedated (needled on inhale and removed on exhale). Points are removed in the opposite order so that the first point to be needled is the last to be removed. The first three points assist with the initial assimilation of gu qi. LI 4 helps to ascend and combust the gu qi, increasing vitality by uniting the earth and metal/air. Additional points are added based upon the point name and its functions. Only add other points outside this model if they are specifically helpful for digestion.

This treatment impacts both emotional and physical inabilities to assimilate. When using SI 2 and BL 66, add points to treat the underlying causes of damp-heat. It assists with promoting balance between wei/ying and the mechanisms required to produce post-natal qi (and blood) under the influence of the Kidney and Spleen yang. Without these mechanisms in place, points like ST 36, Ren 4, and Ren 6 are ineffective. These points add, reduce, or regulate the time that food spends being assimilated in the gut depending on the needling technique used. To these treatments, one can also add Ren 7 and SP 6 to tonify the Spleen and expel damp.

The nervous system and gu

Earlier in this book, I discussed Dr. Shen's Nervous System Tense and Nervous System Weak formulas. To accommodate a diagnosis of gu, I have also created analogous formulas that won't compromise the treatment should gu be present. Each of these formulas maintains the impact on the nervous system, while also taking into consideration each of the five gu treatment strategies. They are as follows:

Nervous System Tense: Gu

Chuan Xiong
Jiang Huang
Bai Shao
Bo He
Gao Ben
Qing Hao
Bai He
E Zhu
Bing Lang

Nervous System Weak: Gu

Chuan Xiong
Jiang Huang
Bai Shao
Bo He
Huang Jing
He Shou Wu
San Qi
Ding Xiang
Huang Qi

Diet

Diet for gu is similar to that for gui. I have provided simply a few foods/categories to avoid as well as some to add into one's diet.

Avoid the following foods: sugar, heat-producing foods, and foods that create phlegm and turbidity such as chicken, duck, shrimp, dates, etc. Jeffrey Yuen has also suggested that a good barometer for determining whether a food is gu-friendly is by considering how difficult it is not to overindulge in it. Foods that we can't easily stop eating and that generate unhealthy cravings are generally gu-friendly candidates. As with the herbal therapics, a rotational diet should be implemented.

Consume more of: spices and vegetables such as tofu, celery, spinach, peppermint, garlic, horseradish, ginger, bitter melon, etc.

PART III

PUTTING IT
ALL TOGETHER

Thus far in this text I have attempted to provide a framework for understanding the complexities of Heart Shock as a systemic diagnosis. In so doing, I have presented my interpretations and synthesis of the Shen-Hammer lineage with that of Jeffrey Yuen's. In Part II, each of the channel systems were discussed, demonstrating their basic usages and energetics, followed by their applications to Heart Shock, and where applicable noting combinations and relationships to other channel systems. Within those chapters a few short vignettes were included from my patients to simply illustrate the particular concept being discussed. This part is tasked with demonstrating the entire process of treating the dynamics of trauma and its sequelae.

As I hope has been made clear, what I have written in this text can be applied more widely than the treatment of trauma. Each chapter in Part II is, in effect, its own teaching, with broad-reaching impact on the various disorders we clinicians face daily within our practices. And as each channel system represents a discrete perspective and lens in which to view our patients and pathology, there is a considerable overlap, and the combinations for their use are manifold. The patient case studies presented herein are simply a variety of what I see daily, and have been chosen to demonstrate particular principles of treatment and those combinations.

In demonstrating the case histories, there is of course the issue of understanding the correlations of the pulse qualities and their interpretations in light of the other pulses and positions that they present in. As teaching how to interpret and analyze the Pulse Record with all its complexities and subtleties is beyond the scope of this book, I will do my best to explain the relationships where possible. For each case I will present my pulse findings in the form of the Pulse Record that I fill out for all my patients. Every quality is important and reflective of some aspect of the patient's physiology/pathology and is considered within the overall treatment plan, though some are more pressing and revealing/important. After explaining the major diagnoses, I will list the priorities as I see them, followed by the treatment strategies. Then, the acupuncture, herbal, and essential oil treatments will be presented.

CHAPTER 10
Case Studies

Patient 1
History

Patient 1 is a 40-year-old male with a chief complaint of chronic lower back pain. As a financial executive, he showed up to the initial evaluation at 11:00am, stressed, already having had 36oz. of "bold" coffee to get him through hours of early morning conference calls. The first prominent sign came immediately from feeling his pulse, which was Ropy and Leather-Hard, with a heart rate of only 40 bpm, and a prominent Rough Vibration.

His history, as one can readily imagine from just the above introduction to his case, contains trauma, the most recent one being the loss of his father, whom he was extremely close to, a few years prior. The loss, of course, is painful enough, but my patient walked in and found his father post suicide. His dad had been severely depressed with major episodes throughout the patient's life (including as a child), and he was his father's major caregiver in his adulthood. An earlier trauma came at the age of five with an abdominal surgery. The patient described it as very traumatic and recounted that he was strapped down, screaming in pain.

Other notable aspects of his pulse were:

Left Distal Position: Primarily absent with an occasional change in qualities to Vague/Tense/Muffled (4–5). As qualities are rated on a scale from (1) being minor, to (5) being severe, this Muffled quality was such that it was extremely unclear and hard to distinguish the vessel boundaries outside of a vague thumping/beating.

Right Distal Position: Same as Left Distal with Muffled (5). It also had an occasional Inflated quality.

Left Proximal Position: Thin Tight, and Feeble.

Looking at just the information provided, Patient 1 demonstrates significant aspects of Heart Shock. The prominent Rough Vibration demonstrates the main pathognomonic finding of trauma, and the Ropy pulse reflects the long-term impact of the stress on the circulatory system and the resultant yin-essence deficiency with heat in the blood. The Leather-Hard pulse is a further depletion of jing-essence and blood; and together with the Ropy pulse suggests jin-ye (hormonal) depletion and insufficiency, including other dense yin fluids such as cerebrospinal fluid, synovial fluids, etc. These deficiencies, of course, impact the circulation (blood to the tissues and muscles, but also nourishment of the spinal segments and their innervations to nerves and sensory motor tracts).

The Muffled qualities in the distal positions suggest deeply suppressed grief and depression, something weighing heavily on the chest. The added Inflated quality in the Right Distal position confirms this trapped grief and inability to let go. The Left Proximal position confirms the yin-blood deficiency impacting the structure (the Kidney yin being the source of the deep hormonal ye fluids). The Feeble nature of this pulse confirms the impact on Kidney yang, and, with the Absent Left Distal position, explains the impact on the heart rate, and overall yang deficiency.

Additional pulse findings

Looking at the Pulse Record, one sees a host of other significant findings on this patient's pulse. They include:

- a Hesitant pulse waveform
- an increase of 26 beats on exertion
- 8x vessel pulses for Du mai and Yin Wei mai
- SM pulses for GB/ST/SI
- Lungs not diffusing their qi
- Spleen/Stomach not ascending to Lungs and chest
- Lungs not descending to Kidneys
- Blood Thick
- blood stagnation and engorgements for the Liver and Gall Bladder (Choppy)
- Thin Tight pulses in the Pelvis/Lower Burner reflecting inflammation (possibly reflecting the pain and stagnation in the lower back)
- diaphragm pulses: (1+) on the left; (2+-3) on the right
- NST
- BL/KI DM.

Ross Rosen, L.Ac., Dipl. O.M. (NCCAOM)
166 Mountain Ave., Westfield, NJ 07090, (908) 654-4333

Name:	Patient 1	Gender:	M	Age: 40	Date:
Chief Complaint: chronic low back pain		Height:		Weight:	Occupation: Finance
Rhythm: Normal				Rate/Min: Begin: 40 End: 40 w/Exertion: 66 ▲: 26 Other Rates During Exam:	

First Impressions of Uniform Qualities	Depths
Tense Robust Pounding (2+) <--> Reduced Pounding Ropy Changing Amplitude (2) Rough Vibration --> Leather-Hard	Wave: Hesitant
	Floating: Tight Rough Vibration Cotton: Qi:
	Blood: Thick Heat / Thick / Unclear
	Organ: O-B: O-S:

Left Side:	Right Side:

PRINCIPAL POSITIONS / COMPLEMENTARY POSITIONS

Dir:	L:	Distal Position	R:	Dir:	L:	Neuro-psychological	R:
Not Expressing Shen	Absent <--> Tense Muffled (4) Vague		Absent <--> Tense Muffled (4) Vague Occas Inflated	Not Diffusing Wei Qi	Doughy Muffled (4)		

Special Lung Position
L: R:
Thin (4) Tight Rough Vibration Feeble   Tense Robust Pounding (4) Rough
Pleura:

SI: Receiving? HT: Empty for 3 hours Floating/Scattering? Nurturing/Calming? SM? Tight Luo? DM? ⊕3	LI: LU: Empty Releasing? Floating/Diffusing? X Descending? Moistening? SM? Luo? DM?	LU not descending to <I

Heart
Mitral Valve: Muffled (4) Rough Vibration
Enlarged: Large Vessel:
Pericardium:

L:	Middle Position	R:	
Tense --> Tight Choppy Reduced Pounding Rough Vibration Y'n portion of wave Muffled Cosine		Tense Robust <--> Reduced Pounding Muffled (1+) Changing Amplitude (1+) Cosine	SP not according to LU

Diaphragm
L: R:
Inflated (1+)   Inflated (2+-3)

GB: Thin Tight Receiving? LR: Rough Vibrat Scattering? Coursing? Discharging? Storing? SM? Luo? DM?	ST: Descending? SP: Ascending? Releasing? Harmonized? SM?Tight ⊕ Luo? DM?

Liver
Engorged: Distal: Inflated (2) Slippery   Ulnar:
Gall Bladder CCPD: Tight Robust Pounding (3) Choppy

L:	Proximal Position	R:
Thin Tight Muffled Rough Vibration Feeble		Tense Muffled (2) Rough Vibration Reduced Pounding Cosine at Blood/Organ depths

Spleen-Stomach
Esophagus: Spleen:
Stom-Pyl. Exten: Tense Robust Pounding Muffled (1+)
Duodenum: Peritoneal Cavity/Pancreas:

Intestines
Large: Small:
Muffled (2+) Tight <--> Tense   Muffled (2) Rough Vibration Changing Amplitude (2+)   Tense Robust Pounding (3)

BL: Receiving? KI: Consolidating? SM? Luo? DM? BL/KI	SJ: Floats? KI/PC: Releasing? Consolidating? SM?Tight ⊕ Luo? DM?

Pelvis/Lower Body
L: R:
Thin Tight Rough Vibration   Tense <--> Tight Rough Vibration Changing Amplitude (1+-2)

L:	8 Extra Pulses	R:
Yin Wei mai		Yin Wei mai
Du mai		Du mai

Tongue:

Coat: Peeled LR/GB

Body: Red Scalloped with deep indentations

Tip red and curled under

Other:

Reminders: (specify side)
Split:
Fan Guan:
San Yin:

△ = Change   (1 —> 5) = low —> high

Additional symptoms

- Achilles pain

- Rotator cuff pain

- Insomnia/Disturbed sleep (wakes often)

- History of IBS/colitis which runs in the family

- Allergies and deviated septum

Surgeries

- Sinus

- Knee

- Hernia (age 5)

Diagnoses

As a Heart Shock case, the main diagnoses in this case all revolve around trauma and the systems most impacted by it, as described in Part I of this text. Under the main diagnosis of Heart Shock, the diagnoses include the following:

Heart Shock and its sequelae

Diagnosis	Pulse quality(ies)
Heart yin-blood deficiency	Hesitant wave, increase on exertion of 26 beats
Heart qi deficiency (severe), moving towards separation of yin and yang	Absent pulse, changing qualities to Muffled/Vague/Tense
Lung qi deficiency, moving towards separation of yin and yang	Absent pulse, changing qualities to Muffled/Vague/Tense
Stagnation of all substances in the chest plus trapped qi/grief	Muffled, Inflated Right Distal, and increased Inflation on right Diaphragm position
Yin-essence deficiency	Ropy
Yin-blood-essence deficiency	Moving towards Leather-Hard
NST	Floating Tight pulse and Tense-Tight pulses throughout the principal positions
Blood stagnation (LR/GB)	Choppy
Kidney yin and yang deficiency	Thin Tight and Feeble
Qi stagnation with heat in the GI (ST/SI/LI) and GB	GB/ST/LI/SI Tense-Tight pulses with Robust Pounding

Trapped qi in the diaphragm	Inflated Diaphragm pulses
Yin Wei mai activity	Yin Wei mai Deep Long pulse in middle and proximal position at 15 beans
Du mai activity	Du mai Long Floating pulse in all three positions at 3 beans
BL/KI DM activity	Divergent pulse in Left Proximal

Patient 1's presentation reflects many of the aspects detailed in Part I of this text. The pervasive Rough Vibration demonstrates the Shock to the deepest yuan level, and from the initial trauma at age five, through the most recent with the violent passing of his father, more than three decades have left its imprint on all aspects of his physiology. The 40 bpm heart rate clues us in to the time lag from the first trauma, as do the Absent pulses in the Left and Right Distal positions. The Feeble Left Proximal position also confirms the detriment to Kidney yang over time, possibly also suggesting a familial history of the depression suffered by his father having been passed down.

Additional common pulse signs of Heart Shock include the Hesitant pulse wave (yin deficiency and obsessive thinking) and the increase on exertion of 26 beats (reflecting Heart blood deficiency and insufficient resources to nourish and calm the shen). The strong Muffled qualities in the Left and Right Distal positions also demonstrate the oppressive sadness weighing on the patient's chest, preventing the po from living in the moment. The inability of the Lung qi to diffuse and the Inflated quality in the Right Distal position also prevent the movement of this weight and the capacity to let go. Instead, the constant vigilance and overworking of the nervous system maintain functioning, but also create tightness and discomfort in the sinews from armoring one's pain. This, coupled with the Heart blood deficiency, the lack of nourishment to the sinews (Liver yin deficiency), and the Feeble proximal pulse, create a weakness and vulnerability to chronic pain especially in the lower back, the home of the Kidneys.

Additional complicating factors include the lack of communication in the Triple Burner due to the trapped qi and blood in the diaphragm and Liver (Inflated Diaphragm and Choppy LR/GB), as well as the chronic inflammation in the gut (Tense-Tight/Robust Pounding pulses in the ST/SI/LI with the history of colitis). This inflammation and underlying weakness (Reduced Pounding in the Right Middle position) demonstrate the impact on the earth and impacts the patient's overall stability.

The three-plus decades of this energetic imbalance have also taken a toll on his resources, creating heat and inflammation in the vessels and a drying out and thickening of his blood, further impacting his circulatory capacity and taxing the Heart (Blood Thick, Ropy, and Leather-Hard pulses). The further depletion on his resources (jing-essence) from accommodating this for so many years shows up in the presence of the BL/KI DM pulse and activity.

The Yin Wei mai and Du mai pulse configurations also demonstrate the depth to which this imbalance has affected Patient 1. The patient has experienced very clear defining moments in his life, from the trauma at age five to the umbilicus (source of pre-natal nourishment), to caring for a mentally ill parent and eventually finding him after he killed himself. I often find that patients tend towards Du mai imbalances when roles reverse requiring quicker than normal individuation, including taking care of one's parent (especially the father), when young. (I often see Ren mai imbalances with bonding and boundary issues with mom.) This individuation has created a strong taxation on yang qi, weakening the structure from the constant heavy burden of caregiving, and eventually even taxed his shoulder (carrying this heavy weight) and his Achilles (influence of Du mai on Yang Qiao mai).

Putting all this information together and weaving the story of this patient's life into a treatment intervention requires prioritizing the diagnoses and understanding how best to proceed. I always create priorities and levels of interventions for all my patients in an outline which reveals all the necessary diagnoses to creating strategies for the patient management. I believe that all diagnoses must be taken into account to allow for the most complete treatments and to prevent unnecessary side effects. In this way, if, for example, communicating Heart and Kidneys is a major treatment principle, but there is also significant blood stasis or diaphragmatic stagnation present, nourishing and anchoring will not be successful without moving the stagnation preventing the communication. Thus, for every treatment strategy, one must search to make sure there is not another diagnosis (even a secondary or tertiary one) preventing its success. Below is the outline for Patient 1.

Priorities and interventions

1. Immediate interventions
   a. Stability
      i. Heart Shock: HT yin, qi, blood deficiency
      ii. Separation of yin and yang
         1. Heart: qi deficiency (severe)
         2. Lungs: qi deficiency (severe)
   b. Circulation/heat/pathogenic factor
      i. Blood stagnation (LR/GB)
      ii. Stagnation of all substances in the chest (LU/HT) (severe)
      iii. Diaphragm trapped qi
2. Root issues
   a. Kidney yin and yang deficiency
   b. Yin-essence deficiency

        c. Yin-blood-essence deficiency

        d. NST

        e. 8x vessel activity

            i. Du mai

           ii. Yin Wei mai

        f. Spleen/Stomach qi-blood deficiency (moderate)

        g. Liver yin, qi, and blood deficiency (moderate)

    3. Secondary issues

        a. Directionality

            i. LU not diffusing wei qi

           ii. SP not ascending to LU

          iii. LU not descending to KI

    4. Tertiary issues

        a. Blood Thick

        b. Qi stagnation with heat GI (ST/SI/LI) and GB

        c. SM activity

            i. GB/ST/SI channels

        d. Pelvic lower body impaired function

Treatment strategies

Based on the foregoing priorities and interventions, my primary strategies included:

1. Nourishing Heart yin and qi

2. Strengthening Kidney qi-yang (and lower back)

3. Opening the chest to allow for HT/KI communication (including helping the Lungs diffuse, and invigorating qi and blood into the diaphragm and LR/GB).

Secondary strategies that needed to be considered included:

1. Nourishing yin-essence and cooling heat in the blood

2. Calming the nervous system and relaxing the sinews

3. Strengthening the SP/ST and moving stagnation.

Treatments
Acupuncture
Acupuncture began with approaching the BL/KI DM, as well as the 8x vessels. The first treatment consisted of:

BL 10, BL 40 DSD

BL 15, 23, 32 DSD

BL 13, 17, 21 SDS

Gua sha from BL 17 to GB 22 area

Left SI 3, Du 4, Shi Qi Zhu Xia extra point

Left PC 6, KI 9

Using the BL/KI DM as the first approach allows for a number of treatment strategies to be implemented. One is strengthening and anchoring the yang-qi back to the Kidneys and Heart with DSD needling. Needling BL 15 and BL 23 further enhances this and nourishes both of these primary organ systems. In addition, the BL/KI DM also allows for the release of the chest and diaphragm, both by using BL 13 and BL 17 with SDS needling, but also by using gua sha on the ring around the chest. As the SI SM pulse was present as well, using gua sha on the taiyang ring helps to release obstructions here (cold), which further hampers yang qi. It also symptomatically addresses the rotator cuff injury. The BL/KI DM provides access to the Bladder shu points, so tapping into whichever organ one wishes is easy to do in conjunction with the treatment principles. Accessing the GI with BL 21 also helps to reduce any stagnation preventing the descension of yang and addresses the inflammatory nature of the patient's colitis.

As I tap into the BL/KI DM and jing-essence, using 8x vessels in conjunction is appropriate as they both address yuan qi. Here, the Du mai was accessed with left SI 3, furthering the impact on yang qi and the spine and lower back. Using Du 4 and extra point Shi Qi Zhu Xia helps to pinpoint the areas of pain and weakness as well as strengthen Kidney yang. And using Yin Wei mai to assist with linking the yin resource of jing-essence was also accomplished with left PC 6 and KI 9 bilaterally to further strengthen and astringe the Kidneys, but also as a point which is noted for rectifying the disjunctive episodes of one's life, and releasing toxins. PC 6 also has the impact of assisting the upper back points and the gua sha for releasing chest oppression, removing dampness, calming the shen, and clearing heat and stagnation in the chest.

Herbal
The initial formula given was:

Xi Yang Shen	9g
Mai Men Dong	9g
Wu Wei Zi	6g
Gui Zhi	9g
Rou Gui	9g
Fu Zi	18g
Sha Ren	9g
Huang Qi	9g
Mu Xiang	9g
Du Huo	9g
Qiang Huo	9g
Sang Ji Sheng	15g
Zhi Gan Cao	5g

The herbal formula consists of a blend of herbs commonly used in the Shen-Hammer lineage with herbs that impact the 8x vessels, and Classical approaches to anchoring yang. The first three ingredients comprise the modified Sheng Mai San (discussed in a previous chapter) and focus on nourishing and astringing Heart yin, and calming the shen (it provides comfort, and treats the insomnia). These three also nourish the earth, as do Sha Ren, Rou Gui, Huang Qi, Zhi Gan Cao, and Mu Xiang, which also prevent any stagnation and have a descending quality. Gui Zhi helps open the diaphragm with Mu Xiang, and with Qiang Huo it helps to open the taiyang "ring around the chest." With Rou Gui, Huang Qi, and Fu Zi, it strongly nourishes the Heart qi. The Du mai is opened with Qiang Huo and Du Huo (which impact the portals via the brain), and Fu Zi with Sha Ren make sure to descend yang back to its home (Fire Spirit School approach). Sang Ji Sheng assists Qiang Huo and Du Huo with ridding wind-cold-damp bi obstruction from the back (caused by the yang qi deficiency), and also nourishes the Liver and Kidney yin, relaxing the sinews. Blood is warmed and moved with Rou Gui and Gui Zhi, and qi is circulated via Mu Xiang, which also relaxes the diaphragm. And lastly, while the formula is not specifically nourishing yin-essence and clearing heat in the blood, it is assisting yin by anchoring yang back to its residence in the lower burner, and astringing yin back to the Heart. By promoting this proper dynamic and relationship, balance should be restored. Future treatments can focus more on nourishing back deficient yin-essence and blood once the Shock is settled.

Essential oils

An essential oil was prepared as a liniment for the patient to massage into his lower back after first applying to left SI 3 to address the Du mai. The four oils below were mixed in rice wine in an 8 percent dilution and applied after friction was created to the points.

Litsea

Cinnamon Leaf

Basil

Camphor

The essential oil blend is highly aromatic, opens the portals as well as Du mai, and regulates the back. Litsea is warming and resolves wind-damp-cold and also strengthens the earth. Basil regulates the Stomach and also opens the nose, as well as strengthening and assisting Kidney yang. Camphor invigorates yang and strongly opens the portals and relieves pain. Cinnamon Leaf assists the yang and movement through the Du mai and Bladder channel.

Patient 2

History

Patient 2 is a 30-year-old female suffering from fainting spells and a tingling sensation throughout her body which produces severe anxiety. Upon feeling her pulse, there were dramatic rate and rhythm fluctuations, the rate ranging from 80 bpm to 100 bpm within a short period of time. The pulse was Interrupted, skipping beats sporadically, was Ropy, and had a prominent Rough Vibration. The Rapid, Rough Vibration, and Interrupted pulse qualities reveal the major systemic imbalance of Heart Shock.

Not surprisingly, trauma has been a companion for Patient 2 since early on in her life, the first coming at birth as a breech presentation that was not discovered until 17 hours into labor. She was born two weeks late via C-section and suffered colic in her early months. Later in life trauma was experienced with witnessing constant parental fighting and via a dysfunctional and abusive intimate relationship that lasted a few years. Her most recent trauma came a few months prior to our initial visit wherein a fall left her with a subarachnoid hematoma (blunt trauma to the area of left BL 10) leaving her unconscious, waking in the hospital a day later. Upon waking she had severe pain in her head, numbness in her face and tongue (left side), low blood pressure, palpitations, and anxiety.

Other notable aspects of her pulse were:

- Empty pulse on the entire left side (Dr. Shen's Organ System): Empty Stage I

- Empty pulse on the entire right side (Dr. Shen's Digestive System, and Triple Burner mechanism): Empty Stage II

- Increased Rate on Exertion of 38–58 beats
- Empty Right Middle Position
- Feeble-Absent Right Proximal Position.

The Empty pulses reflect a significant state of instability, and because they present on both wrists qualify for a "Qi Wild" diagnosis of extreme systemic chaos. The right-sided Empty, while considered the Digestive System by Dr. Shen, in my experience also reflects the Triple Burner mechanism, a major stabilizing force. As a Stage II Empty, the instability is severe.

The increased rate on exertion is quite significant as it is so high; it signifies a very severe Heart blood deficiency. With an increase of 38–58 bpm, Heart blood is insufficient to promote and maintain proper circulation and explains the patient's low blood pressure, tendency towards fainting spells, and her anxiety (and insomnia). As I have noted earlier in this text, a Heart blood deficiency this severe compromises the patient's ability to heal, affecting blood volume (low blood pressure), and how much blood circulation is available to perfuse the tissues with nourishment, and of course overcome any areas of stagnation (especially those caused by traumatic injury).

The Empty Right Middle and Feeble-Absent Right Proximal positions demonstrate the lack of root and foundation, inability to create more blood to be circulated by the Heart, and diminished metabolic energy. These qualities also suggest that they reflect the patient's underlying constitutional weaknesses and have laid a vulnerable foundation with which additional traumas can take advantage of more easily.

Additional pulse findings

Looking at the Pulse Record, one sees a host of other significant findings on this patient. These include:

- Left Neuro-Psychological position Thin Tight/Rough Vibration/Changing Amplitude (3) with the entire position Changing Qualities to Absent
- Left Distal position moving towards a "separation of yin and yang" (Changing Amplitude (3+-4)), along with significant Muffled pulses showing depression and oppression of the chest
- Absent Right Distal position
- Yin Wei mai 8x pulse
- Divergent pulses for the SI/HT, ST/SP, SJ/PC, and LI/LU
- Hesitant and Hollow Full-Overflowing waveform on the left with Floating/Tense/Robust Pounding
- Flooding Deficient waveform on the right
- Blood Thick

- Cotton pulse (2)
- Left Middle position Thin and Tight, with Reduced Substance at the Organ depth
- SM pulses for the GB
- Sticky pulses reflecting phlegm-heat toxins
- Inflated pulse in the Esophagus/Thyroid position
- Inflation and Tight pulses in the Distal Liver Engorgement position
- Changing Amplitude overall
- Ropy pulse.

Ross Rosen, L.Ac., Dipl. O.M. (NCCAOM)
166 Mountain Ave., Westfield, NJ 07090, (908) 654-4333

Name: Patient 2	Gender: Female	Age: 30	Date:
Chief Complaint: Anxiety. Fainting	Height:	Weight:	Occupation:

Rhythm: Rate Change at Rest; Interrupted	Rate/Min: Begin: 80 End: 100 w/Exertion: 138 ▲: 38-58 Other Rates During Exam: 96

First Impressions of Uniform Qualities	Depths
Tense --> Tight Muffled (2+) Rough Vibration Ropy Sticky Robust Pounding (3+-4) Changing Amplitude (2+)	Wave: Left Hollow Full-Overflowing Right Flooding Deficient Floating: Left Tense and Pounding Cotton: (2) Qi: Blood: Thick Heat / Thick / Unclear Organ: O-B: O-S: see sides

Left Side:	Right Side:	
Increased Robust Pounding Empty (Stage I)	Empty (Stage II)	

PRINCIPAL POSITIONS	COMPLEMENTARY POSITIONS

Dir:	L:	Distal Position	R:	Dir:	L: Neuro-psychological R:

Distal Position:
L: Tense / Muffled (3+-4) / Changing Amplitude (3+-4)
R: Absent

SI: / HT: / Floating/Scattering? / Nurturing/Calming? / SM? Luo? DM? SI/HT
LI: Releasing? / LU: / Floating/Diffusing? / Descending? Moistening? / SM? Luo? DM? LI/LU

Neuro-psychological:
Thin Tight Rough Vibration / Changing Amplitude (3+) / <--> Absent

L: Special Lung Position R:

Special Lung Position:
L: Tense --> Tight / Muffled (2) / Rough Vibration
R: Tense --> Tight / Rough Vibration / Pleura: Muffled (1+) Sticky

L:	Middle Position	R:

Middle Position:
L: Thin Tight <--> Tense / Rough / Cosine / Changing Amplitude (2+) / Organ: Reduced Substance
R: Tense / Reduced Substance / Empty

GB: Receiving? / LR: Scattering? / Coursing? Discharging? / Storing? / SM? Luo? DM?
ST: Descending? / SP: Ascending? / Releasing? Harmonized? / SM? Tight Luo? DM? ST/SP @3 beans

Heart:
Mitral Valve:
Enlarged: Large Vessel:
Pericardium:

L: Diaphragm R:

Liver:
Engorged:
Distal: Tight Inflated (1+) Clear:
Gall Bladder CCPD:
Tense Muffled (2) Sticky Rough

L:	Proximal Position	R:

Proximal Position:
L: Tight - Tense / Rough / Changing Amplitude / Squirmy
R: Feeble-Absent

BL: Receiving? / KI: Consolidating? / SM? Luo? DM?
SJ: Floats? / KI/PC: / Releasing? Consolidating? / SM? Luo? DM? SJ/PC

Spleen-Stomach:
Esophagus: Inflated (1+) Spleen:
Stom-Pyl. Exten:
Duodenum: Peritoneal Cavity/Pancreas:

L: Intestines Small:

Large: Intestines   Small:

L: Pelvis/Lower Body R:

Pelvis/Lower Body:
L: Tense - Tight / Rough / Muffled (2)
R: Tense - Tight / Rough / Muffled (3+)

L:	8 Extra Pulses	R:

Yin Wei mai

Reminders: (specify side) Patient Day 23 of menstrual cycle
Split:
Fan Guan:
San Yin: △ = Change   (1 --> 5) = low --> high

Tongue:
Coat: Thick White
Body: Swollen Thick / Red / Tip Red with Petechia
Other: Sublingual veins / thin purple distended

Additional symptoms

- Allergies (mostly seasonal)
- Frequent urgent urination
- Poor balance and coordination
- Insomnia
- Asthma
- Catches colds easily
- Floaters
- Palpitations
- Low blood pressure
- Acne
- Dizziness
- Poor memory

Surgeries

- Abortion

Diagnoses

The main diagnoses revolve around Heart Shock, many actually being instrumental in the formation of Patient 2's constitution due to the early nature of the traumas. Others have been layered in over time from additional traumas, further weakening the system, eventually resulting in the damage done from this last traumatic injury. The diagnoses include the following.

Heart Shock and its sequelae

Diagnosis	Pulse auality(ies)
Qi Wild	Empty qualities bilaterally
Organ System Separation of yin and yang	Left side Empty
Digestive System Separation of yin and yang	Right side Empty, plus Reduced Substance and Empty in Right Middle
Triple Burner instability	Right side Empty and lack of uniformity in left/right pulses in each burner

Heart qi, yin, and blood deficiency (severe) moving towards separation of yin and yang	Changing Amplitude overall (2+), Rate Change at Rest, Interrupted pulse, Increase rate on exertion of 38–58 beats, Changing Amplitude in Left Distal (3+-4)
Kidney qi-yang deficiency	Feeble-Absent Right Proximal
Lung qi deficiency	Absent Right Distal
Liver qi and yin-blood deficiency	Thin Tight Left Middle with Reduced Substance at Organ depth
NST	Floating/Tense on left and Tense-Tight pulses throughout
Yin-essence deficiency	Ropy
Neuro-Psychological inflammation and impaired functioning	Thin Tight/Changing Amplitude and Rough Vibration/Changing Qualities to Absent in Neuro-Psych position
Blood stagnation (Liver)	Distal Liver Engorgement and Rough in Left Middle
Blood Thick	Blood Thick pulse
Wei qi stagnation	Cotton (2)
DM activity (SI/HT, ST/SP, SJ/PC, LI/LU)	DM pulses present
SM activity (GB)	Floating/Tight at 3 beans in Right Middle
8x vessel: Yin Wei mai	Left Yin Wei mai pulse
Depression and Heart oppression	Muffled overall and Muffled Left Distal
Phlegm-heat toxins	Sticky pulse
Esophagus/Thyroid stagnation/trapped qi	Inflated (1+) in Esophagus/Thyroid area
KI yang deficiency with connective tissue/central nervous system weakness	Squirmy pulse in Left Proximal

All of these qualities are significant signs of imbalance that must be addressed within the overall treatment plan for Patient 2. The left Neuro-Psychological pulse demonstrates the area of impact from the most recent trauma and its impact on the circulation and tissues surrounding. But the primary insult is really to the Heart, demonstrating Shock and yin deficiency unable to control yang, but also in its depletion on the qi aspect (Changing Amplitude overall) and its movement towards "separation of yin and yang" (Changing Amplitude in Left Distal). The Muffled pulses overall and in the Left Distal reflect the impact to the shen and oppression in her chest, creating an inability to move past the trauma. The Absent Right Distal also points to a weakness in wei qi and its ability to circulate to the extremities, the head being the fifth limb. Diffusion of Lung-wei qi will be compromised, thus inhibiting the letting go.

The Yin Wei mai pulse informs us of the impact of these traumas, most prevalently in the yin aspect of the Heart (and blood), as well as the need to invigorate blood. The Distal Liver Engorgement and Rough quality in the Left Middle confirm this. The longer-term impact from trauma on her physiology is reflected in the Ropy pulse and yin-essence deficiency as well as the Hollow Full-Overflowing pulse wave (see Figure 10.1) showing heat in the blood, as well as a drying out and thickening of it (Blood Thick). This increased viscosity of blood puts further taxation on the Heart and also contributes to the blood stasis. The DM activity also reveals the damage to the humors in attempting to manage and accommodate the trauma. Both the ST/SP and SI/HT DMs have BL 1 as its upper confluent point and exert a major influence over the head and brain. The ST/SP evidences Digestive System separation of yin and yang as the Empty pulse presents over the entire right side as well as in the Right Middle position, as well as the Flooding Deficient waveform on the right wrist. This weakness also allows for the trapped qi in the throat (Esophagus and Thyroid area). The SI/HT DM also exerts a major influence over the movement of wei qi to the head and face, and plays a role in the patient's allergies, as well as her anxiety, insomnia, fainting, etc. The DM activity also demonstrates a stagnation of the lymph, reflected by the Sticky pulses and phlegm-heat accumulation. Along with the wei qi stagnation, the GB SM reveals activity, furthering the dizziness, floaters, and loss of balance and coordination. The SJ/PC DM further influences the head, as well as damp-heat. The LI/LU DM confirms the weakness of wei qi and yang qi, and contributes to the asthma and allergies.

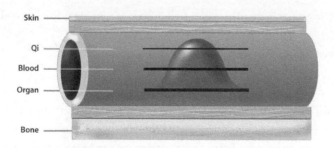

Figure 10.1: Hollow Full-Overflowing waveform
Reproduced with permission from Eastland Press

The patient's emotions are clearly impacted by the trauma, the Muffled pulse showing some depression, and the Cotton pulse (see Figure 10.2) reflecting her resignation and feelings of impotence and vulnerability over her condition and the uncertainty of when she might faint or be overcome with anxiety.

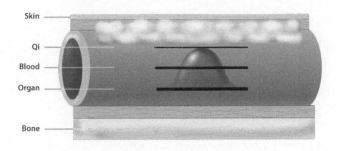

Figure 10.2: Cotton pulse
Reproduced with permission from Eastland Press

Priorities and interventions

1. Immediate

    a. Stability

        i. Qi Wild

            1. Separation of yin and yang

                I. Organ System

                II. Digestive system/Triple Burner

                III. Heart

        ii. Heart Shock

            1. Yin deficiency

            2. Blood deficiency (very severe)

            3. Qi deficiency (moving towards separation of yin and yang)

    b. Circulation/Heat/Pathogenic Factor

        i. Neuro-Psych inflammation and impaired functioning

        ii. Blood stagnation: Liver

2. Root issues

    a. Kidney qi and yin deficiency (including central nervous system impairment)

    b. Yin-essence deficiency

    c. NST

    d. Liver qi and yin-blood deficiency (with blood stagnation)

    e. Lung qi deficiency

3. Secondary

    a. 8x: Yin Wei mai

    b. DM: SI/HT, ST/SP, SJ/PC, LI/LU

    c. SM: GB

4. Tertiary

    a. Blood Thick

    b. Wei qi stagnation

    c. Phlegm-heat toxins

    d. Esophagus/Thyroid

Treatment strategies

Based on the foregoing priorities and interventions, my primary strategies included:

1. Stabilize and anchor Qi Wild by nourishing Heart yin, qi, and blood
2. Nourishing blood and invigorating blood in the head
3. Strengthening the Kidneys and central nervous system
4. Calming the shen.

Secondary strategies that needed to be considered included:

1. Nourishing yin-essence
2. Calming the nervous system
3. Strengthen the digestive system and generating blood and fluids
4. Opening the portals.

Tertiary strategies included:

1. Strengthening the Lungs
2. Clearing wei qi stagnation.

Treatments

Acupuncture

TREATMENT 1

> BL 1, GB 22 DSD
>
> SI 10, SI 16
>
> HT 1
>
> Ren 17, Ren 15
>
> KI 2

Utilizing the SI/HT DM allowed me to accomplish this, along with a number of other Heart Shock strategies. SI 10 and HT 1 are the lower confluents of the SI and HT respectively, and strongly return qi and blood to the chest. HT 1 is also excellent for promoting circulation in the channels and collaterals. SI 16 is a WOS point known to impact the portals, as well as return yin back to the Heart. GB 22 is also an arm yin sinew meeting point and strongly impacts the ye, as well as calming the nervous system. Its influence over blood and the chest is further revealed by it being the original Great Luo of the Spleen. Ren 17 strengthens Heart, Lung, and wei qi, calms the shen, clears heat from the chest, etc., and Ren 15 strongly nourishes yin and is the luo point of the Ren mai, providing additional comfort. KI 2 was utilized to strengthen and anchor Kidney yang and provide the catalyst to support circulation, as well as the digestive system (KI 2 to SP 8 trajectory).

TREATMENT 2

> BL 1, GB 22 DSD
>
> ST 30 DSD
>
> Right SP 4
>
> KI 16, KI 19, KI 25
>
> Ren 17
>
> Left PC 6

The patient responded very well to the first treatment, so the second treatment utilized many of the same principles. A few additions and changes were made, however. The first was to add ST 30 with DSD needling to impact the ST/SP DM. Both the ST/SP and SI/HT DM share BL 1 as the upper confluent, so adding ST 30 seamlessly addresses the digestive system component present in this case. At the same time, right SP 4 was added to incorporate Chong mai which presented on the patient's pulse during this visit. Adding KI 16, KI 19, and KI 25 brought Chong mai's dynamics to the treatment, strengthening the Kidneys, the digestive system, and the Heart. Ren 17 further solidified the impact to the Heart/Pericardium and the treatment was closed with left PC 6, the opening of Yin Wei mai, further influencing the Pericardium and jueyin connection to blood invigoration.

TREATMENT 3

Treatment 2 was repeated.

At this evaluation all Empty pulses had resolved and symptoms were mostly gone. Treatment 2 was repeated to solidify its effect.

Herbal

The initial herbal formula consisted of 13 herbs. As the patient had to make a three-hour journey to see me and could only come monthly for follow-up visits, I thought it prudent to use more herbs and allow for the formula to be received more gently, making consistent progress over time. The patient was also referred to a colleague closer to her home for weekly acupuncture, though finances were a prohibitive factor in that regard. The formula contained:

Sheng Di Huang	9g
Gou Qi Zi	9g
Bai Shao	9g
Dang Gui Wei	9g
Chuan Xiong	6g
Yuan Zhi	6g
Ren Shen	9g
Qiang Huo	6g
Gui Zhi	9g
Ye Jiao Teng	15g
Ji Xue Teng	15g
Suan Zao Ren	9g
Zhi Gan Cao	5g

The initial strategy of anchoring Qi Wild by nourishing the Heart was addressed with Sheng Di Huang, Gou Qi Zi, Bai Shao, Suan Zao Ren, Ye Jiao Teng, and Ji Xue Teng (yin and blood), and Ren Shen and Zhi Gan Cao (qi). Bai Shao and Suan Zao Ren are also sour and help to astringe. These herbs also strengthen the Liver yin-blood, relaxing the nerves. Because of the extreme deficiency, any invigoration must also include nourishment, so Dang Gui Wei, Ye Jiao Teng, and Ji Xue Teng were used. Chuan Xiong also assisted in guiding to the head and the GB SM area. The Kidneys and central nervous system were impacted by Sheng Di Huang, Gou Qi Zi, and Qiang Huo. The shen was calmed by Sheng Di Huang, Bai Shao, Yuan Zhi, Ye Jiao Teng, and Suan Zao Ren.

The secondary strategies used Sheng Di Huang and Gou Qi Zi to nourish yin-essence; Bai Shao, Dang Gui Wei, Chuan Xiong, Qiang Huo, Ji Xue Teng, and Ye Jiao Teng to calm the nervous system; Ren Shen and Zhi Gan Cao to strengthen the GI; and Yuan Zhi to open the portals. Dang Gui, Bai Shao, Gui Zhi, and Gou Qi Zi are also herbs that resonate to the Yin Wei mai.

The tertiary strategies of strengthening the Lungs also relied on Ren Shen and Huang Qi; and wei qi stagnation cleared via Yuan Zhi, Gui Zhi, Qiang Huo, and Chuan Xiong. As the trauma was to the head, the use of Gui Zhi and Qiang Huo also addressed the taiyang zone (BL 10 was the area of impact), and Chuan Xiong addressed the shaoyang GB SM component, which was discussed in Chapter 4. Tian Ma assists these zonal herbs with dispersing any bi-obstruction and also nourishes Liver yin-blood with the other blood tonics above.

The formula was refilled a few times as the patient was unable to return for a follow-up evaluation for approximately three months' time. Upon return, the Right Middle Position was no longer Empty, and the Right Proximal no longer Feeble-Absent. Both had a Reduced Substance quality. Her rhythm had also normalized. All her symptoms were improving. The formula was refilled with the following changes in italics:

Sheng Di Huang	*15g*
Gou Qi Zi	9g
Bai Shao	9g
Dang Gui Wei	9g
Chuan Xiong	*9g*
Yuan Zhi	6g
Ren Shen	9g
Qiang Huo	6g
Gui Zhi	9g
Ye Jiao Teng	15g
Ji Xue Teng	15g
Suan Zao Ren	9g
Zhi Gan Cao	5g
Tian Ma	*9g*

To capitalize on the improvement some changes were made so that it was a bit more aggressive. Sheng Di Huang was increased to 15g to address Heart yin and clear any heat harassing the spirit; and Chuan Xiong to 9g to further invigorate blood in the head and dispel any lingering wind. Tian Ma 9g was added to further address the Liver and control any spasms and headaches with Bai Shao and extinguish wind and pain.

On her visit three weeks later all Empty pulses were resolved and she had no anxiety or panic for the first time since her trauma. The following formula was administered:

Sheng Di Huang	15g
Gou Qi Zi	9g
Bai Shao	9g
Dang Gui Wei	9g
Chuan Xiong	9g
Yuan Zhi	6g
Ren Shen	9g
Qiang Huo	6g
Gui Zhi	9g
Ye Jiao Teng	15g
Ji Xue Teng	15g
Suan Zao Ren	9g
Zhi Gan Cao	5g
~~Tian Ma~~	~~9g~~
Huang Qi	*9g*

Tian Ma was removed and Huang Qi added to further support Heart, Lung, and wei qi, as well as support the GI and Kidney qi/constitution.

Follow up: At her last follow-up appointment, the patient has reported that all symptoms have resolved and that she has become aware that she currently experiences a sense of well-being greater than prior to the trauma. Even prior to the trauma, patient would experience anxiety and panic which have now resolved, demonstrating the thesis as set forth on page 31 from hexagram 51 of the I Jing, that on the other side of trauma, one can find increased joy and wellness.

Essential oils

The oil blend was not administered, but written as:

Angelica

Myrrh

Lavender

Camphor

Safflower Oil carrier oil

Angelica and Myrrh home to the SI/HT DM and help to nourish and invigorate blood and heal traumatic injuries. As a seed, Angelica also supports the constitution, as well as the Lungs and Spleen qi. Lavender directed the blend to the head and assists with regulating qi and blood. Camphor helps to open obstructions and the portals, strengthening Heart and Kidney qi.

Patient 3

History

A 45-year-old female, Patient 3 sought treatment for one-sided constant headaches/ migraines and face pain which radiated to her tongue, neck, and shoulder, and gastritis and reflux with excruciating chest pain causing skipping heartbeats and anxiety. Touching her pulse, the first prominent signs were a Rate Changing at Rest (3+) and an Interrupted pulse, as well as a strong Rough Vibration. Overall, the pulse was Thin and Tight, Changing Amplitude (2), Choppy, and 62 bpm.

Analyzing the above it is clear that this patient was suffering from Heart Shock, and that the trauma had occurred early in life prior to maturation (Interrupted pulse and Slow rate). Additionally, yin and blood were compromised and the nervous system was hypervigilant (overall Thin, Tight). Heart qi was deficient (Changing Amplitude (2), and Slow rate), and there was blood stasis (Choppy).

The progression of Patient 3's illness, like many, began in early life. Her mother, only 18 years old at the time, was emotionally unstable and in a dysfunctional relationship with the patient's father. When she was one year old, they got divorced and the father was awarded custody. Mom became an absentee, and dad deposited her with his parents to be raised, coming in and out of the picture. She experienced lots of physical and emotional abuse, as well as some sexual abuse by her father who would grab her breasts. She was constantly threatened as a child that if she didn't behave she would be sent to live with her emotionally unstable mother. After her grandfather (who raised her) died, she became very depressed, and her husband at the time left her. An additional trauma came in the form of an injury to her jaw which was dislocated and required multiple stitches.

Other notable aspects of her pulse were:

- Heart rate on exertion: increase of 34 beats

- Empty pulse over the entire left wrist

- Empty Left Middle position

- Absent Left Distal position

- Right Special Lung position Full with a Spinning Bean in center

- Left Special Lung position distally Deep and Restricted (early stage)
- Thin Tight/Choppy right wrist.

The heart rate increase of 34 beats on exertion shows a severe Heart blood deficiency. Contributed to by her early traumas and lack of nourishment in her early years, it manifests as the patient's anxiety, insomnia, fatigue, migraines, and palpitations. The Absent Left Distal further confirms the impact of trauma on her Heart and Heart qi deficiency. The Changing Rate at Rest and Interrupted pulses also reveal constant worry and feeling like life is a roller coaster emotionally.

The Empty pulse on the left side confirms the early life deficits and lack of nourishment, and the Left Middle Empty reveals the chaos and lack of stability in the Wood phase, governed by the Liver and Gall Bladder, the other origin of her chief complaints (vertex headache, left-sided pain, and reflux/gastritis, as well as the breast pathology revealed by the pulse). With the nervous system being tense, and the finding of Thin Tight/Choppy pulses on the entire right side, we see the impact of NST overacting on DSW or, in other terms, Liver invading Stomach and the resultant inflammation and blood stasis.

The other very notable finding is in the Special Lung positions, which, when the Liver shows Empty, reveals breast pathology. The Spinning Bean in the center of the Right Special Lung shows a mass on the left breast, which was confirmed via imaging. The Deep and early Restricted pulse in the Left Special Lung shows a burgeoning issue in the right breast which the patient was notified about. She was referred for imaging for a potential breast mass in the right upper lateral breast.

Additional pulse findings

- Flooding Deficient waveform
- Cotton (2)
- Thin (4) Tight pulses in Right Distal position
- Blood heat
- Tight/Rough/Sticky/Cosine Right Middle position
- Tight/Inflated Esophagus pulse
- Tight Stomach-Pylorus Extension position
- Distal Liver Engorgement Inflated (1+)
- Tight/Robust Pounding (3+)/Choppy Gall Bladder
- Medial Thin Tight/Choppy pulses in both Proximal positions
- 8x vessel pulses for Ren mai, Chong mai, and Yin Qiao mai
- DM pulses for ST/SP, SI/HT, LI/LU
- Luo vessel pulses for HT, ST/SP, BL, SJ

Ross Rosen, L.Ac., Dipl. O.M. (NCCAOM)
166 Mountain Ave., Westfield, NJ 07090, (908) 654-4333

Name: Patient 3		Gender: Female	Age: 45	Date:
Chief Complaint: Migraine, Gastritis, Chest pain		Height: 5' 7"	Weight: 180	Occupation: Stay at home mom
Rhythm: Rate Change at Rest (3); Interrupted			Rate/Min: Begin: 66 End: 62 w/Exertion: 96 △: 34 Other Rates During Exam:	

First Impressions of Uniform Qualities	Depths
Thin Tight Muffled (3) Robust Pounding (2+) Changing Amplitude (2) Rough Vibration Choppy	Wave: Flooding Deficient Floating: Cotton: (2) Qi: Blood: Heat Heat / Thick / Unclear Organ: O-B: see sides O-S:

Left Side:	Right Side:
Tense Muffled Increased Pounding Empty	Thinner Tighter Increased Choppy

PRINCIPAL POSITIONS	COMPLEMENTARY POSITIONS

Dir:	L:	Distal Position	R:	Dir:
	Absent		Thin (4) Tight Rough	

SI: Receiving?	LI: Releasing?
HT:	LU:
Floating/Scattering?	Floating/Diffusing?
Nurturing/Calming?	Descending? Moistening?
SM? Luo? HT DM? SI/HT	SM? Luo? DM? LI/LU

L:	Middle Position	R:
Above Qi Tense Tense Cosine Muffled (2+-3) Empty	Tight Muffled (2) Sticky Rough Organ Tense Cosine

GB: Receiving?	ST: Descending?
LR: Scattering?	SP: Ascending?
Coursing? Discharging?	Releasing? Harmonized?
Storing?	
SM? Luo? DM?	SM? Luo? ST/SP DM? ST SP

L:	Proximal Position	R:
Medial Thin Tight Cosine Choppy Muffled (2)	Tight Rough Vibration Muffled (3) Organ Choppy

BL: Receiving?	SJ: Floats?
KI: Consolidating?	KI/PC:
	Releasing? Consolidating?
SM? Luo? BL DM?	SM? Luo? SJ DM?

L:	8 Extra Pulses	R:
Ren mai Chong mai		Yin Qiao mai

Reminders: (specify side)
Split:
Fan Guan:
San Yin: △ = Change   (1 → 5) = low → high

Complementary Positions:

	L:	Neuro-psychological	R:

	L:	Special Lung Position	R:
	Distally Deep and Restricted		Tense-Tight Full Rough Vibration Robust Pounding Middle Spinning Bean Pleura:

Heart
Mitral Valve:
Enlarged: Large Vessel:
Pericardium:

	L:	Diaphragm	R:

Liver
Engorged:
Distal: Inflated (1+)   Ulnar:
Gall Bladder CCPD: Tight Choppy
Robust Pounding (3+) Changing Amplitude (2+)

Spleen-Stomach
Esophagus: tight   Spleen:
Inflated (2)
Stom-Pyl. Exten:
Duodenum: Tight   Peritoneal Cavity/Pancreas:

	L:	Intestines	R:
	Large:		Small:

	L:	Pelvis/Lower Body	R:
	Thin Tight Rough Muffled (2)		Muffled (3) Tense-Tight

Tongue:
Coat: Thick Dry White

Body: Thick Red
Contracted Sides
Dry
Other: Center Crack

Sublingual veins purple

Additional symptoms

- Gastritis/Reflux
- Palpitations and Skipped beats
- Swollen lymph nodes
- Fatigue
- Hair loss
- Itchy skin
- Insomnia
- Allergies
- Anxiety
- Depression
- Alternating constipation and diarrhea
- Recent weight loss of 60 lbs in past year due to GI symptoms
- Back pain
- PMS

Surgeries

- Lymph nodes removed after first pregnancy
- GB removed due to large gall stone
- Tonsils removed

Diagnoses

The early Heart Shock has created multiple issues in this patient's life, affecting multiple systems. They include the following.

Heart Shock and its sequelae

Diagnosis	Pulse quality(ies)
HT qi, yin, and blood deficiency	Changing Rate at Rest, Interrupted pulse, Increase rate on exertion of 34 beats, Absent Left Distal, Changing Amplitude over entire pulse
NST	Thin Tight overall
NST overacting on DSW	Thin Tight/Choppy on Right side

Organ System Separation of Yin and Yang	Empty Left side
Liver Separation of Yin and Yang	Empty Left Middle position
Toxicity	Choppy pulse overall and in Liver Distal Engorgement and Digestive System
Obstruction in breasts	Special Lung positions Spinning Bean and Deep Restricted pulses
Overall qi deficiency (moderate)	Flooding Deficient waveform
Wei qi stagnation, Resignation, Lymph stagnation	Cotton pulse
Lung yin-blood deficiency	Thin (4) Tight pulses in Right Distal
Blood heat	Blood Heat pulse
Inflammation and parenchymal tissue damage in Stomach	Tight/Rough/Sticky/Cosine Right Middle
Trapped qi and inflammation in esophagus	Esophagus/Tight/Inflated pulse
Inflammation in Stomach-pylorus extension	Tight pulse in Stomach-pylorus position
Liver blood stagnation	Distal Liver engorgement
Inflammation, heat, and blood stasis in Gall Bladder channel	Tight/Robust Pounding/Choppy
Yin and blood-essence deficiency in Kidneys attempting latency	Thin Tight/Choppy pulses in Proximal positions that move medially
Chong, Ren, and Yin Qiao activity	8x pulse configuration
ST/SP, SI/HT, LI/LU DMs	DM pulses present
HT, ST/SP, BL, SJ luo vessels	Luo pulses present

While the number of diagnoses are many, as revealed by the pulse, weaving them all together under the Heart Shock diagnosis umbrella and seeing their interrelationships is easy. The long-term burden of accommodating the shock has created a taxation on many resources. Overall, it has left her qi deficient (Flooding Deficient waveform), and has also depleted the Kidney yin (and blood) from overworking of the adrenals, and maintaining a latency of her emotional traumas. The heat from this adrenaline gets metabolized in the blood and has created a Blood Heat pulse, also taxing the LR/GB, creating inflammation and blood stasis (Tight/Robust Pounding/Choppy in GB and Distal Liver Engorgement).

The early traumas and lack of bonding (absentee mother with emotional disability) and boundaries (inappropriate touching from dad), have created a number of adaptations. First, it impacts the first ancestry of 8x vessels associated with boundaries and bonding (Chong and Ren), creating a constant need to find nourishment (patient was 220 lbs), but also impacts the third ancestry and one's self-esteem and worth (Yin Qiao). From a psycho-social developmental and luo vessel perspective, multiple channels are active, most notably the Heart (chest stagnation and betrayal/abuse) and ST/SP (rebellious qi, and gut inflammation), but also the Bladder (headaches) and Triple Burner (depression and hot temper).

The DM activity also reflects the inability to maintain latency in the primary areas of the patient's chief complaints and symptoms: the ST/SP DM and its role of managing the jin-thin fluids and the irritation and inflammation in the gut; the SI/HT DM and the chest symptoms of pain, palpitations, and reflux, along with her allergies; and the LI/LU DM with a major role over Lung/wei qi (allergies, as well as lymph circulation and the Cotton pulse of resignation), but also having a prime role in managing circulation through the breasts (LI DM). In fact, all of these DM channels play a pivotal role in managing lymphatic circulation, as well as traversing the chest and breast region.

Thus, seeing all the interrelationships, one must begin the process of prioritizing and addressing the most immediate priorities, while also considering the root and secondary issues.

Priorities and interventions

1. Immediate
    a. Stability
        i. Heart Shock
            1. Heart yin, qi, and blood deficiency
        ii. Separation of yin and yang
            1. Organ Systems (taiyin, shaoyin, jueyin)
            2. Liver
                I. Qi deficiency
                II. Distal blood engorgement
                III. Qi stagnation
                IV. Neoplastic activity (moderate)
    b. Circulation/Heat/Pathogenic Factors
        i. Chest/Breast: Restricted and Spinning Bean obstructed circulation
        ii. NST overacting on DSW (with blood stagnation)
        iii. Esophagus/Stomach gastritis: yin deficiency and inflammation
        iv. LR/GB wind and heat
2. Root issues
    a. NST
    b. Kidney yin-blood deficiency (and overall yin-blood deficiency)

   c. Lung yin-blood deficiency

   d. Stomach yin deficiency

   e. 8x channels: Ren mai, Chong mai, Yin Qiao mai

   f. DM: ST/SP, SI/HT, LI/LU

   g. Luo vessels: HT, ST, BL, SJ

3. Secondary issues

   a. Blood heat

   b. Wei qi stagnation

   c. GB inflammation (surgery)

   d. Kidney blood stagnation

   e. Stagnation of qi/blood/fluids in middle and lower burner

Treatment strategies

1. Nourish Liver qi and invigorate blood
2. Nourish Heart yin, qi, and blood
3. Open/invigorate blood in chest/breast
4. Calm NST and its overacting on digestive system
5. Regulate qi in Esophagus and Stomach

Treatments
Acupuncture
TREATMENT 1

   Left ST 40 bleeding technique

   Right HT 5

   Right LU 7

   Du 20

   Ren 17

   Ren 12 plus extra point 3 cun lateral to Ren 12

   Left GB 20

   Left GB 34

As the patient presented with Stomach and Heart luo pulses, and her main symptoms are reflective of rebellious qi and circulatory disturbances, I tapped into the luo first. The Stomach luo addresses the root of the internal imbalance in her GI, clearing heat and rebellious qi, and the Heart luo assists with opening the chest and freeing the circulation. It also allows for yin, qi, and blood to return. Second, the patient's presentation of 8x vessel pulses, and in particular symptoms stemming from the vertex and center line, warranted opening Ren mai. Du 20 was chosen as part of Ren mai's secondary trajectory (Du mai), and also as a point to reverse polarity and assist with descending into the abdomen. The Left Middle position was Empty and the Liver governs the vertex and vertex headaches. Its association with the Gall Bladder also is revealed with the patient's pain traveling down the left side of her face and neck/SCM and into her shoulder (GB 20–21 area). To continue the descension of rebellious qi, Ren 17 was needled, which also assists the Heart luo and frees up the chest oppression. Ren 12 helps to anchor the qi to the abdomen and further works to home Ren mai to the SP/ST and source of post-natal nourishment which was lacking from early neglect. I often use Ren mai where parental (especially maternal) influences have been lacking in early life bonding and boundary formation, and, from a DRRBF perspective, that is influenced by the earth. Using Ren 12 as the anchoring point addresses both. Additionally, the use of the extra point 3 cun lateral to Ren 12 taps into and anchors the Liver (a Classical point to treat disparities between the superficial and deep pulses in the Left Middle position). Lastly, left GB 20 and GB 34 were used as sinew points to release the stagnant qi and blood, open the chest, and calm her nervous system.

TREATMENT 2

> Right SP 4
>
> Right LU 7
>
> Yin Tang
>
> Ren 17, 12
>
> KI 25, 19, 16
>
> ST 30
>
> LR 3

The second treatment builds on the first, still focusing strongly on the mother-earth, adding in the Chong mai connection instead of the Stomach and Heart luos. The Chong also provides the relationship to rebellious qi, and taps into the energetics of the Heart via the chest points, and the gut. Additionally, it allowed me to root back into the Liver from Chong's descending pathway to LR 3, which symptomatically helps with the migraines, Liver invading Stomach, and the origin of the Empty pulse. The Ren mai treatment furthers these objectives, and the use of Ren 17 and KI 16 also mimics the lower trajectory of the Heart luo, bringing in that strategy from the prior treatment, and the pulse finding. Both Ren mai and Chong mai focus heavily on the abdomen with the use of Ren 12, KI 19, and ST 30.

At the following visit, the patient reported that she had not experienced heart burn since the second treatment, and her headaches were markedly reduced.

Herbal

The first formula placed a strong priority on invigorating blood and opening the chest/breast due to the significance of the Restricted and Spinning Bean pulses in the Special Lung positions reflecting the breasts. Xue Fu Zhu Yu Tang modified, was prescribed as shown below.

FIRST FORMULA

Xue Fu Zhu Yu Tang jia jian (omissions struck through; additions in italics)

Tao Ren	12g
Hong Hua	9g
Chuan Xiong	~~4.5~~=9g
Dang Gui	9g
Sheng Di Huang	~~9~~=15g
Bai Shao	9g
Chai Hu	3g
~~Zhi Ke~~	6g
Mu Li	*9g*
Gan Cao	3g
~~Chuan Niu Xi~~	~~9g~~
Wang Bu Liu Xing	*9g*
Jie Geng	4.5g
Huang Qi	*9g*
Gui Zhi	*9g*

The use of Xue Fu Zhu Yu Tang as modified allows for a number of treatment strategies to be implemented. First, nourishing the Liver qi and blood is accomplished by Dang Gui and Bai Shao (blood), and Huang Qi and Gui Zhi (qi). Liver blood is invigorated with Tao Ren, Hong Hua, Dang Gui, Chuan Xiong, and Wang Bu Liu Xing. Heart yin is nourished via the large dose of Sheng Di Huang, and its qi strengthened with Huang Qi and Gui Zhi. The chest is opened and blood invigorated by Tao Ren, Hong Hua, Chuan Xiong, Chai Hu, Jie Geng, Wang Bu Liu Xing, and

Gui Zhi. The nervous system is calmed by Chuan Xiong, Bai Shao, Chai Hu, and Sheng Di Huang. The shen is calmed by Sheng Di Huang, Hong Hua, and Mu Li. Mu Li also astringes and anchors the floating yang in the Liver (Floating/Tense pulse in the Above Qi depth), addresses the lymph nodes, and also addresses the patient's gastritis/esophagitis by alkalizing and balancing Stomach fluids. Bai Shao assists treating the gastritis, and also relaxes the nerves and softens spasms and treats the patient's headaches. Chuan Xiong further eliminates the headaches and face/neck pain by invigorating blood and dispelling wind. Tao Ren, Dang Gui, and Sheng Di Huang will help normalize the bowels. Anxiety, palpitations, and insomnia are addressed by the Sheng Di Huang, Mu Li, Hong Hua, Bai Shao, Dang Gui, and Gui Zhi via their impact on the blood and qi. Zhi Ke is removed to allow for more descension, and as Chai Hu is retained to drive to the Liver, its dosage is only 3g. Wang Bu Liu Xing is used instead of Chuan Niu Xi to drive the formula to the breasts and chest. Huang Qi, Gui Zhi, and Jie Geng assist with the allergy symptoms. PMS is addressed via the Liver qi and blood herbs, as is the hair loss. Fatigue and depression are assisted via the invigoration of Liver blood and Heart qi tonification.

Essential oils

Geranium

Angelica seed

Fennel

Sweet almond oil with a few drops of Tamanu oil

Geranium has the functions of nourishing Kidney yin, communicating Heart and Kidneys, calming the shen, and descending the Stomach qi, making it a good oil for the combination of a Ren mai and Chong mai presentation. In addition, it regulates Liver qi, and as a flower impacts the upper part of the body, in particular the breasts (of which it has a primary function), as well as the head for treating headaches. It is analgesic as well as a tonic, and gets rid of varicosities (helping with luo functions). Angelica seed is a favorite oil of mine for trauma as it summons the angelic spirits to treat terror and shock, invigorates and nourishes the blood, calms the shen, strengthens the Lungs and Spleen, and regulates the nervous system overacting on the digestive system. It also opens the diaphragm, regulates qi, and treats pain. Another of my favorite oils, fennel, was used as it exerts a strong influence on the Liver/Stomach dynamic, as well as strengthening HT/KI communication (yang aspect); it strengthens the adrenals, Heart qi, and Liver. Fennel can treat the entire Liver channel, and treat the vertex headache, while anchoring to the lower burner and descending the Stomach. Thus, with this formula, we treat all aspects of Heart Shock—Heart yin, qi, and blood; invigorating blood, strengthening the earth, calming the Liver (nervous system), boosting Kidney yang, opening the portals, and calming the shen—all with oils that also specifically treat the symptomatic presentation and underlying pulse dynamics. Sweet almond oil was used as the main carrier to resonate with LU 7 and open the Ren mai, and Tamanu was used to break up the yin stasis in the chest/breasts. The oils can be applied to the acupuncture points above.

CHAPTER 11
Vignettes

Patient 4

History

Patient 4 was a 61-year-old man who had recently suffered a heart attack, with a right bundle branch block, three blocked arteries, and ventricular tachycardia. At the time of his visit, he wore a pacemaker (set to 60 bpm). He suffered insomnia and sleep apnea, hot flashes, and diverticulitis, with a recent ruptured colon, requiring a colostomy (and eventual reversal). His pulse revealed Rough Vibration, Changing Rate at Rest, and Interrupted pulses, Ropy and Choppy overall. His Left Distal position was Leather-Hard, Tight, Empty, and Changing Amplitude (4); his Right Distal Muffled (5); his Left Middle Empty/Robust Pounding (4) with a Spinning Bean in the proximal aspect; and both Proximal pulses Empty. His heart rate was very difficult to clock due to the severity of the arrhythmia and the premature ventricular contractions (PVCs), but the active functional beats were noted at 36 bpm, with PVCs happening every 7 beats, then every 2–3 beats.

His heart rate presented an unusual circumstance as he was wired with a pacemaker for 60 bpm, which prompted a discussion with him, and then eventually his cardiologist as I was concerned about his Heart health. His cardiologist did not receive my questions well, arguing that he was able to guarantee the 60 bpm from the monitoring of the device. My concern, however, was that the 60 bpm was recording the PVCs in addition to the regular beats, but the PVCs in this patient's case were not functional heartbeats as they would come rapidly after a regular beat and have virtually no amplitude. The beat came so quickly that the ventricle had insufficient time to fill with blood, leading to more of a spasm of the ventricle than promoting any blood flow. This lack of blood flow was contributing to the Leather-Hard pulse in the Left Distal position, demonstrating the Heart becoming deprived of blood. The cardiologist dismissed my concern despite the severity of the patient's symptoms and history, and abruptly ended our conversation. (As a side note, one year later the patient's pacemaker was changed and reset.)

Diagnoses

Patient 4's presentation was positive for Heart Shock (Rough Vibration), and that shock came early in life (Changing Rate at Rest and Interrupted pulses). In fact, he was a victim of abuse in his early childhood. There was significant Heart deficiency and separation of yin and yang in the Heart (Changing Amplitude (4) in Left Distal and Leather-Hard), Liver (Empty Left Middle), and Kidneys (Empty bilaterally in Proximals). There was also severe stagnation in the chest (wei qi, and stagnation of yin/qi/blood), and a hardening of the tissues of the Heart and vessels overall (Leather-Hard and Ropy), with viscous blood (Blood Thick). Pulses for the Yin Wei mai and Chong mai were present as well.

Treatment

Acupuncture treatments varied between addressing the 8x vessels and the primary channels. Few needles were chosen for each treatment as the patient was hypersensitive. Generally, for the primary channels, points were chosen from the Heart and Pericardium channels (HT 3, 5, 6, 7 and PC 3, 4, 6, 7), with Gall Bladder points to open the chest (GB 22, 21, 34), Ren channel points on the chest and associated with the HT/PC (Ren 17, 15, 14), points to set rate and rhythm and wei qi (LU 1, 9), and other chest points influencing Heart blood (e.g., ST 15). 8x channel treatments opened both Chong mai and Yin Wei mai to drive qi, yin, and blood to the chest. And when allowed, I would incorporate a treatment on the SI/HT and GB/LR DM, bringing blood and thicker fluids to the heart and chest.

Herbal medicine treatments were also varied. Many of the herbs used were to strengthen and stabilize the Heart, nourishing its qi, yin, and blood, as well as strengthening and anchoring the Liver and Kidney yang, and opening the chest. They included: Mai Men Dong, Wu Wei Zi, Xi Yang Shen, Chen Pi, Fu Ling, Fu Zi, Sha Ren, Chai Hu, Yin Yang Huo, Mu Xiang, Ren Shen, Xiang Fu, Zhi Gan Cao, Hu Po, Dai Zhe Shi, Tian Ma, etc.

Essential oils used included: Angelica seed (strengthening Heart blood, communicating to the Kidneys, nourishing the Lungs and Spleen, invigorating blood, addressing negativity and perverse qi and fright that damages self-worth, and opening the diaphragm), Benzoin (strengthening and astringing the Heart while diffusing Lung qi and ridding damp from chest), Geranium (nourishing Heart blood, communicating Heart/Kidneys, addressing damp-heat stagnation in the chest, and invigorating blood), Fennel (strengthening the Heart and Kidney yang, moving the Liver, and strengthening the Stomach), and Orange (clearing heat from the chest which creates the PVCs).

Changes

Over the course of a few months the patient's sleep had dramatically improved and his hot flashes were virtually non-existent. Bloodwork and physical, including the nuclear stress test, were all normal, with no blockages and no evidence of ventricular tachycardia. His cardiologist gave him a clean bill of health and the patient discontinued his treatments. Despite the significant changes in the patient's symptoms, the Interrupted pulse was still present, as were the PVCs as per pulse diagnosis, albeit to a much lesser degree. Follow-up treatments and herbal care were still warranted from my perspective as the duration of treatment was insufficient to fully address the root causes.

Patient 5

History

Patient 5 was a 50-year-old female suffering from insomnia, day-time fatigue, depression, anxiety, Celiac disease with bloating and chronic constipation, Hashimoto's thyroiditis, and an inability to focus and concentrate. Her pulse had a profound Rough Vibration, was Ropy, Tense-Tight, and Choppy overall, with a Blood Unclear finding. Her heart rate was 60 bpm with an Absent Left Distal position (and an inability to express her shen), Empty Left Middle position, Muffled (3+) in the Right Distal with an inability to diffuse Lung qi, and approaching Empty in the Right Middle and Left Proximal positions (Blood and Organ depths were Reduced Substance). Her pulse also revealed sinew (Gall Bladder) and luo vessel (Liver and Spleen) activity, as well as divergent meridians (ST/SP and SI/HT). 8x vessels present included Dai mai and Yin Qiao mai.

Her history was significant for trauma, being raised in a turbulent home, neglected by mom, and sexually abused by an alcoholic dad. As a teenager, she was further sexually assaulted by a medical professional, and was involved in multiple dysfunctional relationships, all of which created poor self-esteem, self-loathing, and suicidal ideations.

Diagnoses

Patient 5's pulse and history confirm trauma (Rough Vibration) and the resultant impact on her nervous system causing anxiety and hypervigilance (Tense-Tight pulse, including on the Floating and Qi depths, and sinew pulse), Heart qi deficiency (Absent Left Distal and 60 bpm), and overall instability (Empty Left Middle, and Blood and Organ depth Reduced Substance in the Right Middle and Left Proximal). Yin-essence has been depleted with resultant inflammation and heat in the blood (Ropy), as well as damage to her self-image (Yin Qiao mai), which includes a feeling of being unworthy and toxic (Blood Unclear finding and Choppy overall) to the point of having suicidal ideations (Liver luo). The weakness in Kidney and Spleen qi damaged her middle, creating a burden and an inability to process and assimilate nourishment (history of neglect and abuse), and also creating an active Dai mai and Spleen luo with dampness congesting the middle and lower burners. Opening one's Heart and chest were impaired, as trust and vulnerability issues were profound (Heart not expressing shen, Lung not diffusing wei qi, Muffled (3) Right Distal).

Treatment

Treatments varied considerably over the course of time that I treated Patient 5, depending on the urgency of the pulse findings in any given treatment day, and as a process of first creating stability and comfort, then attempting to further move and unblock. Some of the acupuncture visits included the following:

- HT 3, Ear Shenmen, SI 16, KI 25, Ren 15, Ren 6, LR 3
- PC 6, Ren 17, KI 25, LR 14, Ren 12 plus extra point 3 cun lateral, ST 25, SP 6, LR 3
- GB 13, HT 3, PC 7, Ren 17, LR 14, Ren 6, LR 3
- BL 1/GB 22 DSD, SI 18, Ren 17, Ren 12, Ren 4, SI 3
- GB 1/Ren 2 DSD, BL 1/GB 22 DSD, Ren 17, LR 14, LR 13, GB 25.

Herbally, I began with the following formula (subsequent changes are shown with italics and strikeouts):

Bai Zi Ren	9g
Xi Yang Shen	9g
He Shou Wu	15g
Xiang Fu	9g
Chuan Xiong	6g
Ren Shen	9g
Xuan Shen	9g
Mu Xiang	9g
Hou Po	9g
Sheng Di Huang	9g
Gan Cao	5g

With this first formula, focus was given to stabilizing the Heart and Liver, while opening the middle to allow for assimilation, ridding her burden, and allowing for the anchoring.

Bai Zi Ren	9g
Xi Yang Shen	9g
He Shou Wu	15g
Xiang Fu	9g
Chuan Xiong	6g
Ren Shen	9g
Xuan Shen	9g
Mu Xiang	9g
Hou Po	9g
Sheng Di Huang	9g
Gan Cao	5g
Zhi Shi	*6g*

This modification was to continue moving the middle and unblock what was preventing her from receiving nourishment and comfort.

Bai Zi Ren	9g
Xi Yang Shen	9g
He Shou Wu	15g
Xiang Fu	9g
Chuan Xiong	6g
Ren Shen	9g
~~Xuan Shen~~	~~9g~~
Mu Xiang	9g
~~Hou Po~~	~~9g~~
Sheng Di Huang	*15g*
Gan Cao	5g
Zhi Shi	6g
Gui Zhi	*9g*
Si Ni Bei or Fu Zi	*30g*

This next formula removed the Hou Po as her bowels had freed up, and her boundaries were improving. Xuan Shen was removed as she became more able to voice her trauma, having gone deep into the darkness, finding a way to open her heart, and relaxing the restriction in her throat. Gui Zhi and Si Ni Bei/Fu Zi were added to more strongly nourish and strengthen her Heart, Liver, Stomach, and Kidney qi-yang.

Changes

Patient 5 and I worked together for approximately six months before a job change relocated her, making it difficult to come for visits. In that period of time, however, she experienced many changes. Sleep and energy improved, depression resolved, and she was able to get off Western medications. She learned to assert her boundaries more effectively in her relationships, and she entered into an intimate relationship wherein she was able to receive love and affection while still being able to communicate her needs. She was referred to a colleague to continue the good progress she had achieved.

Endnotes

1   Lonny Jarrett's *Nourishing Destiny* by Spirit Path Press is a premier text on this topic and has influenced the author since its publication. In addition, his landmark three-part article series, Betrayal of Intimacy was my first exposure to the concepts of trauma and shock as a systemic etiology. It was these articles and text that led me to seek out study with Dr. Hammer and the Shen-Hammer pulse lineage. Jarrett's *The Clinical Practice of Chinese Medicine* similarly explores this topic.

2   While not diagnostic in the following quote, the term for shock is first mentioned in Chapter 5 verse 6 of the Su Wen (China Science and Technology Press; Wu and Wu). 天有四时五行，以生长收藏，以生寒暑燥湿风。人有五藏，化五气，以生喜怒悲忧恐

3   Su Wen Ch. 21 (China Science and Technology Press; Wu and Wu).

4   Ibid, Ch. 8.

5   Hammer, Leon I. and Rotte, Hamilton, *Chinese Herbal Medicine: The Formulas of Dr. John H.F. Shen*, Thieme, 2013.

6   Yin and Yang as representation of the Heart-Kidney axis; Su Wen Ch. 2 states: "The growth and development of all things on earth depend on the intercrossing of the energies of Yin and Yang. If the two energies fail to communicate, all things on earth will lose their source of nourishment." Su Wen Ch. 2 (China Science and Technology Press; Wu and Wu).

7   The Triple Burner, an energetic organ system without form, has multiple roles within Chinese medicine, including mediating the movement of yang qi up the Du mai to disseminate yuan qi to the organ systems, regulating fluid metabolism through the three burners, assisting overall thermodynamics, autonomic and hormonal functions, and much more. A detailed exploration of the Triple Burner is outside the scope of this text, but more information can be found throughout this book in terms of its relationship to the sinew, luo, primary, and divergent channel systems.

8   Hammer, Leon I. and Rotte, Hamilton, *Chinese Herbal Medicine: The Formulas of Dr. John H.F. Shen*, Thieme, 2013.

9   Often found with Choppy and/or Liver Engorgement and Diaphragm pulses. These latter two involve positions in the Shen-Hammer lineage wherein one rolls fingers between the distal and middle positions looking for inflations representing trapped qi and blood.

10   Hammer, Leon I. and Rotte, Hamilton, *Chinese Herbal Medicine: The Formulas of Dr. John H.F. Shen*, Thieme, 2013.

11   Ibid.

12 Ibid

13 Ibid.

14 Ibid.

15 Levine, Peter, *In an Unspoken Voice, How the Body Releases Trauma and Restores Goodness*, North Atlantic Books, 2010, p.23.

16 Ibid, pp.31–32.

17 Lynn, Richard John and Wang, Bi, *The Classic of Changes: A New Translation of the I Ching as Interpreted by Wang Bi, Translated by Richard John Lynn*, Columbia University Press, 1994.

18 Legge, James, *Sacred Books of the East, Yi King, Volume II, Part II*, Oxford University Press, 1882.

19 Levine, Peter, *In an Unspoken Voice, How the Body Releases Trauma and Restores Goodness*, North Atlantic Books, 2010, p.48.

20 Ibid.

21 Su Wen Ch. 39 (China Science and Technology Press; Wu and Wu).

22 Ibid, Chs. 5 and 19.

23 Ibid, Ch. 67.

24 Ibid, Ch. 39.

25 Ling Shu Ch. 8 (China Science and Technology Press; Wu and Wu).

26 Ibid.

27 Ibid.

28 Ibid, Ch. 6.

29 Su Wen Ch. 3 (China Science and Technology Press; Wu and Wu). I am making a correlation here to invasion by cold, and invasion by fear.

30 Ibid, Ch. 70.

31 Ibid, Ch. 17.

32 Ibid, Ch. 39.

33 Ibid, Ch. 5.

34 Ibid.

35 Ling Shu Ch. 19 (China Science and Technology Press; Wu and Wu).

36 Luo Xiwen, *Synopsis of Prescriptions of the Golden Chamber with 300 Cases*, New World Press, 1995, p.187.

37 Su Wen Ch. 43 (China Science and Technology Press; Wu and Wu).

38 Ling Shu Ch. 8 (China Science and Technology Press; Wu and Wu).

39   Mitchell, Craig, Ye, Feng and Wiseman, Nigel, *Shang Han Lun: On Cold Damage,* Paradigm Publications, p.28.

40   Ling Shu Ch. 47 (China Science and Technology Press; Wu and Wu).

41   Levine, Peter, *In an Unspoken Voice, How the Body Releases Trauma and Restores Goodness*, North Atlantic Books, 2010, pp.13–14.

42   Ibid, p.13.

43   Ibid, p.15.

44   Su Wen Ch. 5 (China Science and Technology Press; Wu and Wu).

45   Levine, Peter, *In an Unspoken Voice, How the Body Releases Trauma and Restores Goodness*, North Atlantic Books, 2010, p.16.

46   Lynn, Richard John and Wang, Bi, I Jing, *Hexagram 51*, Columbia University Press, 1994.

47   Ibid.

48   Ibid.

49   Wilhelm, Richard, *I Ching*, 1950. Available at www2.unipr.it/~deyoung/I_Ching_Wilhelm_Translation.html#51, accessed on January 22, 2018.

50   Some circulatory imblances can create different rates between the sides, and it is possible to perceive different rates in the neuro-psychological positions where there is increased electrical activity in the brain (e.g., seizures).

51   This is different from normal heart rate variability wherein when the lungs are fully expanded there tends to be a little bit of a speeding up as we breathe in and a little bit of a slowing down when we fully expire.

52   Note that this image depicts a Hollow pulse that is also Yielding at the qi depth.

53   This denotes a sense of urgency; see also Ying Huang, William Morris, Peng Wan, TCM Case Studies: Dermatology, People's Medical Publishing House, 2014, p.149.

54   Hammer, Leon I. and Rotte, Hamilton, *Chinese Herbal Medicine: The Formulas of Dr. John H.F. Shen*, Thieme, 2013.

55   Ibid.

56   Ibid,

57   Fisher, Sebern, *Neurofeedback for the Treatment of Developmental Trauma: Calming the Fear-Driven Brain*, W.W. Norton & Co., 2014, p.52.

58   The following list of etiologies have been adapted from my article co-authored with Brandt Stickley and Hamilton Rotte "Expressions of the Heart," Chinese Medicine Times, Vol. 3, Issue 1, 2008 as well as Hammer, Leon I. and Rotte, Hamilton, Chinese Herbal Medicine: The Formulas of Dr. John H.F. Shen, Thieme, 2013.

59   Su Wen Ch. 39 (China Science and Technology Press; Wu and Wu).

60   See Buhner, Stephen Harrod, *The Secret Teachings of Plants: In the Direct Perception of Nature*, (Bear & Company 2004), wherein he describes the power of the circulatory pumping heart having the pressure to shoot water 6 feet into the air (p. 72), the heart's action as an endocrine gland (p. 78), its role in the central nervous system (p. 82), it's role in perception and communication (p. 89), its communication with the brain (p. 102), and of course its spiritual components (p. 116), etc.

61   Hammer, Leon and Bilton, Karen, *Handbook of Contemporary Chinese Pulse Diagnosis*, Eastland Press, 2012, Ch. 3 (edited by Ross Rosen).

62   Su Wen Ch. 24 and Ling Shu Ch. 78 (China Science and Technology Press; Wu and Wu).

63   Ling Shu Ch. 8 (China Science and Technology Press; Wu and Wu).

64   Many of the Heart patterns are found in the following article: Rosen, Ross, Stickley, Brandt, with Rotte, Hamilton, "Expressions of the Heart," *Chinese Medicine Times*, Vol. 3, Issue 1, 2008. It is available on my website at http://rossrosen.com/document/Expressions_of_the_Heart.pdf.

65   Tài shàng lǎo jūn shuō cháng qīngjìng jīng, *The Scripture of Constant Clarity and Stillness as Spoken by Taishang Laojun (deified Laozi)*, translated by Josh Paynter and Jack Schaefer.

66   Roth, Harold, *Original Tao: Inward Training (Nei-Yeh)*, Columbia University Press, p.72. While Roth translates the heart radical as "mind," I have added Heart in brackets.

67   Van Der Kolk, Bessel, *The Body Keeps the Score: Brain, Mind, and Body in the Healing of Trauma*, Penguin Books, 2014, p.21.

68   Levine, Peter, *In an Unspoken Voice, How the Body Releases Trauma and Restores Goodness*, North Atlantic Books, 2010, pp.74–75.

69   Hammer, Leon I, *The Patient–Practitioner Relationship in Acupuncture*, Thieme, 2008.

70   Jeffrey Yuen, lectures (Luo Vessels, 2007).

71   Personal communication with Dr. Hammer.

72   Van Der Kolk, Bessel, *The Body Keeps the Score: Brain, Mind, and Body in the Healing of Trauma*, Penguin Books, 2014, pp.30–31.

73   Ibid, p.31.

74   Satprem, *Sri Aurobindo or the Adventure of Consciousness*, Discovery Publisher, 2015, p.190.

75   Ibid, p.191.

76   Sri Aurobindo and the Mother, compiled by A.S. Dalal, *Powers Within, Selections from the Works of Sri Aurobindo and the Mother*, Lotus Press, 2002, p.10.

77   Ibid, p.24.

78   Ibid, p.23.

79   Satprem, *Sri Aurobindo or the Adventure of Consciousness*, Discovery Publisher, 2015, p.251.

80   Ibid, p.250.

81   Van Der Kolk, Bessel, *The Body Keeps the Score: Brain, Mind, and Body in the Healing of Trauma*, Penguin Books, 2014, p.27.

82   Hammer, Leon I., *Dragon Rises, Red Bird Flies, Rev. Ed.*, Eastland Press, p.3.

83   Van Der Kolk, Bessel, *The Body Keeps the Score: Brain, Mind, and Body in the Healing of Trauma*, Penguin Books, 2014, p.37.

84   Ibid, p.37.

85   Ibid, p.38.

86   Hammer, Leon I., "Psychotherapy and Growth," *Contemporary Psychoanalysis*, Vol. 10, No. 3, 1974.

87   Su Wen Ch. 13 (China Science and Technology Press; Wu and Wu).

88   Ibid, Ch. 14.

89   Hammer, Leon I., *The Patient–Practitioner Relationship in Acupuncture*, Thieme, 2008.

90   Hammer, Leon I., *Dragon Rises, Red Bird Flies, Rev. Ed.*, Eastlands Press, p.11.

91   The 3 beans will reflect the yang sinews, the 6 beans will reflect the yin sinews.

92   David Berceli PhD coined the name Tension and Trauma Release Exercise (TRE) which "is an innovative series of exercises that assist the body in releasing deep muscular patterns of stress, tension and trauma" which "safely activates a natural reflex mechanism of shaking or vibrating that releases muscular tension, calming down the nervous system" (see Dr. Berceli's website www.traumaprevention.com for more information). Liz Koch also discusses and teaches about the psoas muscle and its importance in the fight/flight/freeze response (see www.coreawareness.com for more information). Koch, along with others, such as Shaye Molendyke of Yogafit for Warriors, utilizes yoga and somatic exercises to release this important muscle (see www.yogafit.com).

93   It should be noted that the illustration of the Choppy pulse is an approximation and often will not have the variations of amplitude as shown in the figure.

94   The Rough pulse is similar to the Choppy but the points are more rounded than sharp.

95   The Sticky pulse is a quality that I have found beginning around 2010. The primary sensation of this pulse is that it feels waterlogged or rubbery or sticky in that the pulsation of the artery seems to linger on your fingertip. It is a quality of the vessel and its texture and is distinguished from the Leisurely pulse which feels as if its movement is slowed down or exaggerated. One of my colleagues helped describe it as the "Peanut Butter" quality as your finger sticks to it. I consider the Sticky pulse to be a progression and accumulation of phlegm-heat. In the Liver, it can reflect phlegm-heat toxins; in the Stomach and Spleen potentially candida and malabsorption and gluten intolerance (manifestations of gu). It is most often found in the middle positions, but I have found it mostly everywhere by now. I consider this pulse quality a more recent expression of toxicity in general whereby the lymphatic system attempts to trap pathogenic (including gu) influences (rather than Choppy which is influencing the blood circulation).

96 The Blood Thick quality is found by releasing pressure from the organ depth up to the qi depth. If there is a significant expansion and/or pounding in the vessel as one lifts, and that continues up past the blood depth to the qi depth (often beyond), it is a Blood Thick quality suggesting excess heat in the blood which has dried the fluids, creating more viscous blood.

97 Levine, Peter, *In an Unspoken Voice, How the Body Releases Trauma and Restores Goodness*, North Atlantic Books, 2010, pp.71–72.

98 Ling Shu Ch. 22 (China Science and Technology Press; Wu and Wu), p.614.

99 Levine, Peter, *In an Unspoken Voice, How the Body Releases Trauma and Restores Goodness*, North Atlantic Books, 2010, p.82.

100 It should be noted that, prior to engaging in this discussion, I had known the patient for some time and had already established an intimate patient–practitioner relationship.

101 Jeffrey Yuen, Luo Vessels lectures.

102 Personal communication, July 2017.

103 The character traits I present from DRRBF are but a small piece of what Dr. Hammer details in his groundbreaking text. The reader is referred to the book for the full clinical picture and psychological profiles.

104 Ni, Yitian, *Navigating the Channels of Traditional Chinese Medicine*, Oriental Medicine Center, San Diego, 1996, p.24.

105 Hammer, Leon I., *Dragon Rises, Red Bird Flies, Rev. Ed.*, Eastland Press, Ch. 12.

106 Ibid, Ch. 11.

107 Jarrett, Lonny S., *The Clinical Practice of Chinese Medicine*, Spirit Path Press, 2003, p.625.

108 Hammer, Leon I., *Dragon Rises, Red Bird Flies, Rev. Ed.*, Eastland Press, Ch. 10.

109 Jarrett, Lonny S., *The Clinical Practice of Chinese Medicine*, Spirit Path Press, 2003, p.340.

110 Ibid, p.60.

111 Hammer, Leon I., *Dragon Rises, Red Bird Flies, Rev. Ed.*, Eastland Press, Ch. 8.

112 Hammer, Leon I., *Dragon Rises, Red Bird Flies*, Eastland Press, p.103.

113 Jarrett, Lonny S., *The Clinical Practice of Chinese Medicine*, Spirit Path Press, 2003, p.439.

114 Ibid, p.440.

115 Jeffrey Yuen, Primary Channel lectures.

116 Hammer, Leon I., *Dragon Rises, Red Bird Flies*, Eastland Press; p.404.

117 Su Wen Ch. 74, line 6 of the 19 lines (China Science and Technology Press; Wu and Wu).

118 Hammer, Leon I., *Dragon Rises, Red Bird Flies, Rev. Ed.*, Eastland Press, Ch. 10.

119 Ibid, pp.461–462.

120 Jeffrey Yuen, Primary Channel lectures.

121 Hammer, Leon I., *Dragon Rises, Red Bird Flies, Rev. Ed.*, Eastland Press.

122 Jarrett, Lonny S., *The Clinical Practice of Chinese Medicine*, Spirit Path Press, 2003, p.467.

123 Ibid, p.478.

124 Jeffrey Yuen, Primary Channel lectures.

125 Ibid.

126 Jeffrey Yuen, Primary Channel lectures.

127 Jarrett, Lonny S., *The Clinical Practice of Chinese Medicine*, Spirit Path Press, 2003, p.492.

128 Jeffrey Yuen, Primary Channel lectures.

129 Jarrett, Lonny S., *The Clinical Practice of Chinese Medicine*, Spirit Path Press, 2003, p.492.

130 Jarrett, Lonny S., *The Clinical Practice of Chinese Medicine*, Spirit Path Press, 2003, p.495.

131 Hammer, Leon I., *Dragon Rises, Red Bird Flies, Rev. Ed.*, Eastland Press, Ch. 9.

132 Hammer, Leon I., *Dragon Rises, Red Bird Flies, Rev. Ed.*, Eastland Press, Ch. 9.

133 Hammer, Leon I., *Dragon Rises, Red Bird Flies, Rev. Ed.*, Eastland Press, Ch. 9.

134 Jarrett, Lonny S., *The Clinical Practice of Chinese Medicine*, Spirit Path Press, 2003, p.545.

135 As taught by Jeffrey Yuen.

136 Jeffrey Yuen, Alchemy lecture.

137 Jeffrey Yuen, Alchemy lecture.

138 All of Dr. Shen's formulas can be found in the following text by Dr. Hammer and Hamilton Rotte: Hammer, Leon I. and Rotte, Hamilton, *Chinese Herbal Medicine: The Formulas of Dr. John H.F. Shen*, Thieme, 2013.

139 Drs. Shen and Hammer tended to use Fu Zi in very small dosages due to its toxicity. I use the Fu Zi provided by Classical Pearls and Heiner Freuheuf in dosages beginning with 18g and moving up from that baseline as needed. Typically, this is combined with Sha Ren or the like to assist with its descent into the lower burner.

140 Luo Xiwen, *Synopsis of Prescriptions of the Golden Chamber with 300 Cases*, New World Press, 1995, p.188.

141 Jeffrey Yuen & Kathryn White, Introduction to Divergent Meridians lecture, 2004.

142 Ibid.

143 See my article co-written with Dr. Hammer on the impact of radiation on our physiology: Hammer, Leon MD and Rosen, Ross LAc, "The Pulse: The Electronic Age and Radiation—Early Detection," *American Acupuncturist* (Spring 2009).

144 Jeffrey Yuen & Kathryn White, Introduction to Divergent Meridians lecture, 2004.

145 Ibid.

146 Ibid.

147 Ibid.

148 Yang of yang is the skin and sinews; yin of yang is the bones and joints; yang of yin is the fu organs; and yin of yin is the zang organs.

149 Jeffrey Yuen & Kathryn White, Introduction to Divergent Meridians lecture, 2004.

150 Ibid.

151 Ibid.

152 Pathways for the channels in this chapter were adapted from Jeffrey Yuen & Kathryn White, Introduction to Divergent Meridians lecture, 2004.

153 Ibid.

154 Indications for the channels in this chapter were adapted from Jeffrey Yuen & Kathryn White, Introduction to Divergent Meridians lecture, 2004.

155 The DM personalities presented are as learned from Jeffrey Yuen, but the many similarities to Dr. Hammer's DRRBF Five Phase presentations should be noted.

156 Ni, Yitian, *Navigating the Channels of Traditional Chinese Medicine*, Oriental Medicine Center, San Diego, 1996, p.70.

157 Shima, Miki and Chace, Charles, *The Channel Divergences: Deeper Pathways of the Web, Rev. Ed.*, Blue Poppy Press, 2001, p.20.

158 Ibid.

159 Jeffrey Yuen, Divergent Meridian lecture.

160 Ibid.

161 Ibid.

162 Ni, Yitian, *Navigating the Channels of Traditional Chinese Medicine*, Oriental Medicine Center, San Diego, 1996, p.84.

163 Jeffrey Yuen, Divergent Meridian lecture.

164 It is unclear if taiyang refers to the temples or the taiyang Bladder and Small Intestine which governs the area of the upper back and the posterior aspect of the Lungs.

165 Hammer, Leon I., *Dragon Rises, Red Bird Flies*, Eastland Press, Ch. 13.

166 Based on notes from a lecture given by Sheila George on material from Jeffrey Yuen, at the American University of Complementary Medicine.

167 See Hammer, Leon I. and Rotte, Hamilton, *Chinese Herbal Medicine: The Formulas of Dr. John H.F. Shen*, Thieme, 2013.

168 This Daoist cosmological understanding is as learned from Jeffrey Yuen.

169 Legge, James, *Sacred Books of the East, Yi King, Volume II, Part II,* Oxford University Press, 1882.

170 Liu Yousheng, translated by Liu Zuozhi and Wilms, Sabine, *Let the Radiant Yang Shine Forth: Lectures on Virtue,* Happy Goat Productions, 2014, pp.43–44.

171 Ibid.

172 As Lung qi descends to the Kidneys, the breath moves to ming men fire. As the oxygen (Lung qi) stokes the ming men fire, Kidney essence is burned to vapor which rises along the Du mai, irrigating the back shu points with yuan qi.

173 By age seven or eight, children began more formalized learning, taking them away from the parental influence. By 14 or 16, children were often married. By 21 or 24 they themselves have had children of their own, etc.

174 Wang Shu-he, translated by Yang Shou-zhong, *The Pulse Classic: A Translation of the Mai Jing,* Blue Poppy Press, 1997, p.54.

175 Wang Shu-he conceived of the Chong mai as the deeper pre-natal central channel, thus putting it at the deep level. Li Shi-zhen places it on the moderate depth as a reflection of its post-natal attributes.

176 *Chen Ke-zheng,* published by Chinese National Chinese Medicine & Medicinals Publishing Co., Beijing, 1995; Maciocia, Giovanni, Diagnosis in Chinese Medicine: A Comprehensive Guide, Churchill Livingstone, 2004, pp 998-1005; Tian De Yang, The Herbs of the Eight Extra Meridians, www.acupuncture.com/herbs/eightextraherbs.htm

177 Consolidates yang from deficiency caused by yin stasis.

178 Flaws, Bob, translator, *Chen Ke-zheng,* published by Chinese National Chinese Medicine & Medicinals Publishing Co., Beijing, 1995.

179 Maciocia, Giovanni, *Diagnosis in Chinese Medicine: A Comprehensive Guide,* Churchill Livingstone, 2004, p.1005.

180 The description and content of these concepts and treatments identified below have been culled from multiple courses and study with Jeffrey Yuen.

181 Jeffrey Yuen letcture on Chinese psychology: Sun Si-miao perspective.

182 Heiner Freuheuf also teaches and writes on the subject of gu syndrome, and the strategies listed by Jeffrey Yuen (as they both originate from Daoist teachings) are virtually the same, with some slight changes in category names. For the purposes of this section, the strategies and herbs listed are a combination of both sources.

183 Jeffrey Yuen lecture on Chinese psychology: Sun Si-miao perspective.

Subject Index

Author Index

Berceli, D. 129*n92*
Bilton, K. 69*n61*
Buhner, S.H. 67*n60*

Chace, C. 298*n157*, 298*n158*

Dalal, A.S. 87*n76*, 87*n77*, 87*n78*

Fisher, S. 65*n57*
Flaws, B. 384*n178*
Freuheuf, H. 409*n182*

Hammer, L.I. 22*n5*, 26*n8*, 26*n10*, 26*n11*,
    27*n12*, 27*n13*, 27*n14*, 60*n54*, 60*n55*,
    61*n56*, 65*n58*, 69*n61*, 81*n69*, 82*n71*,
    88*n82*, 89*n86*, 90*n89*, 90*n90*, 212*n105*,
    217*n106*, 225*n108*, 231*n111*, 231*n112*,
    238*n116*, 243*n118*, 244*n119*, 245*n121*,
    253*n131*, 259*n132*, 260*n133*, 267*n138*,
    290*n143*, 319*n165*, 326*n167*

Jarrett, L.S. 12*n1*, 221*n107*, 226*n109*, 230*n110*,
    233*n113*, 234*n114*, 245*n122*, 246*n123*,
    247*n127*, 248*n129*, 248*n130*, 260*n134*

Koch, L. 129*n92*

Legge, J. 31*n18*, 333*n169*
Levine, P. 30*n15*, 30*n16*, 31*n19*, 32*n20*,
    38*n41*, 39*n42*, 39*n43*, 40*n45*,
    81*n68*, 183*n97*, 188*n99*
Luo, X. 34*n36*, 280*n140*
Lynn, R.J. 31*n17*, 41*n46*, 41*n47*, 41*n48*

Maciocia, G. 385*n179*

Mitchell, C. 35*n39*

Ni, Y. 211*n104*, 297*n156*, 305*n162*

Rosen, R. 75*n64*, 290*n143*
Roth, H. 76*n66*
Rotte, H. 22*n5*, 26*n8*, 26*n10*, 26*n11*, 27*n12*,
    27*n13*, 27*n14*, 60*n54*, 60*n55*, 61*n56*,
    65*n58m*, 75*n64*, 267*n138*, 326*n167*

Satprem 84*n74*, 84*n75*, 87*n79*, 88*n80*
Shima, M. 298*n157*, 299*n158*
Stickley, B. 65*n58*, 75*n64*

Van Der Kolk, B. 78*n67*, 82*n72*, 82*n73*,
    88*n81*, 88*n83*, 88*n84*, 88*n85*

Wang, B. 31*n17*, 41*n46*, 41*n47*, 41*n48*
Wang, S. 344*n174*, 344*n175*
White, K. 290*n141*, 290*n142*, 291*n144*, 292*n145*,
    292*n146*, 292*n147*, 292*n149*, 292*n150*,
    294*n151*, 295*n152*, 295*n153*, 295*n154*
Wilhelm, R. 42*n49*
Wiseman, N. 35*n39*

Ye, F. 35*n39*
Yousheng, L. 333*n170*, 333*n171*
Yuen, J. 81*n70*, 195*n101*, 236*n115*,
    245*n120*, 246*n124*, 246*n125*, 247*n126*,
    248*n128*, 261*n135*, 261*n136*, 263*n137*,
    290*n141*, 290*n142*, 291*n144*, 292*n145*,
    292*n146*, 292*n147*, 292*n149*, 293*n150*,
    294*n151*, 295*n152*, 295*n153*, 295*n154*,
    300*n159*, 300*n160*, 301*n161*, 307*n163*,
    332*n168*, 407*n181*, 410*n183*